A DOCTOR'S GUIDE TO ALTERNATIVE MEDICINE

What Works, What Doesn't, and Why

MEL BORINS, MD, FCFP

Foreword by Dr. Bernie Siegel

With contributions by: Heather Boon, BScPhm, Phd;
Carol Chan, BScPhm, ACPR, RPh; Jennifer Fink, MD;
Scott Forman, MD; Jason Mackie, BSc; Linda Rapson, MD;
Cherry Tanega, BSc; Cheryl Tyler, BScPhm

LYONS PRESS
Guilford, Connecticut
Helena, Montana
An imprint of Rowman & Littlefield

Lyons Press is an imprint of Rowman & Littlefield

Distributed by NATIONAL BOOK NETWORK

Portions of this text were originally published by the author in a slightly different form in *Canadian Journal of Diagnosis*, *Patient Care* magazine, *Canadian Family Physician*, and *Postgraduate Medicine*, a JTE Multimedia publication.

British Library Cataloguing-in-Publication Information available

Library of Congress Cataloging-in-Publication Data available

ISBN 978-1-4930-0595-6 (paperback)

∞™ The paper used in this publication meets the minimum requirements of American National Standard for Information Sciences—Permanence of Paper for Printed Library Materials, ANSI/NISO Z39.48-1992.

The case histories used in this book are mainly taken from my clinical practice in Family Medicine. Names and details have been changed to protect the confidentiality of my patients.

This book is not intended to diagnose or treat conditions and should only be used under the supervision of your doctor. Each person's situation is unique and requires personal medical attention. The author assumes no responsibility for the consequences of applying information in this book.

CONTENTS

CONTENTS

FOREWORD

The Importance of Integrative Medicine

Alternative Medicine is no longer really alternative. It is just that it has not been integrated into classical medical information and training, and so it is seen as alternative. We, as physicians, receive a great deal of information during our training, but we need to be better educated about what would open our minds and orient us to the patient's experience and potential to heal. All living things have the ability to overcome various afflictions. It is built into us so we can survive, and when we open our minds we can integrate all these therapies and natural gifts and use them to help us overcome a variety of health problems, diseases, and bodily wounds. I have experienced first-hand how acupuncture, chiropractic, homeopathy, and herbal therapies can heal and cure when I have had to live with back pain and chronic Lyme disease. What I experienced has made me a believer and aware of the benefits of alternative and integrative medicine.

I feel that too often the body is treated as a house that we reside in. If your house has a problem you call the appropriate therapist: the electrician, plumber, roofer, or carpenter. They can repair the problem without knowing about or paying any attention to the other systems. The human body is not like that. It is an integrated system where psyche and soma interact and affect one another, and so our therapies cannot be disassociated. They must be integrated so the entire patient's life, body, and experience are included in the therapy.

This book speaks the truth from a well-grounded and holistic physician, Mel Borins. When the body and mind are seen as a unit and one's mind remains open to the various therapeutic modalities, then true health care occurs. Rather than seeing it as alternative, let us see it as integrative and accept as therapeutic whatever is beneficial to our health care.

We all need to keep an open mind—not close it based upon our beliefs, and risk refusing to experience the potential benefits of alternative therapies. When health care providers open their minds, medicine will truly progress as a healing occupation and not one just focused on battling a disease and empowering the enemy. We need to help our patients to heal and find peace and not fight wars. One of my patients was told by an oncologist that his treatment would kill his cancer. He responded, "I am a conscientious objector. I don't kill anything." He walked out of the office to pursue alternative therapies and lived for over twelve years.

What I have learned from my life is to live by my experience and not let beliefs close my mind. My wife Bobbie was diagnosed with MS many decades ago and this led me to become a member of the American Holistic Medical Association. She is still with me, far exceeding any expectations of her neurologist. At one of the American Holistic Medical Association meetings a healer, Olga Worral, gave a lecture on hands-on energy healing. At the time I had a leg injury incurred while training for a marathon. My wife suggested I ask Olga to help me. My reaction was that what she had to say did not make sense and was hard for me to accept. So Bobbie asked Olga to come over and help me. She placed her hands on my leg and the heat from her hands was incredible. Five minutes later I stood up and walked away, pain free and completely healed.

We also need to explore inner space and understand the body-mind interactions and holistic, integrative, and alternative therapies. This can open the way to offering patients lessons in survival behavior rather than saying I cannot accept that, or to see a recovery as a case of self-induced healing versus spontaneous remission. Patients, too, have much to teach us, but so many doctors will say, "You are doing well. Keep doing what you are doing," rather than ask the patient to tell them what they are doing that had been so effective.

In my reading I have come across many therapeutic modalities that were never discussed in medical school and it made me angry. I don't want to have to discover on my own what benefits my patients. This is why Mel's excellent book is a resource I can appreciate.

It is very important to create a compassionate team for the patient because patients of compassionate doctors recover faster. We need to listen to patients' stories and learn from them to help us to explore new and integrative modalities. Death will not be the enemy and disempower us. Healing will become our goal and we will help patients to integrate all the factors in their life into their treatment. Reading about integrative medicine can open us to new potentials for our patients and make the process easier for us all.

So read on and utilize Mel's open-minded approach to medicine to empower you to seek safe, alternative treatments that better serve your health needs. All healing is scientific even when we can't explain the mechanisms. The human body is intelligent and we need to both create and become a member of an open-minded healing team ready to accept the science of integrative medicine. We need to explore and learn about our inner space more than we do outer space. The solution lies within Dr. Mel Borins' experience and wisdom and what he shares in his well-written book.

—Dr. Bernie Siegel

ACKNOWLEDGMENTS

Many people have been instrumental in the making of this book.

I would like to thank Heather Boon, Carol Chan, Jennifer Fink, Scott Forman, Jason Mackie, Linda Rapson, Cherry Tanega, and Cheryl Tyler, who each helped co-write a chapter of this book.

Craig Saunders, Jason Kalra, and Paul Lima made helpful corrections to a few of the chapters. Marie Claire Boyle, Aileen Burford-Mason, Rick Glazier, Deborah Kopansky-Giles, Laurie Obornick, Susan Schelberg, Morris Sherman, Caroline Smoyer, Jerry Steinberg, Howie Vernon, and Margaret Yanicki all read versions of the manuscript and made helpful corrections and suggestions.

Thanks to my agent Katie Reed and my book consultant Andrea Hurst for their assistance in getting this book published. Also a special appreciation to Brandon LaFave for his help along the way.

Mary Norris and Ellen Urban from Globe Pequot Press were wonderful to work with and assisted me in so many ways.

Librarians Rita Shaughnessy and Barbara Iwasiuk aided in the literature searches and finding the articles upon which the book is written. I was so fortunate to have them helping me.

A special thanks goes to Cindy Hurn who did an incredible job editing this book and making it more accessible to the general reader.

In the interests of transparency I would like to disclose that over the years I have received an honorarium from PharmaCare Canada, Ferring, MFI Pharma, and Boiron to give talks to community physicians about natural health products.

Finally I would like to acknowledge my wife, Bonnie, who has been an amazing supporter and cheerleader through this long project. She has edited every version of every chapter from the very beginning. She is the person whose opinion I cherish the most.

INTRODUCTION

After finishing medical school and completing a grueling internship, my wife, Bonnie, and I packed up our apartment, said goodbye to relatives, friends, material possessions, and responsibilities, and set off for a fourteen-and-a-half-month sabbatical around the globe. It was during this journey that I was introduced to alternative medicine. Halfway through our trip, we were living in Kashmir, Northern India, on an ornately hand-carved wooden houseboat in Nageen Lake with our friends Lynn and Jack. All was going amazingly well until one morning when Jack woke up with severe pain in his back.

"This isn't the first time it's happened," he said nonchalantly. "I have a chiropractor who fixes my 'tricky back' with just a few physical manipulations." There was a slight problem with Jack's plan, because his chiropractor was on the other side of the world. Even though I was a medical doctor at the height of my training, I knew absolutely nothing about spinal manipulation. Without access to analgesics, anti-inflammatories, muscle relaxants, and physiotherapy, the only advice I could offer to Jack was bed rest. But Jack was not a bed rest kind of guy. He came up with another solution.

"I'll show you what my chiropractor does, and then you can do the manipulation." He stretched out on the thick Indian carpet, rolled over, and told me where to place my hands. Then he directed me to push here and apply force there, but nothing I did could get his spine back into position. I remember thinking: after all those years of medical training, without drugs and therapy equipment, I can't do a thing to help my friend. I felt helpless and inadequate. Jack did the best he could to ignore his back, but for the next few days, he was still in severe pain, so we went to the houseboat owner, Ali Major, and asked for his advice. He recommended a visit to the local healer.

I was nervous for my friend. What kind of a quack might he end up with, and what would this person do to him? I decided to go with Jack and make sure he was okay. We hired a horse and buggy and clip-clopped our way into the small town of Hazratbal on the outskirts of Srinagar. Nothing makes a ride seem longer than when you see your friend wince each time the buggy lurches and jolts over a rutted road. We finally reached the town and asked some locals where we might find the healer. They led us to a distant sidewalk where we observed a short, bearded man surrounded by a small crowd.

Jack climbed out of the buggy and approached the healer. Now, Jack is a six-foot-four giant, and that man on the sidewalk was no more than five-foot-two at best. Jack stood out like a tree in a cornfield. The healer motioned for Jack to step forward and said something we couldn't understand. With no common language, Jack pointed to his back, grimaced, and made the universal sounds for pain. The short, relaxed man deftly wheeled Jack around, placed his knee against Jack's back, lifted him off the ground, and with one manipulation, dropped Jack back onto his feet. With his spine back in alignment, Jack's pain was completely gone.

Until then, I had no experience with chiropractors, for my training had been very orthodox. I had lumped spinal manipulation into the quackery category. But the incident with the healer on the street made me question, why would there be so many people going to chiropractors if it didn't work? How could I, with all my training, not be able to help my friend, yet this healer could alleviate his pain in a matter of seconds?

After I returned home, I met a chiropractor for the first time. Dr. Don Vigianni didn't have horns or a long tail, and he impressed me with his knowledge, skill, and desire to help people. We started talking, and over time we established the Toronto Holistic Health Association. Every month, we'd bring in a speaker who was trained in a different kind of healing approach. Through these seminars, I was introduced to therapies such as iridology, homeopathy, cranial sacral work, and massage, along with many other alternatives. I began to learn everything I could about them.

I have no bones to pick with modern medicine; in fact, quite the opposite. I'm a conventional physician, and I rely on the pharmaceutical industry and modern medical practices to deal with the great majority of problems that I see. Modern drugs and treatments are, after all, the mainstay of modern medicine. During the last century, advancements such as antibiotics, immunization, new surgical techniques, X-rays, and scanning devices have relieved suffering, saved lives, and helped us to achieve the highest standards of health ever known in the history of mankind. Despite these advances, modern medicine is still far from perfect. Treatments are sometimes fraught with side effects and for all of the benefits we have received through modern medicine, there are still many illnesses for which conventional methods are simply not effective. Perhaps this is one reason why so many people are continuing to turn to alternative medicine for help.

Nearly one in three North Americans routinely use alternative treatment or take natural health products and supplements. Therapies such as acupuncture, cranial sacral therapy, massage, nutritional therapy, therapeutic touch, Shiatsu, Ayurveda medicine, and Traditional Chinese Medicine have become popular. Increasingly, some alternative therapies and treatments are accepted and covered by insurance companies. Physicians want to be educated about alternatives because their patients are often asking questions about which alternatives work and which don't.

For the last three decades, I have plowed through massive amounts of scientific research related to the use of alternative medicines. I have spent a considerable amount of time lecturing to physicians and writing in medical journals about the scientific evidence that is available, yet I still get the sense that even though so much has been written, the scientifically supported evidence doesn't get out there to the general public. All too often misinformation, conflicting opinions, and half-truths about alternative medicine and practices make it difficult for doctors and confusing for patients when trying to decide on safe and effective alternative options.

Physicians' Concerns

It is not uncommon for me to hear patients talk about an article they read lauding an "alternative" treatment, or that they spoke to their herbalist or salesperson in the health store who recommended taking this or that supplement. Sometimes my patients are taking a shopping bag full of vitamins and supplements, which brings up the question, do these really help or are they causing more problems? There is good reason to be concerned about scientifically unproven treatments.

Doctors worry that their patients may get into difficulty when taking an alternative or unregulated drug or they may delay receiving medical treatment that could improve their health or even be lifesaving. Take Sam, for example, a seventy-six-year-old patient of mine who was having trouble with constipation. He delayed seeking medical help because he had decided to self-treat with herbs. When Sam came to see me, he explained he'd been taking an over-the-counter, cathartic herbal formula that relieved his constipation, but as soon as he stopped taking the product, his irregularity became increasingly worse. Rather than cure the problem, the herbs merely relieved the symptoms. I ordered a blood test and found that Sam's hemoglobin was low. In a man of his age, this can be a serious marker for bleeding. I sent him for a barium enema, and he was found to have cancer of the colon. Luckily for Sam, he hadn't delayed too long. With surgery, Sam's cancer was cured and his problem with constipation resolved.

Sales pitches for these products and treatments may reasonably be compared to the snake oil salesmen of the Old West who traveled from town to town touting tinctures and potions and claiming they'd cure everything from scabies and rabies to colicky babies! Physicians are all too familiar with the stories of people who had faith in a particular treatment, spent a bunch of money, and then received no benefit from it at all. Nothing we take internally is without risk. Even water when taken to excess can be harmful. Many physicians know of relatives or friends or patients who were harmed by alternative medicine.

Placebo

It is important to realize that people may feel better from a treatment just because they believe it will help. Ted Kaptchuk, a researcher who is interested in the placebo effect,[1] did a randomized clinical trial involving 270 people suffering from musculoskeletal pain. Half the subjects received fake or placebo pain-reducing pills while the other half got fake or sham acupuncture treatments. Many of the patients reported real relief and reported side effects that were exactly what patients had been warned that their treatment might produce.

Researchers have found that placebo treatments can stimulate real physical changes in the body. Placebos have caused changes in heart rate, blood pressure and chemical activity in the brain in cases involving pain, depression, anxiety, fatigue, and even symptoms of Parkinson's disease.

Sometimes a placebo can make people feel better even though objectively a patient may be getting worse. The worry of some physicians is that using alternative treatments that make the person feel better subjectively may delay those from getting help when in fact they were not getting better at all.

Studies have shown that even if patients were told they were getting a placebo, they did better than patients who received no treatment. It may have been the expectation of the benefit that led to the same chemical response in the placebo group. Similar chemical changes on brain imaging tests were seen with placebo in studies of pain and in studies of depression. In the studies of Parkinson's disease and of pain, the more severe the disease symptoms and the more dramatic the treatment, the more likely the subjects were to experience benefit with placebo treatment.[2] It appears that when patients expect to get better the same natural pathways in the brain as medications are activated.

It is difficult for consumers to make informed decisions. Although the medical literature includes increasingly more studies on alternative medicine, there is still a paucity of scientific trials for alternative treatments.

The Science of Medicine

What does it mean when we say a treatment is supported by science? There are many ways for doctors to decide what treatments work, but the gold standard in medicine is to use data that have been collected from randomly assigned, double-blind, controlled trials.

Imagine for a moment that a five-year-old girl falls down on the pavement, scrapes her knee, and starts to cry. The child's father picks her up and whispers comforting words of reassurance. Then he takes the child into the house and washes the injury with soap and water. He gently applies a bandage while telling his daughter funny stories, assuring her that he loves her and remarking what a brave girl she is.

What if we wanted to scientifically discern what was the most important ingredient that affected the child's healing? Was it the soap, water, and clean bandage? Or was it the father's comforting behavior and words? There's also the possibility that the cut may have healed no matter what the parent did. We would have to examine every aspect of the treatment to find what influenced the healing and how much each factor influenced it. We'd also have to repeat the study, using thousands of children receiving different combinations of this care to reach a statistical analysis based on all the factors to form a scientific conclusion.

The same questions arise when we take a natural health supplement like glucosamine or use a treatment such as acupuncture. How do we know if the product or treatment really was effective? Would healing have taken place without any intervention? Or was there simply a placebo effect? Doctors have been known, when nothing else was available, to give patients sugar pills and call them anti-nausea pills or pain medication—and the patient's discomfort goes away. When a substance has no medicinal properties, but the person taking it gets relief from their symptoms, they are experiencing the placebo effect and the pills they took are the placebo.

Let's imagine that health-food stores have recently been stocking capsules of a powdered root, one known to be used in ancient times for aching joints. The manufacturer of the capsules claims this is a wonder cure, and people are flocking in to buy it and try it. Let's name this imaginary product TX-2. Some customers may have reported that TX-2 did relieve their pain, but we don't know if it is due to the powdered root or their belief that the powder works—the placebo effect. We want to know whether TX-2 is effective, what the optimum dose is, and if there are any side effects or interactions it may have with other foods, drugs, or the environment. Rather than rely on hearsay and customer feedback, we need to test the product in scientifically controlled conditions.

Now let's imagine that we designed a research trial to test TX-2, using 3,000 of the 8,000 volunteers who responded to a television advertisement. These 3,000 volunteers were chosen because they complained of mild to moderate pain in hips, knees, or hands and they had no other serious medical conditions. These volunteers range widely in age, gender, and socioeconomic status. A self-reported pain scale (of 1 through 10, with 10 representing extreme pain and 1 representing very little pain) is used, along with a visual assessment of joint function. We designed our trial to be conducted with randomized, double-blind, placebo-controlled methods. What does that mean?

Random assignment (randomized) means that when people take part in a trial, they are assigned to specific condition groups, not by choice, but by chance, such as the toss of a coin or picking their number from a hat. Let's say that in our study, when volunteers entered the building, our researchers counted them out as one, two, and three. All the ones were directed to Room 1; the twos directed to Room 2; and the threes went to Room 3. The chance that any specific individual went to a specific room was completely random.

A *controlled* trial means that other factors such as smoking, age, and blood pressure were reviewed, and when volunteers were randomly assigned, people with those factors would have been spread evenly amongst the groups in order not to skew the results of the trial. This means that although the volunteers were assigned randomly, various key factors were controlled. If Room 1 had a majority of the smokers or people with hypertension, then that group might have done worse than the others no matter what treatment was given. The other requirement of a controlled trial is that (at least) one group is treated differently (the experimental group), and one group (the control) receives no treatment at all, whether by placing them on a wait list for treatment, using sham (fake) treatment, or by giving them a placebo. In our trial, people in Room 1 were given capsules containing 25 units of TX-2. People in Room 2 were given capsules containing 50 units of TX-2. People in Room 3 (control group) received capsules containing only cornstarch and were not expected to show any relief from joint pain.

A *blind* trial means that the volunteers did not know whether they were receiving capsules containing some amount of TX-2 or capsules containing only cornstarch.

A *double-blind* trial means the researchers who gave out the capsules, and those who later collected data from the volunteers, also did not know which capsules each of the groups was assigned to receive.

Baseline—All three of our groups received a health check at the beginning of the trial and their data (levels of pain and function) was recorded. This gave researchers a *baseline* to make "before and after" comparisons.

Method—The *method* of the trial was that volunteers received identical instructions for taking the capsules, (i.e., take one capsule with eight ounces of water, daily upon rising). Every month they filled in and returned a questionnaire, and at three, six, and twelve months, they underwent another health check where pain level and function were recorded.

All of the collected data was analyzed using statistical mathematics. If a mathematically significant difference in pain and function levels was found between the control and experimental groups, researchers would then conclude that data supported the theory that TX-2 was effective for joint pain. If no significant difference in pain and function level was found, they would conclude that the data did not support the theory. A scientific paper would usually be written and presented for publication in a peer-reviewed recognized journal. This report would give clear, precise information about all aspects of the trial, enabling other scientists to replicate the experiment and test again under similar circumstances. Any side effects experienced would also be included and recommendations made for further studies.

There are many more factors involved in the design and methodology of scientific trials, but the basic elements we've just discussed, of a randomized, double-blind, controlled trial, are relatively effective in making sure that: (a) volunteers are divided into groups which are similar in content; (b) neither volunteers nor researchers can influence or bias results due to awareness of which treatment participants are receiving; and (c) one group receives no experimental treatment, to provide untreated data for comparison with experimental condition data.

Another form of accepted research is called a *meta-analysis*. This involves the careful selection of several peer-reviewed, published research trials. A comparison of the multiple studies is made, taking into consideration the various trial designs, elements, data, results, and conclusions. Finally, the review authors will summarize, state their conclusions, and make recommendations.

As with any endeavor, attempts to study people using scientific methods can meet with varying levels of success. Even randomized controlled trials can vary in quality from providing poor evidence that is badly biased to strong evidence that is rigorous and credible. For reasons that are not always clear, there is a tendency for studies that are funded by product manufacturers to show more positive results than studies paid for by third parties.

As you can imagine, unless you are used to devouring medical journals or science magazine articles, research can make rather dry reading. There are no heroes, no villains, no sex or violence—not even a hair-raising car chase. The language of scientific papers resembles nothing like the climax of a thriller or resolution of a love story, so the reader is left without the satisfying feeling of a Friday night at the movies. Even the most well-written research could dull the taste of hot buttered popcorn if you dared to snack while reading, so it's no wonder that the general population does not make a habit of reading scientifically supported research on alternative medicine.

Choosing the Material

After the editors of the *Canadian Journal of Diagnosis* received numerous queries from physicians wanting reliable information about alternatives for their patients, the *Journal* editors approached me and asked if I would write a monthly column with evidence-based reviews on alternative medicines and therapies. This book has evolved from those original articles. I have also extended the number of topics to include those that I have attempted to learn and digest to better help my patients. I will share practical information about vitamins, herbs, and other treatments that, with your physician's approval, you could potentially use in your life right away, especially if you understood their benefits and possible pitfalls.

There are many millions of websites offering advice on health and many are misleading people to make poor therapeutic choices. When a meta-analysis or review is undertaken, the way that the authors of the review searched for the research studies is always included in the Method section of the paper. So I think it is important for me to share how I found the studies I am quoting in this book. Fortunately I am an associate professor at the University of Toronto, so I had the availability of an amazing librarian named Rita Shaughnessy who did the literature search on many of the articles I was writing about. Because I am on active staff at St. Joseph's Health Center, I was also able to have our librarian, Barbara Iwasiuk, get the hard copy of the articles for me to review. However, most of you have no access to a librarian, and it might be helpful to know how you can search for credible material. I recommend you use US National Library of Medicine National Institutes of Health or www.ncbi.nlm.nih.gov/pubmed/ to search for credible studies. Another reliable site is www.naturalstandard.com. Most of the journals that are included in Pub Med are peer-reviewed and uphold a minimum level of quality. However, the quality of research even in this source may vary widely.

There are many physicians who feel that alternative medicine is quackery, a waste of time, and totally unscientific. On the other hand, there are many alternative health care practitioners who believe that all alternative medicine is good, has few if any side effects, and is the way of the future. I stand somewhere in the middle. Just because something is natural does not mean it is entirely safe or useful. So no, it's not all quackery; there is science to it, but there are many treatments out there that have no scientific support.

Please be aware that a lack of published research on a specific treatment does not automatically imply that it doesn't work or that it is not a safe treatment; all it means is that it cannot be *scientifically* supported as of today, due to the lack of scientifically conducted trials. Many successful treatments and medicines have been around for thousands of years and were adopted without the benefit of modern research methods. Observation that takes place over the long term is sometimes considered good enough. In order to be most helpful to readers, I have attempted to focus only on therapies and treatments that do have scientific support.

I hope this book will provide you with a user-friendly, critical analysis of research data and give you an objective perspective about things you've previously been unclear about. Only the key points of the trials and their results will be given in short summaries, hopefully saving you hours of plowing through technical material. When researchers' conclusions from multiple trials are not in agreement, I attempt to give both sides and end with my own conclusions and advice. I may not be able to give thrilling scenes of sex and car chases, but I do include historical background, curious folklore, and patients' anecdotal accounts, which will provide some entertainment as you become increasingly familiarized and comfortable with the language and methods of science. I hope I can help to dispel some myths and misunderstandings in the area of alternative medicine.

Feel free to accompany your reading with a bag of popped corn, or better yet, some fresh fruit. Whether you are a patient or a doctor, I encourage you to use *A Doctor's Guide to Alternative Medicine* as a guide for exploration. I am confident that it will enable you to make better-informed decisions about what is useful and what is not. Good health to you.

Section I: Traditional Healing and Herbal Remedies

Do you remember your mother using a family remedy when you were ill as a child? Perhaps she gave you a glass of ginger ale when your stomach was upset, or, when you had a fever and swollen glands, she might have swabbed your forehead and throat with an astringent of witch hazel. Ever since recorded time, people have taken herbs for health. Western medicine tends to adopt a rather ethnocentric point of view, believing that our modern way must be the only "right" way, and we all know this is not true. When looking at the scope of human history, modern medicine is in its infancy; people have survived for thousands of years with traditional healing practices.

It wasn't until I began to travel extensively around the world that I saw for myself how health care is (or isn't) distributed to populations. The World Health Organization reports claimed that the majority of the world's inhabitants do not have access to modern medicine and pharmaceuticals. Throughout India, Asia, China, Africa, and developing countries across the world, a shortage of physicians and medical centers, as well as the prohibitive cost of drugs and treatments, mean that accessibility, especially in rural areas, is almost nonexistent.[1, 2]

Some years ago, I decided to merge my love of long-journeyed travels with my sincere desire to become more familiar with the world's approach to healing and health—what type of services there were and how much accessibility existed for people in different countries and cultures. I wanted to observe how doctors and healers in other countries worked with the resources they had. While we have made leaps and bounds in our knowledge about disease and the body, improved treatments, and designed surgical techniques, equipment, and preventive measures, we still have much to draw upon and learn from the apothecaries and practices of our ancestors.

So in 1981, my wife Bonnie and I set out again, only this time we took our three-year-old son, Larry, and we traveled for nearly ten months, going from Fiji and Raratonga to New Zealand, then up to Indonesia, Thailand, Japan, India, Sri Lanka, and Kenya. The Canadian government was instrumental in the success of our journey, putting me in contact with officials in countries where healing practices were outside the realm of Western medicine. Through these dedicated people, I was able to meet and observe healers of many different disciplines.

Of the traditional folk healers, I met bonesetters, herbalists, spiritual healers, and those that combined all three. Particularly in rural areas, these were the mainstay of health care and medicine, and they provided similar care to what a medical doctor does in our culture. In other countries, such as Japan, China, and India, I met medical doctors who practiced Western medicine, as well as those who worked within other well-organized systems of healing and medicine, some of which date back thousands of years. Traditional Chinese Medicine, Ayurvedic, Unani, Siddha and other disciplines mirrored ours, with universities, medical schools, research facilities, hospitals, and outpatient clinics.

CONDITIONS AND PHILOSOPHIES

In many countries, where the majority of the population lives in rural areas but most physicians live in the cities, governments have come to recognize the advantage of using what is available locally. In Thailand, for example, the Ministry of Health developed and distributed a handbook with a chapter on indigenous herbs that would help to alleviate common medical problems—and they encouraged people to grow and use them. The health ministry thus capitalized on three main advantages of using herbs: They can be grown locally in remote areas; people trust their effects; and they generally require less medical supervision than drugs.

Traditional folk healers use herbal remedies that were handed down within families from one generation to another.[3] They use the leaves, root, bark, berries, and flowers of natural growing substances to relieve symptoms, and they frequently ask their patients to gather the herbs themselves. The herbs are picked fresh and are usually combined into teas or concoctions.

Practitioners claim that although their method of preparation is somewhat primitive and slow, the natural substances in each plant maintain their activity and purity, and the essence of the herbs is not destroyed. The traditional practitioners that I interviewed in the South Pacific and India believed that Western synthetic drugs are not compatible with the human constitution. One of their major complaints was how modern physicians also apply Western concepts to ancient traditions when they use natural substances. The Western focus has been to isolate the active ingredient in plants and use this as the sole remedy. But processing deranges the plant's basic cellular structure and this, the traditional practitioners believe, accounts for the problems and side effects that accompany the use of modern drugs. They believe the body repels synthetic drugs, resulting in many iatrogenic diseases (illness caused by a drug, treatment, or physician). They insist that by isolating the active ingredient in an herb, you go against the basic philosophy and traditions of healing.

In modern medicine we might use two or more drugs to treat a medical condition. For example, for congestive heart failure we might use a diuretic that acts on the kidney, an ACE inhibitor or digoxin that acts on the heart, and potassium to ensure there is no electrolyte (mineral salts) imbalance. Similarly, a traditional healer might use five or more herbs in combination, believing that each herb acts on a different organ system. The herbs are mixed together for the specific ailment and symptoms exhibited by the patient. Although the recipes are handed down from generation to generation, they are often altered to fit the constitution of the individual.

ATTITUDES TO RESEARCH

In India, the healing disciplines of Ayurveda, Siddha, and Unani use herbal formulas that have been passed down for hundreds of years. Journals of Ayurvedic and Unani medicine contain many articles describing double-blind studies of herbal formulas that have successfully treated conditions like asthma, vitiligo (loss of skin color or depigmentation), and rheumatoid arthritis. But many of these trials are ignored by modern medicine mainly because the trials were not done in western countries under controlled conditions.

Researchers in China have also published scientific studies that confirm the efficacy of herbs for many medical conditions. With more than five thousand kinds of Chinese medicinal herbs, more than seven hundred patent Chinese medicine factories, and more than fifteen hundred factories of Chinese herbal pills and decoctions, one can easily see that the practice of Traditional Chinese Medicine is firmly established.

Many technologically advanced countries like the United States, Japan, Britain, and Germany are interested in studying herbal formulations to isolate the active and toxic ingredients. Pharmaceutical companies will then develop synthetic drugs that mimic the plant's action. Although this research has helped to create more medications, it does little good for developing countries. The synthetic drugs are so expensive that people in developing countries can't afford them. This doesn't only apply to pharmaceuticals, as herbal companies are also becoming more sophisticated. Instead of manufacturing crude natural substances and mixing herbal formulations in the traditional way, they are mimicking the drug companies and producing expensive medicaments in controlled factory environments.

Japan's Toyama Medical and Pharmaceutical University's Research Institute for Wakan-Yaku [Oriental Medicines] has an extensive library, sophisticated research equipment, and both inpatient and outpatient departments for treating all kinds of diseases exclusively with herbs. When I visited the institute, Dr. Terasawa, a physician of Oriental medicines, explained that herbs seem to be most successful for disorders such as headaches, gastrointestinal disturbances, chronic fatigue, and low energy. Not only do they give relief from the chronic pain of rheumatoid arthritis, neuralgia (nerve pain), and headaches, but the herbs seem to deal with the cause of the problem as well. Herbs are especially useful in patients who cannot tolerate conventional pain medication, and they have helped to alleviate chronic infections such as pneumonitis, chronic vaginitis, and recurrent urinary tract infections.

VISION FOR THE NEW MILLENNIUM

You may be wondering by now why we don't incorporate more traditional herb remedies into modern medicine. It sounds reasonable, doesn't it? But because modern medicine is based on science that involves experimental trials under controlled conditions, gathering and recording data, and comparing results, we have been slow to adopt folk traditions that have not been proven in western trials. Before western consumers can judge which herbal medications are effective, scientific trials need to be performed with crude substances as well as the extracts or synthetics. Yet because trials require a huge investment of time and funding, most of the time the pharmaceutical companies cannot afford to research herbs that they cannot patent to get a return on their investment.

It makes sense to me that herbal formulations that have seemingly proven successful for generations should be tested to support their continued use in their natural form. If we did this, people in developing nations could be encouraged to collect and grow the plants. We should also be collaborating with poorer countries to support their healing traditions and investigate their practices in a more scientific way—which might be better than using expensive, processed drugs. Collaboration between developed countries' funding and scientific resources on the one hand, and underdeveloped countries' generational knowledge, natural resources, and motivation on the other, has to be a win-win situation.

Another major concern for today's world is that thousands of plants are becoming extinct each year. We need to ensure that great care is taken to preserve species that have served mankind for thousands of years. Herbs that have been used by human beings for such a long time have great potential for use by modern medical doctors. We should be teaching the uses, benefits, and side effects of commonly used herbs in all modern medical schools, and we need to encourage and support research that taps this age-old approach to medicine.

When people from older cultures come to North America, they bring their own belief systems and methods of healing; eventually they blend old practices and beliefs with modern medicine. Patients, especially those from Europe and Asia, will often take herbs before they visit their doctor.

Some herbs are also prescribed by western physicians, such as ginger for nausea and senna for constipation. There has been a continual increase in the use of herbs by many segments of the North American population.[4,5] For example, of 114 randomly selected patients attending a university-based AIDS clinic, 22 percent reported using one or more herbal products in the three months prior to the survey.[6]

In the next few chapters, we will look at some of the most commonly used herbs on which randomized, double-blind, controlled trials have been published. I will conclude the herb section of this book by reviewing some of the major concerns doctors have about the use of these herbs— not to frighten or dissuade you, but to help you make informed decisions and to seek advice from people specifically trained in the use of nature's bounty. I hope that by reading this section on herbal medicine and following the recommendations at the end you will have a safer experience with positive results.

CHAPTER 1
ST. JOHN'S WORT FOR DEPRESSION

If I was commanded by the master of all healing to seek an herb that contained the magical properties of the sun—whose blossoms exuded robust energy and unbridled cheer—I would likely return with an armful of St. John's wort. Clusters of this herb's pale stamens upon golden blossoms burst skyward like raised arms that dance in celebration, regardless of their surroundings. They capture the epitome of a positive mood. Perhaps it is no wonder then, that of all the herbs studied by modern clinical trials, St. John's wort, *Hypericum perforatum*, has clearly been shown to be most useful in treating mild to moderate depression.

When I say mild to moderate, I'm not talking about feeling the blues on the odd occasion, or about enduring weeks of suicidal ideation. Mild to moderate levels of depression refers to losing the ability to feel joy; having problems with sleep, concentration, appetite, and weight; and each day becomes a continuous uphill struggle, sometimes to the point where it is difficult just to get out of bed. Depression can negatively impact your life and can even become debilitating, so treatment is highly recommended.

For patients struggling with depression, I recommend taking a serotonin reuptake inhibitor (SSRI) or one of the other new antidepressant medications. I find that these drugs are effective and usually have minimal side effects. I also recommend that my patients have psychotherapy in addition to the drugs. But some people don't want to take antidepressants or they cannot tolerate them. In such a case, St. John's wort may be a useful alternative to discuss with your primary care physician.

THE SCIENCE BEHIND ST. JOHN'S WORT

The majority of St. John's wort trials have conclusively found that its overall antidepressant effect is comparable to that of conventional drugs but without the same side effects.[1, 2, 3, 4, 5]

Two clinical trials have shown that St. John's wort is not effective in the management of severe depression (defined as scoring twenty or greater on the Hamilton Depression Scale), and so the herb is currently only recommended for mild to moderate depression. At the same time, it is important to note that some of the trials for modern antidepressant drugs show them to also be sometimes ineffective in treating severe depression. When a patient is suffering severe depression, a completely different treatment approach needs to be considered with the help of a doctor.

There are also some preliminary trials that show St. John's wort may be helpful in treating other emotional disorders.

SIDE EFFECTS OF ST. JOHN'S WORT

Patients taking St. John's wort have reported side effects. In some cases it has caused drowsiness, sensitivity to the sun, gastrointestinal upset, restlessness, confusion, and skin rashes. There have also been reports that it may exacerbate psychosis in patients with schizophrenia, induce mania and hypomania, and cause serotonin syndrome (a potentially life-threatening drug reaction that is a result of the body having too much serotonin).

One of the concerns physicians have in prescribing St. John's wort for a long length of time is that none of the research has followed patients for more than a year. So doctors are naturally cautious about prescribing something that has not been tracked over the long run.

DRUG INTERACTIONS WITH ST. JOHN'S WORT

Certain components of St. John's wort may interfere with enzymes that metabolize food and drugs in the body, especially one of the main cytochrome P450 isoenzymes, called CYP3A4. Put more simply, St. John's wort speeds up the body's metabolizing action, which can decrease the effect of several prescribed drugs. A few examples of these medications are: digoxin (heart medication), indinavir (used for treating HIV disease), cyclosporin (prevents heart transplant rejection), warfarin (blood thinner), simvastatin (cholesterol reduction), oral contraceptives (birth control), and anti-epileptic (seizure) medication. I would not recommend taking St. John's wort if you are on those medications unless your doctor can adjust the dosage.

St. John's wort should probably not be combined with other modern antidepressants because the interactions have not been well-studied, and side effects and the serotonin syndrome could be triggered.

The best rule of thumb is to check with your physician before taking St. John's wort, especially when taking any other medication. This way you can monitor your health and avoid drug interactions.

ADVANTAGES OF ST. JOHN'S WORT

People who cannot afford health insurance often can't afford the cost of antidepressant drugs either. Even those who are insured may feel the bite when they pull out their wallet to cover the co-pay or they haven't reached their deductible for that year. The cost of St. John's wort, on the other hand, is relatively low; people without drug plans may find it more affordable.

A certain segment of the population suffering with depression is afraid of taking drugs; they may worry about the side effects or don't want to put anything unnatural into their system. On the other hand, out of 3,250 patients who took St. John's wort, only 2.4 percent reported adverse effects. There may be less sedation, dry mouth, gastrointestinal disturbances, and sexual dysfunction with St. John's wort compared to modern synthetic drugs. This lack of side effects could also make it more likely that people will continue taking the herb for the length of time required to prevent relapse.

St. John's wort can be purchased at health-food stores without a prescription. There is still some shame attached to mental and emotional health issues in our society. For a few people, taking a prescription antidepressant may bring up feelings of failure, or being labelled mentally ill, whereas taking over-the-counter herbs would have fewer negative connotations. Other people may worry about filling in insurance forms or job applications that ask whether the applicant is being medically treated for any mental illness such as depression.

SELF-MEDICATION PITFALLS OF ST. JOHN'S WORT

Jane is a forty-three-year-old secretary who became quite depressed and was not getting any better. I recommended that she take a serotonin reuptake inhibitor because she was not functioning, had thoughts of suicide, and was not responding to psychotherapy. Her mother had been psychotically depressed and had ended up in a psychiatric facility. Depression can often be hereditary. When Jane was a teenager she visited her mother in the hospital and remembers seeing her "all doped up" and in bad shape. Jane vowed never to end up like her mother and refused the medication I prescribed. She was very interested in natural forms of healing, however, and was willing to take St. John's wort. Over the next few weeks Jane improved; soon all her symptoms of depression disappeared, and she was in remission.

When prescribing a drug for depression, many physicians advise patients to stay on the medication for nine to twelve months in order to prevent a relapse of depression. The same probably holds true for St. John's wort, and I advised Jane to stay on the herb for at least one year. Regrettably, she ignored my advice, and as soon as she felt better, she stopped taking the herb. After a few months, Jane relapsed into another state of depression.

With all medicines there is a minimum dosage required to achieve results. When people don't take enough of a dose, or discontinue its use too soon, they will not achieve the results they want. Some people change the dosage depending on how they feel that day; many more are apt to stop taking over-the-counter medication as soon as they feel better. What they don't realize is that depression is not like a headache, which can be treated with one pain pill. The causes of depression can be deep rooted and involve physical and chemical structures in the brain that take time to grow or readjust.

MEDICINAL NOTES ON ST. JOHN'S WORT

When taking St. John's wort for depression, it is best to use a standardized extract of *Hypericum perforatum* at a dose of 300 mg, taken three times a day. The therapeutic effect may depend on the hyperforin content—the greater the amount, the more effective it seems to be. Be aware that, just as in treatment with antidepressant drugs, when using St. John's wort, there is a delayed effect. It may take two to four weeks before there is a clinical improvement in the mood disorder.

When starting treatment, it is sometimes important to take an adequate dose for at least four weeks before any decisions can be made about how effective the herb has been. People need an objective person who is qualified to help them make this decision. Those who are self-medicating should see a practitioner frequently to make sure they are taking the right dose and are not stopping the herb too soon. It is also beneficial to receive psychotherapy for depression in addition to taking the herb. Your doctor can often help you create a treatment plan that meets your condition.

CONCLUSION

St. John's Wort is one herb that has many scientific trials that support its usefulness for the treatment of depression. Using this herb under the supervision of your health care practitioner and adding psychotherapy as an additional therapeutic modality can help deal with mild to moderate depression.

CHAPTER 2
ECHINACEA FOR UPPER RESPIRATORY INFECTIONS

Do you remember your last cold, and how everyone you met offered some advice or had a folk remedy that was sure to cure the virus? A typical scene might unfold like this:

You call your boss to say you're not well and when she hears the sound of your runny nasal passages and chesty cough she replies, "Take the day off, go to bed, and drink lots of liquids." Then Grandpa, who recently moved in with the family, suggests his own remedy, "Eat garlic. That always scares the colds away, and it works on vampires too." You frown at Grandpa, wondering just how many vampires he's been fighting off lately. You shuffle slowly up the stairs, climb into bed, and soon your daughter enters, bearing two glasses, each one filled with a suspicious-looking liquid. "My biology teacher," she announces brightly, "said we should gargle with salt water when we have a cold and we should drink apple cider vinegar every morning." You reply, "No thanks, Honey," to the proffered glass of diluted vinegar, but seeing the hurt look on your daughter's face, you agree to gargle with the (extra salty) salt water.

Dragging yourself out of bed, you shuffle to the bathroom, gargling glass in hand. Your body aches, and your chest hurts when you cough, and all you really want is a rum hot toddy and someone to give you a mentholated chest rub along with lots of sympathy. Finally, your spouse comes in and hands you a glass of water with a cheery, "I put a few drops of echinacea in it. Drink up!" Two days later, you begin to feel much better and you go back to work. Your spouse attributes your speedy recovery to the echinacea supplied every eight hours. So what's the verdict? Did the echinacea do the job or was it the Vicks on your chest?

THE HERB ECHINACEA

Echinacea is one of the most commonly used herbs in North America. The name, of Greek origin, means hedgehog—a good choice for a plant whose prickly characteristics somewhat resemble the animal. The flower boasts hot-pink or purple daisy-like petals that surround a prominent conical center of dark orange; the blossom sits upon a tall, robust stem with coarse, fuzzy leaves. If anything could tackle a cold, this sturdy plant looks like it has a winning chance.

There are nine known native species, of which *Echinacea purpurea*, *Echinacea angustifolia*, and *Echinacea pallida* are most commonly used. The plant also goes by the name of coneflower, purple coneflower, and American coneflower. The aboveground parts of the plant are used either fresh or dried to make teas, and they can be crushed (expressed) to make extracts. Anecdotally, many of my patients rave about its ability to decrease or stop the symptoms of upper respiratory infections.

EFFICACY OF ECHINACEA

Some of the difficulty scientists have had with evaluating whether this herb is effective stems from the different varieties of echinacea used; whether the whole plant, the roots, just the flowers or leaves, or a combination of these have been used; and also, how the herb's medicinal constituent is extracted. Sometimes the extractions are done with alcohol and other times with water. But along with support from many generations of folk medicine use, there is some laboratory evidence that echinacea strengthens our immune system.

Controversy in the scientific literature over results of trials makes it downright confusing and you might ask, why can't the scientists agree? But science isn't a matter of opinion. Scientists report on data collected from trials, and using statistical math upon this data they can tell you only whether the results are significant (it appears to work) or that they don't support the hypothesis about the plant having healing properties. Risking some readers' frustration on how divergent scientific conclusions can be, I will present the opposing sides, each one supported by clinical trials. Don't worry if you feel thoroughly mind-boggled with the debate. I will conclude this chapter with my own opinion, based on my interpretation of these results as well as the subjective and anecdotal experiences of my patients.

RESEARCH THAT SHOWS ECHINACEA IS HELPFUL

Ninety-five subjects with early symptoms of cold or flu either received Echinacea Plus tea at a dose of five to six cups per day, or a placebo. Result: In the Echinacea Plus group, there was a statistically significant decrease in cold and flu symptoms in a shorter period of time than with the placebo group. There were no side effects reported by any of the subjects in either group.[1]

In another study, out of 282 participants between eighteen and sixty-five years of age, and with a history of two or more colds in the previous year, 128 contracted a common cold. At the onset of the first cold symptoms the participants received either echinacea, from freshly harvested *Echinacea purpurea* plants (commercially available as Echinilin), or a placebo. They took ten doses on the first day, and four doses per day on the subsequent seven days. The severity of their symptoms and dosing were recorded daily. A nurse examined the subjects on days three and eight after the onset of infection. Result: The total daily symptom scores were found to be 23.1 percent lower in the echinacea group than in the placebo group. Throughout the treatment period, the response rate to treatments was greater in the echinacea group. A few side effects were observed in both groups.[2]

A third study included 430 children, aged one to five years, who were randomized to receive a placebo or an herbal extract preparation called Chizukit. This contained 50 mg/mL of echinacea, 50 mg/mL of propolis (plant resin collected by honeybees), and 10 mg/mL of vitamin C. Of those who received Chizukit, children in the group aged one to three years were given 5.0 mL, and those in the group aged four to five years were given 7.5 mL. Preparations and placebo were given twice daily as preventive medication for twelve weeks. Result: In the Chizukit group, there was a 55 percent reduction in the number of illness episodes, a 50 percent reduction in the number of episodes per child, and a 62 percent reduction in the number of days with fever per child. The total number of illness days and the duration of individual episodes were also significantly lower in the Chizukit group. Adverse drug reactions were rare, mild, and transient.[3]

A 2006 Cochrane review, which is a well-designed analysis of scientific studies, looked at trials comparing echinacea to a placebo. The trials were double-blinded and of good quality. A significant effect was found in nine trials, a trend was found in one trial and no effect was found in six trials. The authors concluded that there is some evidence to suggest that preparations made from the aerial parts of *Echinacea purpurea* might be effective in the early treatment of the common cold in adults. The review found it difficult, however, to compare individual echinacea trial results, as the preparations varied greatly.[4]

Shah and his colleagues did a meta-analysis of fourteen studies on the prevention and treatment of echinacea for the common cold. They concluded that the published evidence supports echinacea's benefit in decreasing the incidence and duration of the common cold.[5]

However a more recent 2014 Cochrane review[6] reports that results from prevention trials suggest that a number of echinacea products slightly reduce the risk of getting a cold in healthy individuals. They stated that although it seems possible that some echinacea products also have effects over placebo for treating colds, the overall evidence for clinically relevant treatment effects over placebo is weak.

RESEARCH THAT SHOWS ECHINACEA DOES NOT WORK

Four hundred and thirty-seven young adults were divided into four groups. Each group received either placebo or one of three extractions of *Echinacea angustifolia* roots with distinct phytochemical profiles. The extractions were made using one of three methods: extraction with supercritical carbon dioxide, with 60 percent ethanol, or with 20 percent ethanol. The volunteers were then subdivided into seven groups that received the various echinacea combinations and/or a placebo. The trial was performed in two phases: a prophylaxis (preventive) phase and a treatment phase.

The prophylaxis phase lasted seven days. On the seventh day, the already-treated volunteers were exposed to a nasal mist containing the common cold (rhinovirus). Result: There were no statistically significant effects of the three echinacea extracts on rates of infection, severity of symptoms, or virus titres (the lowest concentration of virus that still infects cells).[7]

In another study, 128 patients were given either placebo or 100 mg of *Echinacea purpurea* as freeze-dried, pressed juice made from the aerial (aboveground) portion of the plant. The treatment was taken three times daily within twenty-four hours of the onset of a cold until cold symptoms were relieved or until the end of fourteen days, whichever came first. Symptoms were scored subjectively by the patient and recorded daily in a diary. Result: There was no statistically significant difference between groups for either total symptom scores or the duration of symptoms.[8]

Four hundred and seven healthy children, two to eleven years old, were given either echinacea or placebo for up to three upper respiratory infections over a four-month period. Study medication was begun at the onset of symptoms and continued throughout the upper respiratory infection, for a maximum of ten days. Result: There was no statistically significant difference in the duration or severity of symptoms. There was no difference in the rate of adverse events, but rash occurred in 7.1 percent of the children treated with echinacea and only 2.7 percent of those treated with placebo. There was a significantly lower incidence in subsequent upper respiratory infections in those children receiving echinacea.[9]

Finally, 148 students were given *Echinacea* in an encapsulated mixture (25/25/50) of unrefined *E. purpurea* herb and root and *E. angustifolia* root from Shaklee Tecnica. Doses of 1 g were given six times per day on the first day and three times per day for up to nine more days, or placebo, for the treatment of the common cold. Results: No significant difference was found on any outcome measures including cold duration and symptom severity.[10]

In a structured review of 322 articles related to echinacea and colds, nine placebo-controlled, clinical trials were found. Of the nine studies, only two were judged to meet all the criteria of a well-designed, unbiased study. The results of these two studies did not support echinacea's efficacy as a cold remedy. Of the remaining seven studies, the criterion most

16

commonly missing was proof of double-blinding. Six of the seven trials reported positive results, and only one was judged to have negative results. This structured review suggested that the possible therapeutic effectiveness of echinacea in the treatment of colds has not been established.[11]

SIDE EFFECTS

It is usually advised that echinacea not be used in people with immune dysfunction or autoimmune disorders like multiple sclerosis, tuberculosis, AIDS, or lupus because it has not been properly studied in these kinds of conditions. It should probably not be used if you are on immune-modulating drugs like cyclosporine or prednisone. Although adverse reactions are uncommon there have been reports of allergic reactions, which may vary from mild to anaphylactic. Safety in pregnancy has not been established.

CONCLUSION

When trials of echinacea did not show positive findings, the poor outcomes were often blamed on a variety of reasons: using the wrong part of the herb; using inadequate concentrations; using the wrong echinacea variety; or because taking the preparations began too late after the beginning of the infection. There is also controversy about the different methods of extraction and the impact of the extraction type on the results of studies.

Although the scientific evidence is mixed, from my years of clinical experience, I do believe echinacea works for the treatment of the common cold. I take it myself when I feel a cold coming on. At the first sign of infection, I use echinacea and vitamin C. I get feedback from my patients that using echinacea seems to stop that recurring cold situation.

If you are interested in using this herbal alternative, I recommend that you take a tincture of echinacea manufactured from a water extraction method and not an alcohol-based extraction, as some researchers have said that alcohol kills the active ingredient. You should take ten to twenty drops in water every few hours at the first sign of a cold.

CHAPTER 3

GINGER FOR NAUSEA AND VOMITING AND MENSTRUAL PAIN

Had I but one penny in the world, thou shouldst have it to buy gingerbread.

—**SHAKESPEARE**

Few medicinal herbs have a history as colorful and well traveled as the tropical herbaceous ginger, *Zingiber officinale.* No one knows for certain where the plant originated, although many botanists believe it came from India, since that is where most biologically diverse varieties of ginger are found. The part of the plant used for culinary and medicinal purposes is the rhizome, a thickened underground stem, from which roots and shoots appear.

Ginger was mentioned in literature as far back as the fourth century BCE, in the Indian epic *Mahabharata*, as one of the main flavorings used in stewed beef. In the fifth century AD, if you traveled on a merchant ship in the South China Sea or Indian Ocean, you might have seen potted ginger plants with their reed-like leaves and strange blossoms on board being transported to distant lands. During the thirteenth and fourteenth centuries of medieval England, the cost of one pound of preserved ginger was equivalent to the price of a whole sheep.[1]

Farmers and country folk have used the root for centuries to brew ginger beer in England and to make ginger wine in Europe. Many Asian dishes contain fresh, candied, powdered, or marinated ginger root. The traditional and much-beloved pumpkin pie that is served at Thanksgiving would not taste so exquisite without a teaspoon of powdered ginger added to the recipe. For many people, the very mention of ginger brings decorated gingerbread cookies and houses to mind, particularly

18

at Christmas. One youngster asked his schoolteacher for the meaning of the word *cannibal.* When she explained that it meant "people who eat people," he thought about it for a moment, his brow fixed in a worried frown. Suddenly, with a look of great relief he said, "Oh, we eat people at Christmas! Grandma makes them for us. I like to eat the legs first and then I bite off his head." And so the homely looking rhizome is treasured and loved the world over.

GINGER FOR NAUSEA

While ginger has a long culinary history, it has also been used traditionally for healing, most notably in ancient China and India. Perhaps the best-known medicinal use for ginger today is for antinausea treatment. From ginger ale to ginger tea, ginger biscuits or ginger extract—all of these are used by people to settle the stomach.

Diane is a friend who developed intolerance to onions. She suffers with severe stomachache whenever she eats anything with fresh, cooked, or dried onions in it. Diane accidently discovered that when she drank ginger tea or took a ginger capsule before eating at a restaurant, or prior to eating any prepared food that might contain onion, she no longer experienced the gastric discomfort. Was it just coincidence, or does ginger really have antinausea properties? Let's have a look at the science and see what the trial results have shown.

GINGER FOR SEASICKNESS

There have been a number of randomized, double-blind controlled trials for nausea and vomiting. In a systematic review of trials[2] published in 2000, researchers found that 1 gram of ginger powder, given as a single dose to eighty cadets, decreased seasickness compared to placebo. The powdered rhizome of ginger also reduced the symptoms of motion sickness better than dimenhydrinate or placebo in patients that were experimentally provoked by a revolving chair.

GINGER FOR PREGNANCY

A meta-analysis looked at six randomized, double-blind, controlled trials with a total of 675 participants. Four of the six trials showed superiority of ginger over placebo; the other two trials indicated that ginger was as effective as the reference drug (vitamin B6) in relieving the severity of nausea and vomiting episodes. There was an absence of significant side effects. No spontaneous or case reports of adverse events happened during ginger treatment in pregnancy or adverse effects on pregnancy outcomes. The authors concluded that ginger may be an effective treatment for nausea and vomiting in pregnancy. They recommended more observational studies, with a larger sample size, to confirm the encouraging preliminary data on ginger safety.[3]

The Society of Obstetrics & Gynecology of Canada also recommends ginger's use for nausea of pregnancy at a dose of 250 mg four times per day.[4]

GINGER AFTER SURGERY

A meta-analysis of five randomized trials totaling 363 participants was pooled for analysis of preventing postoperative nausea and vomiting. This review demonstrated that a fixed dose of at least 1 gram of ginger is more effective than placebo for the prevention of postoperative nausea and vomiting, as well as for treatment of nausea and postoperative vomiting. Only one side effect, abdominal discomfort, was reported. They concluded that the use of ginger for reducing postoperative nausea and vomiting is effective.[5, 6, 7]

Another study looked at the use of ginger aromatherapy in an outpatient surgical unit in North Carolina. After surgery, out of 1,151 postoperative patients, 303 reported having nausea. Patients with nausea received a gauze pad saturated with a randomly chosen aromatherapy agent and were told to inhale deeply three times. They were given one of four substances to inhale: (1) essential oil of ginger, (2) a blend of four essential oils: ginger, spearmint, peppermint, and cardamom, (3) isopropyl alcohol, or (4) saline, which was used as the control. A significant improvement in the level of nausea was recorded for the blend and for ginger, but not for the alcohol. The number of antinausea medications requested by patients after aromatherapy was also significantly reduced when the ginger or ginger blend was used versus saline.[8]

GINGER AFTER CHEMOTHERAPY

Despite the widespread use of antiemetics (antinausea and vomiting drugs), post-chemotherapy nausea and vomiting continue to be reported by up to 70 percent of patients after treatment. In a 2009 study, 644 patients who had experienced nausea following any chemotherapy cycle, and who were scheduled to receive at least three additional cycles, volunteered and were randomized into four groups: Group One received a placebo; Group Two received 0.5 g ginger; Group Three received 1.0 g ginger, and Group Four received 1.5 g ginger. All patients took three capsules of ginger or placebo twice daily for six days, beginning three days before each of their next two chemotherapy cycles. On days one to four of each treatment cycle, patients reported the severity of nausea during the morning, afternoon, evening, and night using a seven-point scale (1 = no nausea and 7 = extremely nauseated). Results: All doses of ginger significantly reduced nausea. The largest reduction occurred with 0.5 g and 1.0 g of ginger. Researchers concluded that ginger supplementation at a daily dose of 0.5 g to 1.0 g significantly aids in reduction of nausea during the first day of chemotherapy.[9]

GINGER FOR MENSTRUAL PAIN

Another traditional use of ginger is the relief of menstrual cramps. Primary dysmenorrhea is menstrual pain that is not associated with obstruction or disease. Many women experience cramps during menses.

One trial was conducted with 150 medical university students. Participants were divided into three groups, with Group One receiving 250 mg capsules of ginger rhizome powder four times a day for three days from the start of their menstrual period. Groups Two and Three received 250 mg mefenamic acid, or 400 mg ibuprofen capsules, respectively, using the same protocol. Comparison between groups was made after one menstruation. Results: All groups reported a decrease in pain and no significant differences were found between the groups. No severe side effects were reported. Researchers concluded that ginger was as effective as mefenamic acid and ibuprofen in relieving pain in women with primary dysmenorrhea.[10]

Another study, based on 120 university students with moderate or severe primary dysmenorrhea, divided subjects into two equal groups, one for ginger and the other for placebo. Both groups were divided into two treatment protocols with monthly intervals. In the first protocol, groups received 500 mg capsules of ginger root powder or placebo three times a day. Treatment was given two days before the onset of the menstrual period and continued through the first three days of the menstrual period. In the second protocol, ginger and placebo were given only for the first three days of the menstrual period. Results: Significant differences were recorded in the severity of pain in both treatment protocols between placebo and ginger groups. The duration of pain was significantly reduced in the treatment group who received ginger root powder before the onset of the menstrual period, but not in the group who received ginger only for the first three days of the menstruation. Researchers concluded that students who received ginger for five days (beginning two days before menses onset) had a statistically significant reduction in primary dysmenorrhea.[11]

CONCLUSION

Research suggests ginger can be useful for nausea and vomiting due to seasickness, anesthesia, pregnancy, and chemotherapy. Few side effects are linked to ginger when it is taken in small doses. Side effects most often reported are gas, bloating, heartburn, and nausea. These effects were mostly associated with powdered ginger.

With your doctor's approval I recommend taking 250 to 500 mg of powdered ginger root two to four times per day for nausea and vomiting. A glass of ginger ale or ginger tea may also help gastric discomfort. Of course it is always imperative that the cause of the nausea be determined. Ginger may be a safe alternative for menstrual pain (primary dysmenorrhea).

CHAPTER 4

BLACK COHOSH FOR MENOPAUSAL SYMPTOMS

Imagine a warm glowing sensation rising in your chest. Suddenly the heat becomes much more intense, as if an inner microwave had been turned on to the high setting, and you can't turn it off. It climbs from your chest to your neck and face, and you want to rip your clothes off. You look at the fridge, wondering if there is room on the shelf for you to climb in. Does that sound familiar? If the answer is yes, you may be a woman between the ages of forty and fifty-five experiencing one of the common symptoms of menopause. You may also have noticed untypical mood swings, inability to concentrate, vaginal dryness, and other changes that make you wonder where your old self went.

Symptoms of menopause do not just belong to the realm of modern women. Hormonal changes that bring about the end of childbearing years have been happening since the days of Eve. Historically, menopause has affected women's social roles as well as their physical bodies.

A BIT OF HISTORY

Aboriginal women across the world have practiced many rituals surrounding the female cycles. During the four heaviest days of their menses, many Native American women would retreat and stay in a menstrual hut, away from the men. It has long been observed that women who live in close quarters and in small communities often regulate to each other's cycles. It is likely, then, that the menstrual hut hosted more than one woman on a regular basis. Familiarity with each other's cycles would quickly make it apparent to the group when one of the women missed her menses. Perhaps the women would nod and smile, hoping the missing woman was with child. When an older woman stopped coming to the menstrual hut,

23

she gained new respect. Her status rose to that of Wise Woman and she would often be consulted by the younger members of the community.

Some of the earliest records of natural remedies in North America are found in the journals and sketchbooks kept by herbalists and botanists of the eighteenth century. These early collectors of indigenous plants often relied upon Native Americans who generously shared their knowledge with the explorers and settlers. In Northeastern America, one of the most common herbs recommended for "female problems" was black cohosh, sometimes referred to as snake root. People dug the plants up in the autumn after the leaves fell, when the root was thickest and therefore considered to be stronger medicine. The root was used for a variety of women's conditions, from painful menses to childbirth and menopausal symptoms. They also used it to relieve the pain of rheumatism, reduce fevers, and as a tonic. Eventually, black cohosh became one of the most commonly used herbs and was listed as an official drug in the *United States Pharmacopoeia* from 1820 to 1926.[1, 2]

THE BLACK COHOSH PLANT

Black cohosh, *Cimicifuga racemosa*, is a perennial herb that grows to four feet. Its twelve-inch spikes of flowers burst open with fluffy white stamens as they rise above the lush, green foliage. Many gardeners plant the herb in mixed borders of shrubs and perennials to achieve a striking effect of soft color and texture, against the rigorous beauty of its leaves. The plant grows naturally in deciduous forests and on the shady edges of meadows in Eastern North America. When the plant is dug up, its roots hang in long bunches, almost like a handful of young garter snakes, hence its common name, snake root.

The rhizome of the true black cohosh, *Cimicifuga racemosa*, is used in Traditional Chinese Medicine as an anti-inflammatory, analgesic, and anti-fever remedy. The herb is often confused with blue cohosh, *Calophyllum thalictroides*, and is also mistaken for *Cimicifuga foetida*, another Chinese medicinal herb, which is used for different purposes.

A MODERN ALTERNATIVE TO BLACK COHOSH

In more recent times, hormone replacement therapy (HRT) became the medicine of choice to replace female hormones that are no longer produced by the ovaries. Were you one of the women taking HRT in 2002? You may remember the announcement in the news that the Women's Health Initiative, a massive research trial, was cancelled before its planned completion date due to the finding of a significant association with breast cancer, stroke, blood clots, and heart disease in women who were taking HRT therapy. Overnight women across the western world stopped taking their HRT treatment. Doctor's offices were suddenly flooded with patients' complaints of extreme hot flashes and other sudden onset menopausal symptoms that came with unusual vigor after the women stopped taking replacement hormones. These women were asking for safe, natural alternatives. Since then, some have turned to herbal remedies for relief of menopausal symptoms. Black cohosh is one of the most commonly used alternatives, especially for hot flashes.

THE SCIENCE BEHIND BLACK COHOSH

Remifemin, distributed by GlaxoSmithKline, is the name given to black cohosh extract, an herbal remedy corresponding to 20 mg of crude drug, and standardized to 1 percent of 27-deoxyacetine.

Borrelli and Ernst did a review of six randomized, double-blind, controlled trials on Remifemin involving a total of 1,112 women. While evidence gathered does not consistently demonstrate an effect of black cohosh on menopausal symptoms, a beneficial effect of black cohosh on symptoms was found for women in perimenopause. The authors of this review concluded that the efficacy of black cohosh as a treatment for menopausal symptoms is uncertain and further rigorous trials seem warranted.[3]

A Cochrane review of sixteen studies that included 2,027 women found insufficient evidence to support the use of black cohosh for menopausal symptoms. The authors felt that the quality of most of the studies was quite poor and, of course. further good quality research is necessary to say whether black cohosh is useful for menopausal symptoms. They felt there was not enough evidence to either support or oppose the use of black cohosh for menopausal symptoms.[4]

Researchers from Germany report that an aqueous/ethanolic extract of black cohosh and other European preparations reduced major climacteric complaints as effectively as conjugated estrogens and significantly more than placebo. They believe that some US preparations were ineffective most likely because of the too high doses used or due to the adulteration with Asian cimicifuga preparations.[5] Other reviewers challenge the results of the *Cochrane Review* and when analyzing the same data find that black cohosh had a significant effect better than placebo.[6]

A study at the Mayo Clinic in Scottsdale, Arizona, examined the safety and effectiveness of black cohosh in reducing hot flashes. Out of the twenty-one women who completed the study, weekly hot flash scores were reduced by 56 percent among the women who received black cohosh. Researchers noted that previous studies have reported relatively high placebo effects in tests of treatments for hot flashes, but in this trial, the control group experience of placebo effects ranged from 20 to 30 percent. "The efficacy found in this trial seems to be more than would be expected by a placebo effect," reported the researchers. Women taking black cohosh in this study also reported less trouble sleeping, less fatigue, and less sweating.[7]

SAFETY OF BLACK COHOSH

Black cohosh does not appear to contain the isoflavonoid phytoestrogens (plant-based hormones) that are contained in hormone replacement medications. Most studies suggest it has no effect on hormone levels and little or no effect on the lining of the vagina. It appears that black cohosh did not hook up with estrogen receptors, suggesting that black cohosh may not increase the risk of cancer of the uterus. There is also a lack of bad effects on estrogen-sensitive breast cancer cells, suggesting a favorable safety profile. Moreover, it appears that black cohosh enhances the effect of Tamoxifen, a drug used to treat cancer of the breast.[8]

A published review took into account all forms of black cohosh post-marketing surveillance and adverse-report data from the FDA and the World Health Organization. Looking at 2,800 women's responses, it found a low incidence of adverse events (5.4 percent), most of which were mild, such as stomach upsets.[9] Adverse reactions such as nausea, vomiting, headaches, dizziness, mastalgia (breast pain), and weight gain have been observed in some clinical trials. However, the safety of black cohosh is inconclusive.

CONCLUSION

In my clinical practice I have found quite a variable response to the use of black cohosh for menopausal symptoms, with some of my patients saying it was helpful while others found it was not useful at all. There may be a large placebo effect. Generally, at least four to twelve weeks of treatment may be required before any therapeutic benefits become apparent, so do not expect your hot flashes to disappear after taking one dose of the herb. Because isolated reports of liver toxicity have been made, it is advisable, before using the herb, to tell your doctor, who may wish to order a regular blood test to monitor your liver enzymes.

CHAPTER 5

RED CLOVER FOR MENOPAUSAL SYMPTOMS

The state flower of Vermont, red clover, *Trifolium pretense*, is native to Europe and Asia and belongs to the pea and bean family, *Leguminosae*. Red clover successfully migrated to the New World and quickly became a naturalized citizen, populating pastures, lawns, and garden paths as well as tilled fields. Farmers and allotment gardeners refer to it as one of the best green manure crops, for the deep-rooted perennial extracts nitrogen from the air and stores it in little nodules attached to its roots. When these are dug into the soil, nitrogen is released, providing an excellent, cheap fertilizer for leafy green plants, such as spinach, and for brassicas, like broccoli and Brussels sprouts. Red clover's pink tufts sit like upturned shaving brushes upon three-leafed ground-covering stems.

MEDICINAL PROPERTIES OF RED CLOVER

Red clover belongs to a group of herbs that contain compounds called isoflavones. These compounds function like the female hormone, estrogen, but they are phytoestrogens (plant-origin) versus endogenous (produced in the body). The phytoestrogens bind to estrogen receptors in the body and fool the body into acting as if it had received more estrogen. When phytoestrogens were first observed in 1926,[1] it was unknown whether they had any effect upon human or animal metabolism, but in the 1940s, farmers began to notice that sheep grazing in fields of red clover were producing greater numbers of lambs.[2]

Red clover has been used traditionally for the treatment of menopausal symptoms and a good number of studies have been done to test its efficacy. Many patients report anecdotally that red clover is helpful. Aida is typical of women in their forties and early fifties. In her own words, she shares what she was experiencing:

> *About three years ago, I started getting hot flashes really, really bad. I would get red in the face and people would think I was blushing. But I was in my early forties, and I thought I was too young for menopause. So I went to my family physician and she did a blood test. Checking the results, she said, "Yes, you are in menopause."*
>
> *The most frustrating symptom was the hot flashes. I would get hot flashes every half hour, no matter if it was the middle of the day or the night, and I did not like waking up in the middle of the night. When the hot flash would pass, I'd be wet and cold. Then there were the mood swings.*

Aida discussed treatment options with her doctor. Due to recent findings on possible risk factors with HRT, Aida preferred to try a natural supplement first. Her doctor recommended red clover. Aida was able to purchase the herbal remedy without a prescription from her favorite health food store. Here's what she reported:

> *After one month, I experienced a change. The hot flashes were less severe and less frequent. After four months, it was working even better. I've been taking natural supplements now for three years. Sometimes I forget that I could still have symptoms, and I'll stop taking the supplements. When I do, usually by the third day, I start to get the hot flashes again.*

THE SCIENCE BEHIND RED CLOVER

In a 2007 Cochrane review of seven randomly controlled trials, no significant difference was found in five of the trials in overall frequency of hot flashing between Promensil (red clover extract) and placebo. In two trials, no significant difference was found in the percentage of hot flash severity reduction between Promensil and placebo. Reviewers felt there was a strong placebo effect (up to 59 percent).[3]

One of the studies in another Cochrane review assessed an unspecified red clover extract (not included in the previous meta-analysis), and this study reported a benefit for hot flash and night sweat severity. After treatment, only 15 percent of women taking red clover reported hot flashes compared with 98.1 percent of women taking a placebo; values for night sweats were recorded as 30.2 percent for women taking red clover and 92.5 percent for those on the placebo.[4]

Howes et al. did a meta-analysis in 2006 and reported that isoflavones may produce a slight to modest reduction in the number of daily flashes. They found that women who regularly experienced a high number of flashes per day received the most benefit.[5]

Coon et al. also did a meta-analysis. They reported that there is evidence of marginally significant effect of red clover for treating hot flashes in menopausal women.[6]

Another study not included in the Cochrane review found that daily treatment with 80 mg red clover isoflavones (Promensil) resulted in a significant reduction in hot flushes from baseline, and there was a significant decrease in hot flushes of 44 percent between the active and placebo group, demonstrating the effectiveness of Promensil in the management of hot flushes.[7]

A study reported in *Gynecological Endocrinology* found that 80 mg of red clover isoflavones per day caused a significant reduction of hot flashes and night sweats compared to placebo.[8]

One more study found that 80 mg of red clover isoflavones per day caused a significant reduction of depression and anxiety compared to placebo in menopausal women.[9]

SAFETY OF RED CLOVER

The majority of the research seems to indicate that red clover is relatively safe from the standpoint of stimulating endometrial lining and breast tissue. There does not seem to be the same risk as taking hormone replacement therapy.

At least forty-five studies of over 430,000 women exposed to preparations containing isoflavones seem to suggest that red clover either has cancer-preventive effects or does not have cancer-promoting effects (breast and endometrium) and that there is no increased cancer risk. A meta-analysis showed that there was a 16 percent reduction in cancer or relative risk per each 10 mg of isoflavones/day.[10]

The Shanghai Breast Cancer Survival Study followed 543 women after breast cancer therapy. At five years follow-up they found exposure to isoflavones reduces mortality.[11]

There is some evidence that red clover may decrease triglyceride and LDL (bad cholesterol) and increase HDL (good cholesterol) levels. One study seems to indicate that red clover improves blood pressure and the lining of the uterus in menopausal patients with Type 2 diabetes.[12]

CONCLUSION

Red clover products are usually standardized to contain 40 mg of total isoflavones (genistein, daidzein, biochanin A, and formononetin). I generally recommend 80 mg of red clover to my menopausal patients who are experiencing distressing symptoms. Some of my patients have found taking 80 mg of red clover per day helpful. Note: It is important to take the herb for at least four weeks before any benefit can be assured.

CHAPTER 6
GINSENG FOR WHOLE BODY HEALTH

The most widely known types of ginseng are Asian ginseng (*Panax pseudoginseng*), American ginseng (*Panax quinquefolius*), and Siberian ginseng (*Eleutherococcus senticosus*), which has similar medicinal properties, but comes from a different genus of plants. This chapter will focus on the two *Panax* species, which contain similar active ingredients.

ASIAN GINSENG

This story dates back thousands of years, with the first written version appearing in the Chinese Herbal: *Shen-nung pen-ts'ao-ching* (an encyclopedia of medicinal herbs from the first century AD). The Herbal stated that the roots of the plant "schinseng," (meaning man-form or man-shape) boosted longevity, increased endurance, enlightened the mind, increased wisdom, and functioned as an aphrodisiac. The herb was considered so valuable that powerful lords and even centralized government armies fought for and maintained control over ginseng-growing territories.[1] It baffles the mind to think of armies fighting over a plant root rather than gold or diamonds, but the all-body miracle worker was highly prized.

Ancient cultures across the world independently adopted the belief that the shape of plants or shape of their parts determined what part of the body they could cure. It was as if nature had assigned the plant's shape as a hint to man of its healing properties. People believed that if a plant's use was revealed by its physical attributes, surely God had placed his signature upon the plant, a philosophy often referred to as the Doctrine of Signatures. This doctrine was well established by the time the Greek physician Dioscorides (surgeon for Nero's army 50–70 AD) was practicing in Rome. In the case of ginseng, the roots of a mature plant look like a man with arms and legs. Herbalists and physicians believed, therefore, that it could be used to heal the whole man, or that it could make a man whole.

AMERICAN GINSENG

In the New World, American ginseng, *Panax quinquefolius*, which is closely related to the Asian species, was also used by Native Americans for whole-body purposes. Menominee hunters chewed the aromatic root to attract deer, while the women of Meskwaki and Pawnee nations used it to attract a lover or husband. Penobscot women drank an infusion of the root to increase their fertility, and Ojibwa hunters carried it for a good luck charm. The Iroquois used it as eyewash for infants' sore eyes, and an infusion was drunk to alleviate body sores. The pulverized root also was a treatment for asthma by some tribes, while the Delaware used the roots and other plant parts as a general tonic.

Native Americans collected ginseng root in late summer to early autumn, just before the ripened red berries were ready to drop off the umbrella-shaped flower stems. Stewards of their environment, each time native people dug ginseng root out of the earth, they dropped an umbel of ripened berries into the remaining hole, and firmed the soil upon it. This ensured the survival of the plant species, while providing another crop that would be harvested three to five years later.[2]

Unfortunately in China, years of over-harvesting Asian ginseng (*Panax pseudoginseng*) almost decimated the plant in the wild, and a new supply was eagerly sought. In the eighteenth century, Canadian Jesuits became the first exporters of American ginseng to China.[3] It was in 1714 that Father Jartoux, a Jesuit priest living in China, sent Father Lafitau, a Canadian Jesuit, a dried specimen of the Chinese root and herb and asked him if it grew in the New World. Father Lafitau searched for and found the closely related American ginseng (*Panax quinquefolius*). He shipped several pounds of the dried root to China and was delighted to receive a whopping five dollars per pound in return.

Word of the lucrative market soon spread, and a North American cash crop was born. Daniel Boone was one of many colonists who supplemented their incomes by digging, drying, and selling American ginseng roots. Even Thomas Jefferson listed it in his inventory of native plant resources. In 1824, an all-time record of 750,000 pounds of ginseng root was shipped from the United States to China.[4]

American ginseng was nearly wiped out of its wild habitat, an area that ranged from the Maritime Provinces of Canada to the Appalachian and Blue Ridge Mountains, where it grew in humus-rich soil in the deep shade of deciduous hardwood forests. To protect the few remaining plants, members of the United States Convention on International Trade in Endangered Species (CITES) listed *Panax quinquefolius* as one of six North American medicinal plants protected under Wild Fauna and Flora regulations. The U.S. Fish and Wildlife Service also passed a law requiring that wild plants must be five years or older before harvesting.[5]

Due to environmental interventions, some eastern states have reported increasing wild growth of American ginseng and landowners keep a close watch on their wild crops. In West Virginia, a lack of digging over several years has given the herb a reprieve, and in the 2000–2001 growing season, 8,600 pounds of wild ginseng roots were collected, earning from three to four hundred dollars per pound.[6] Today, much of the American ginseng on the market has been cultivated in conditions that mimic the wild.[7]

MEDICINAL PROPERTIES OF GINSENG

What are the facts about ginseng's efficacy as a medicine? Herbalists classify ginseng as an adaptogen, a term that refers to the plant's ability to help the body cope more effectively with stress. Herbalists believe that adaptogens generate a substance that brings the body back into balance and exerts a normalizing influence on the body, neither overstimulating nor inhibiting any of the normal body functions. Specifically, they believe that adaptogens may recharge the adrenal glands, which are the body's mechanism for responding to stress and emotional changes.

American ginseng is grown commercially mainly in the Canadian provinces of British Columbia and Ontario and in Wisconsin, the largest producer of American ginseng in the United States. The products are usually standardized to their ginsenoside (or panaxoside) content. Most often the active ingredient is extracted from the root of the plant, but the berries and leaves, which also contain active ginsenosides, may be used. Other names for American ginseng include: Anchi ginseng, Canadian ginseng, North American ginseng, Ontario ginseng, *P. quinquefolium,* red berry, ren shen, sang, Tienchi ginseng, and Wisconsin ginseng.

THE RESEARCH ON GINSENG

In the journal *Public Health Nutrition,* Kitts and Hu[8] summarized the various research studies of ginseng in animals and humans. They felt there may be differences in pharmacological properties between different species of ginseng. Using the traditional Asian concept of the complementary forces of yin and yang, American ginseng (*Panax quinquefolius*) provides a cooling effect with yin conditions that offset stress, while the Asian ginseng (*Panax pseudoginseng*) provides warmth, with yang conditions to counterbalance stress. The reviewers believed that these apparent differences in the cause and effect properties of ginseng may be related to the different composition of ginsenosides present in these two sources of the herb.

Kitts and Hu state that Panax (both varieties of ginseng) has been shown to have metabolic effects that account for its antioxidant activities. It has been shown to enhance oxygen uptake and cellular glucose uptake, have a stimulatory effect on the brain's neuronal activity (increased brain cell activity), and to lower blood glucose (esp. *P. quinquefolius*). It has also been shown to have impact on the adrenal glands through enhanced adrenocorticotrophin secretion (moderates the body's stress hormone release), increased plasma cortisone (hormone that combats inflammation), and a reduction of ACH-evoked catecholamine release (reduced fight or flight symptoms).

They also report that Panax also seems to have a positive effect on immune function. This is believed to be mediated through its positive effect on white blood cells, an increase in T-helper cells, macrophages, and a reduction in leukotriene release. Some research suggests that Panax ginseng may also have a positive effect on the cardiovascular system. This potentially may include the ability to enhance recovery of heart and brain cells that suffered reduced blood supply and the inhibition of platelet aggregation (cells responsible for increasing clotting of our blood, which can lead to heart attacks and strokes).

There is also preliminary research showing ginseng may have anti-cancer properties.[9]

AMERICAN GINSENG'S EFFECT ON TYPE 2 DIABETES MELLITUS

American ginseng has a positive impact on the way the body handles sugar. It is believed to slow down the absorption of sugar, increase the ability to move glucose into our cells, and increase the body's ability to store glucose for later use. It may also help with insulin secretion.

A double-blind, placebo-controlled study was done at St. Michael's Hospital in Toronto with nineteen patients (ten healthy; nine diagnosed with Type 2 diabetes). Patients were given 3 g of ginseng daily, either forty minutes before, or together with, a 25 g oral glucose (sugary drink) challenge.[10] In patients with diabetes, there was a significant reduction (19 to 22 percent) in postprandial glycemia (rise in blood sugar) versus placebo regardless of when the ginseng was taken. In healthy patients, the effects were only seen if ginseng was ingested forty minutes before the glucose challenge.

Another study at the same institution found that American ginseng, 3 g, 6 g, or 9 g, given to non-diabetic patients, improved glucose tolerance when taken 40, 80, or 120 minutes before a glucose challenge.[11]

One more study looked at ten Type 2 diabetic patients who were randomly administered 3 g, 6 g, 9 g, or 0 g (placebo) of ground American ginseng root in capsules at 120, 80, 40, or 0 minutes before a 25-g oral glucose challenge. Capillary blood glucose was measured before ingestion of American ginseng or placebo and at 0, 15, 30, 45, 60, 90, and 120 minutes from the start of the glucose challenge. The conclusion was that American ginseng reduced postprandial glucose irrespective of the dose and the time of administration.[12]

GINSENG FOR CHEMOTHERAPY OR RADIATION-INDUCED CHRONIC FATIGUE

After receiving chemotherapy or radiation therapy, many patients suffer from long-term, debilitating fatigue. Although fatigue decreases in time, some patients may not return to their old level of energy. A trial led by Mayo Clinic researchers studied 340 patients who had completed cancer treatment or were being treated for cancer at one of forty community medical centers. Participants received a placebo or 2 g American ginseng a day administered in capsules containing pure, ground American ginseng root. At four weeks, the pure ginseng provided only a slight improvement in fatigue symptoms. At eight weeks, ginseng offered cancer patients significant improvement in general exhaustion (described as feelings of being "pooped," "worn out," "fatigued," "sluggish," "run-down," or "tired") compared to the placebo group. No apparent side effects were reported.[13]

COLD-FX, FOR COLDS

Cold-FX is made from poly-furanosyl-pyranosyl-saccharide-rich extract from roots of American ginseng. In a randomized, controlled trial, 323 patients aged eighteen to sixty-five took placebo or Cold-FX twice a day for four months. In the Cold-FX group, there was a reduction of the mean number of colds per person, and in the proportion of people that had two or more colds; a reduction was also noted in severity of symptoms, and in the number of days that cold symptoms were reported.[14]

In another trial, 783 community living adults received American ginseng or a placebo over a six-month period. Upper respiratory infections were lower in the treated group, and there was a reduction of the severity and duration of upper respiratory infections.[15] Two randomly assigned double-blind controlled trials were done on 198 institutionalized patients in long-term care settings that included a nursing home and assisted living centers. Patients given 200 mg of Cold-FX twice a day during the flu season significantly reduced the incidence of acute respiratory infections compared to placebo.[16]

SIDE EFFECTS AND DRUG INTERACTIONS OF GINSENG

Few side effects and drug interactions have been documented with American ginseng. Reports of hypertension, gastrointestinal disturbances, insomnia, depression, confusion, and nervousness have been reported with high doses of different species of ginseng. Long-term use (twelve weeks) of 3 g of American ginseng seems to have no effect on twenty-four-hour blood pressure and kidney function in hypertensive (high blood pressure) individuals.

Ginseng/drug interactions have been observed with phenelzine, a monoamine oxidase inhibitor, and it reduces the effect of warfarin.

There have been isolated reports in the literature suggesting various ginseng products may have estrogen-like effects, may prolong the QT interval (a measurement of time between heart waves on electrocardiogram), decrease white blood cells, have manic effects, and increase bleeding.

Traditional healers and Traditional Chinese Medicine practitioners tend to use ginseng in combination with other herbs so its exact impact is hard to measure. Safety in pregnancy and lactation has not been established.

DOSAGE OF GINSENG

One of the biggest problems in the use of ginseng is determining dosage. A survey of fifty commercial ginseng preparations from eleven different countries demonstrated that greater than 90 percent of the preparations varied between 2 and 9 percent in total ginsenoside content, and some preparations contained no ginsenosides at all. Generally 100 to 200 milligrams of a standardized ginseng extract (4 percent ginsenosides) taken by mouth once or twice daily has been used in studies for up to twelve weeks. Some other studies have also used 0.5 to 2 grams of dry ginseng root, taken daily by mouth in divided doses.

CONCLUSION

Ginseng is a popular herbal medicine that is used worldwide for improving well-being in many different kinds of health problems. Ginseng appears to be relatively safe but the quality of most of the research is poor.[17] Although there is some controversy about the use of American ginseng in the prevention of colds[18, 19, 20], if you are getting frequent colds each year, then taking American ginseng in the form of Cold-FX may help to prevent recurrent upper respiratory infections. It appears to be relatively safe.[21]

CHAPTER 7
FEVERFEW FOR MIGRAINE

For such a humble relative of the common daisy, feverfew, *Tanacetum parthenium,* boasts an incredible number of names. Bachelor buttons, featherfoil, mother herb, flirtwort, midsummer daisy, and febrifuge are among the dozen or more aliases. Historically the herb's botanical name was listed as *Chrysanthemum parthenium,* but in recent times it was recategorized to the Aster family and listed as *Tanacetum parthenium.*

As with most herbs, feverfew has a rich history of folklore and stories. In medieval times, when the fearsome plague loomed as a genuine threat, people might have worn an amulet of feverfew, believing its long-lasting, strong aroma would ward off evil spirits while cleansing the putrid smell of death from their nostrils. Originally native to the Balkans, feverfew was spread by deliberate planting throughout Europe and the Americas. Today organic gardeners plant feverfew around vegetable beds to act as a natural barrier against pests such as white fly, cabbage moth, and other destructive insects, while a sachet of the dried leaves hung in the closet is reputed to be an effective moth repellent.

Historically, feverfew has been used to prevent severe headaches, stimulate appetite, reduce tinnitus and dizziness, induce abortions, regulate menstruation, and relieve muscle cramps. A tincture of the herb was commonly used to treat insect bites.

THE SCIENCE BEHIND FEVERFEW

Scientific research on the plant was almost nonexistent until an interesting chain of events and characters connected in a fine display of symbiosis. It was in the 1970s that the chief medical officer of England's National Coal Board told his colleagues about his wife's frequent and debilitating migraines. A sympathetic coal miner suggested that she try an old folk remedy that had worked for him. "Tell her to chew two leaves of feverfew each day in order to prevent migraines," he said. Much to the chief medical officer's delight, when his wife tried the folk remedy, her migraines disappeared almost completely. The CMO shared his remarkable story with Dr. E. Stewart Johnson of the London Migraine Clinic, who then offered the feverfew remedy to ten of his patients for migraine treatment. The positive results observed by Dr. Johnson from that experiment led to some of the British studies described below.

FEVERFEW FOR MIGRAINES

Interest in feverfew increased with the results of two double-blind, placebo-controlled trials that were published in the *Lancet* and the *British Medical Journal* showing the herb's usefulness in the prevention of migraines.

In the Lancet study,[1] fifty-nine people took part for eight months. For four months, half received daily an 82 mg capsule of powdered leaves; the other half took placebo. The groups were then switched and followed for an additional four months. Treatment with feverfew produced a 24 percent reduction in the number of migraines and a significant decrease in nausea and vomiting during the headaches.

A double-blind study[2] of seventeen people who suffered migraines was reported in the *British Medical Journal*. Experimental subjects were given powdered, freeze-dried feverfew leaves amounting to 50 mg per day. The study found that use of feverfew leaf could decrease the severity of migraine headaches. Unfortunately, this trial did not report whether there was any change in the frequency of migraines; it is possible, therefore, that this study actually showed a symptom-reducing effect rather than a preventive benefit.

Some migraine sufferers experience a mild headache before the onset of their full-blown migraine. In 2011, a randomized trial involving sixty such patients found that a sublingual (placed under the tongue for rapid absorption) combination of feverfew and ginger, taken at the onset of this early headache, helped to reduce or eliminate pain for at least two hours. Researchers concluded that sublingual feverfew/ginger appears safe and effective as a first-line abortive treatment for a population of migraine sufferers who frequently experience mild headache prior to the onset of moderate to severe headache.[3]

A Cochrane review looked at five trials involving 343 patients. Results from these trials were mixed, and the authors did not feel that the evidence was convincing enough to establish that feverfew is efficacious for preventing migraine.[4] Inconsistencies in the results of those studies were probably related to wide variations in the strength of the active ingredient (parthenolide) and differences in the stability of feverfew preparations.

In 2002, a more stable feverfew extract (MIG-99) was evaluated in a placebo-controlled trial involving 147 patients. Although none of the doses significantly reduced the number of migraine attacks (compared with baseline) in the last month of the three-month study relative to those in the placebo group, a subset of patients with high frequency of migraine attacks did seem to benefit.[5]

In a 2005 follow-up multicenter, double-blind, placebo-controlled study with 170 participants, investigators evaluated the dosage of 6.25 mg of MIG-99, taken three times a day, versus placebo, and reported a statistically significant and clinically relevant reduction in migraine frequency in the MIG-99 group compared with placebo.[6]

HOW DOES FEVERFEW WORK?

Feverfew is thought to have anti-inflammatory and analgesic properties. It may reduce the release of inflammatory substances from your blood cells and slow down your body's production of histamine, a chemical transmitter. This may play an important role in how your immune system works, how your pain is transmitted, and how you feel pain.

DOSAGE RECOMMENDATIONS FOR FEVERFEW

Patients in the United Kingdom who self-medicate generally eat two to three leaves daily, taken with food or sweetener to relieve the bitter taste. In Canada, where feverfew is approved by Canada's Health Protection Branch, it is marketed as Tanacetum at a recommended dosage of 125 mg/

CAUTION

As with any herbal remedy, consult your own doctor before starting treatment. Because feverfew might slightly inhibit the activity of blood-clotting cells known as platelets, it should not be combined with anticoagulants or blood thinners, such as aspirin, warfarin (Coumadin), or heparin, except on medical advice. It may also interact with anti-inflammatory drugs like ibuprofen and other anti-migraine medications. Feverfew should not be used by pregnant or lactating women.

Feverfew is related to ragweed and so has the potential to cause allergy symptoms. Mouth ulcerations are a very common side effect and sometimes a more widespread mouth inflammation can occur. If you are suffering from kidney, liver, or cardiovascular disease, you should get your physician's clearance before taking any herb.

If you decide to stop taking feverfew, it is best to decrease the amount you take and gradually phase it out. Some people who have suddenly stopped taking it after several years have experienced a return (rebound) of their previous level of migraines along with other symptoms such as nausea, anxiety, and insomnia.

day. Four to six weeks are required to notice a response. Since therapeutic efficacy has been demonstrated for preparations of feverfew that contain the ingredient parthenolide, it is suggested that when buying feverfew it may be helpful to make sure that the product contains parthenolide.[7]

CONCLUSION

If you suffer from migraine headaches, feverfew may be a prevention remedy to try with your physician's supervision.

CHAPTER 8

GINKGO BILOBA FOR DEMENTIA, VASCULAR DISORDERS, AND STROKE

In the Western world, *Ginkgo biloba* is called the maidenhair tree, but the Japanese commonly refer to it as *I-cho*, "tree with leaves like a duck's foot."[1] This tree stands over one hundred feet tall at maturity. Its graceful, pale green leaves resemble those of the maidenhair fern, delicate fan shapes that flutter in the wind, and in autumn, leave thick yellow carpets beneath gently skirting branches.

The small, pale, plum-shaped fruit of ginkgo are considered a delicacy in many countries, but when left to rot on the ground, they emit an odor that some liken to rancid butter or vomit.

A friend in California had one growing in her front yard. For a few days each year, she was aware of an unpleasant odor but had no idea where it came from. One autumn she spotted a coyote eating something that lay amongst the fallen ginkgo leaves. After the coyote left, she went outside to investigate, and discovered it had been feasting upon the rotting fruit of her favorite tree. "When I picked up the fruit," she said, "I suddenly realized that's where the awful smell was coming from! It was such a pleasure to watch the coyote through my window at close range; I've forgiven my tree for the annual stink."

The ginkgo is extraordinary in many ways. It is the only surviving tree out of the group called Ginkgoales. Fossils of leaves that look eerily similar to today's ginkgo may be found today across Eurasia and in parts of North America. The trees whose leaves imprinted upon those stones grew during and before the Jurassic period. Imagine walking beneath a tree today whose ancestors became fast-food delicacies for dinosaurs!

Ginkgo biloba nearly succumbed to the extinction of its cousins. When natural conditions that helped ginkgo seed to disperse and germinate in the wild were no longer there, tradition says that ancient Japanese and Chinese monks cultivated it for their temple gardens, inadvertently rescuing it from oblivion. Many generations later, it was adopted as an ornamental tree for gardens and cities in Europe and in the New World. Today ginkgo is mostly found in cities of temperate climates. Its natural resistance to pollution and pesticides has made it a popular choice for economic as well as aesthetic reasons.[2]

Ginkgo biloba has become a popular herb in the lay press, and its consumption by the general public is increasing. It is interesting that a tree with such close roots to the prehistoric world is used today by those hoping to preserve memory, increase mental acuity, and decrease the obstruction of life-giving blood to the body's extremities.

THE *GINKGO BILOBA* EXTRACT

EGb 761 Formula is the name of the standardized extract made from the dried leaves of *Ginkgo biloba*. It contains 24 percent ginkgo-flavonol glycosides and 6 percent terpene lactones, such as ginkgolides A, B, C, and J, and bilobalide.

GINKGO BILOBA FOR DEMENTIA

Perhaps the most famous ginkgo study was a randomized double-blind placebo-controlled trial reported in the *Journal of the American Medical Association* (*JAMA*) that looked at the effects of ginkgo in a multi-centered sample of patients with dementia.[3] Multi-centered refers to a study of subjects from many different cities. This reduces the possibility that the variables affecting one particular population (such as local pollution) could skew results.

Patients were assigned to receive either 40 mg of EGb 761 (ginkgo extract) three times a day before meals or a placebo, and they were monitored every three months with outcome evaluations performed at twelve, twenty-six, and fifty-two weeks. Cognitive impairment was assessed by a performance-based test that tested memory, language, praxis (sensory-motor capacity), and orientation (awareness of one's environment with reference to time, place, and people). Daily living and social behavior was assessed by a forty-nine-item inventory that was completed by the caregivers. General psychopathology (signs of mental illness, distress, abnormal or mal-adaptive behavior) was measured by an interview-based global rating that quantified clinicians' judgment in the amount of change in overall impairment compared to the baseline. Results: From 309 patients who began the study, only 202 were followed for fifty-two weeks. Patients on ginkgo showed improved cognitive performance and social functioning compared to the placebo group. There seemed to be no difference in the side effect profile of the EGb 761 patients when compared to the placebo group.

Although the study seemed to show that ginkgo was effective, there were major criticisms of the study. Because there was a large dropout rate, only 202 out of the original 309 patients completed the study, bringing the whole reliability of the results into question. Also, since no significant difference was noted in the clinicians' global impression of change, there did not seem to be actual significant measurable clinical real-life improvement in impairment.

In a double-blind, placebo-controlled trial, 309 patients with mild to severe Alzheimer's disease were treated with 40 mg of EGb 761 three times a day over twenty-six weeks. In the 244 patients who completed the study, there was a slight improvement on cognitive assessment, as well as daily living and social behavior compared to a statistically significant worsening in the placebo group. There was no difference in the side effects between the two groups.[4]

In another study, 160 patients with mild cognitive impairment were given *Gingko biloba* (EGb 761) daily 240 mg per day for twenty-four weeks or placebo. EGb 761 improved neuropsychiatric symptoms and cognitive performance in patients compared to placebo. The drug was safe and well tolerated.[5]

A review of four randomized, controlled trials investigating the efficacy of *Ginkgo biloba* extract EGb 761 in elderly patients with Alzheimer or vascular dementia with neuropsychiatric features found that patients treated with EGb 761 showed improvements of cognitive performance and behavioral symptoms that were associated with advances in activities of daily living and a reduced burden to caregivers.[6]

GINKGO BILOBA FOR PERIPHERAL VASCULAR DISEASE AND INTERMITTENT CLAUDICATION (LEG PAIN)

People with blocked arteries and impaired circulation in their legs often get pain in their legs when they attempt to walk even a short distance. The sensation may be as mild as discomfort and tiredness during exercise, up to a painful, burning sensation in their calves. At night, they may wake with severe aching in their toes. In North America, this condition affects more than 20 percent of patients over seventy years of age. Risk factors are: smoking, diabetes, high blood pressure, high cholesterol, and advanced age.[7]

Researchers reviewed eight randomized, double-blind, placebo-controlled trials using ginkgo for intermittent claudication. They found a significant difference in the increase of pain-free walking distance for patients who used ginkgo compared to those who took the placebo. Adverse effects were rare, mild, and, transient.[8]

Schweizer and Hautmann compared the effect of ginkgo biloba extract (EGb 761) over a 24-week period, in seventy-four patients with Fontaine's stage IIb peripheral arterial occlusive disease (the narrowing, hardening, and obstruction of arteries supplying legs and feet, which are not within the coronary, aortic arch vasculature, or brain). Volunteers were divided into two groups, one receiving dosages of 120 mg/day and the other receiving 240 mg/day. Although walking distance improved in both groups of patients, those who received the 240 mg dosage had a statistically significant increase in pain-free walking. Also recorded was a mean increase of 60.6 meters in the group who received 120 mg compared to a mean increase of 107 meters in those who took 240 mg. Both treatments were considered safe and well tolerated.[9]

GINKGO BILOBA FOR STROKE

Although ginkgo is widely used in China for the treatment of stroke, a meta-analysis of randomized, controlled trials failed to show a significant improvement in the treatment of stroke with ginkgo as compared to placebo. Fourteen trials were identified, of which ten trials (792 patients)

47

were included in the analysis. In those ten trials, follow-up was performed at fourteen to thirty-five days after the stroke. In all studies, neurological outcome was assessed but none of them reported on disability (activities of daily living function) or quality of life. Only three trials reported adverse events during the trial period.

Result: Nine out of the ten trials (all of which were assessed to be of poor quality) reported that *Ginkgo biloba* extract was associated with a significant increase in the number of improved patients. The placebo-controlled trial (the only one assessed to be of good quality) reported that there was no improvement in neurological deficit at the end of treatment. The authors concluded there was no convincing evidence from trials of sufficient methodological quality to support the routine use of *Ginkgo biloba* extract to promote recovery after stroke. High-quality and large-scale randomized controlled trials are needed to test its efficacy.[10]

SIDE EFFECTS OF GINKGO BILOBA

Sometimes gastrointestinal upsets, dizziness, headaches, and allergic skin rashes can occur with the use of ginkgo.[11] There is also a concern about spontaneous bleeding, especially in patients taking aspirin or Coumadin, which is a blood thinner. Ginkgo is believed to decrease platelet aggregability (clumping) and fibrinogen. There have been reports of subarachnoid hemorrhage (bleeding between brain and the thin tissues that cover it), intracerebral hemorrhage (stroke) on warfarin, spontaneous subdural hematoma (bursting of a blood vessel in the brain), and one of hyphema (bleeding into the eye).

CONCLUSION

Scientific studies to date do not provide any certainty that *Ginkgo biloba* works for conditions like the effects of stroke. But there is some evidence that Gingko may be helpful for intermittent claudication (leg pain) and mild to moderate dementia. Most neurologists I have spoken with do not feel that there is any benefit to using Gingko for dementia. My advice is to discuss it with your doctor before taking this herb. Patients who are taking aspirin or blood thinners should not take ginkgo at the same time. Treatment with ginkgo probably should be stopped before surgery as it may prolong the bleeding time.

CHAPTER 9

HORSE CHESTNUT SEED EXTRACT FOR VEINS

Horse chestnut, *Aesculus hippocastanum*, is one of the world's most beautiful trees, particularly when it bursts into flower with majestic twelve-inch candles of white or red blossoms. After the leaves fall, leaf stalk scars remain on the twigs in a distinctive horseshoe shape, complete with seven nail holes. These unique marks may have given rise to the tree's name. Growing up to one hundred feet at maturity, the tree's candelabra branches have towered over gardens and parks for many years. Although native to the Balkan Peninsula (Greece, Romania, Albania, etc.) the horse chestnut is one of the most beloved trees in the British Isles, Europe, and in temperate climes of the New World.

HISTORY OF HORSE CHESTNUT SEED EXTRACT

French and Swiss cloth makers washed natural fibers of hemp, wool, flax, and silk in a strained soapy liquid made from crushed, soaked horse chestnuts in order to whiten the cloth and remove spots and stains. Older residents of Fredericksburg, Virginia, boasted about having thirteen horse chestnuts that were imported and planted by George Washington who named them after each of the thirteen colonies. Alexander Hamilton also planted them outside his home in New York. In July 2004 the last of George Washington's standing horse chestnuts was felled and removed for safety concerns.[1] Another horse chestnut in Amsterdam received notoriety through Anne Frank's diary where she referred to it as her "beautiful tree." Sadly, the diseased tree succumbed to a strong wind in the summer of 2010.[2]

When the horse chestnut's prickly green fruit drops to the ground in the autumn, it cracks open, exposing a hard brown nut called a conker. The first record of the game appeared in the Isle of Wight in 1848. Today the annual World Conker Championships are held in Northamptonshire, and they attract thousands of people and participants from all over the world.

Unfortunately the centuries-old game is now under real threat along with the magnificent horse chestnut tree and its fruit, due to an invasion of alien moths that entered England "on the back of a lorry." First reported near London in 2002, a leaf miner attack has spread at the rate of thirty-seven miles per year. These moths, a species of the *Cameraria* genus that was unknown until 1978 when it was discovered in Macedonia, lay eggs on the underside of the horse chestnut leaf. The eggs hatch into tiny caterpillars called leaf miners; these don't kill the tree, but their feeding causes the leaves to prematurely brown in midsummer and drop off, making the tree vulnerable to disease. Pesticides have not been successful either in control or eradication.

As a result of their weakened state, more than half of Britain's horse chestnuts have become infected with bleeding canker, a deadly disease that leaves weeping sores on the bark. Local governments have been removing horse chestnuts from parks and roadsides for fear of diseased branches falling and injuring passersby.

MEDICINAL PROPERTIES OF HORSE CHESTNUT SEED EXTRACT

There are two principal ingredients in the horse chestnut seed. Aescin is believed to affect capillary permeability, making it harder for fluid to leak out of veins and capillaries, and it may strengthen and improve tone of the walls of veins. Aesculin thins the blood, improving its viscosity.

A standardized extract from the horse chestnut seed has been used in Europe for many years in the treatment of symptoms of poor circulation (chronic venous insufficiency) and venous diseases such as varicose veins, hemorrhoids, tiredness, itching, swelling in the legs, edema (water retention), and swollen veins (phlebitis—inflammation of the veins). Aesculus preparations are used orally and externally (in the form of ointments and gels).

CAUTION

Do not use raw or unprocessed horse chestnut seeds, leaves, bark, or flowers. They contain aesculin, which is poisonous and can cause death when taken by mouth. When properly processed, horse chestnut seed extract contains little or no esculin and is considered generally safe when used for short periods of time. Signs of poisoning include stomach upset, kidney problems, muscle twitching, muscle weakness, loss of coordination, enlarged eye pupils, vomiting, diarrhea, depression, paralysis, and stupor. Immediate medical attention should be sought if there has been an accidental ingestion of horse chestnut. Incidences of children being poisoned by eating the seeds or making tea from the leaves have been recorded.

HORSE CHESTNUT SEED EXTRACT FOR VENOUS INSUFFICIENCY

Poor blood flow in the veins of the legs is a condition that can develop with inactivity and older age. When severe enough, it can result in a condition called chronic venous insufficiency. People with the condition may suffer a host of symptoms such as nocturnal leg cramps, pruritus (itchiness), hardening or scaling of the skin, redness, and edema (swelling from water retention) along with a sensation of heaviness in the legs when walking. Wearing compression bandages or stockings is one of the more traditional solutions that can be helpful, but these are uncomfortable for some people. I find patients are often non-compliant with this treatment because of the difficulty of putting them on as well as their unsightly appearance.

Treatment

In Germany, Commission E (equivalent of the U.S. Food and Drug Administration) approved the standardized powdered extract of horse chestnut seeds adjusted to an aescin content of 16 to 20 percent as an appropriate treatment for conditions of the veins of the legs, such as pain, feelings of heaviness, nocturnal calf muscle spasm, itching, and swelling.

Dosage

For chronic venous insufficiency: 300 mg of horse chestnut seed extract containing 50 mg of aescin, the active ingredient, taken twice daily by mouth.

THE SCIENCE BEHIND HORSE CHESTNUT SEED EXTRACT

In 2006, scientists with the Universities of Exeter and Plymouth in England sifted through years of studies and selected the best randomized, controlled trials for a meta-analysis in the well-respected *Cochrane Database of Systematic Reviews.*

Leg pain was assessed in seven of the placebo-controlled trials. Six reported a significant reduction of leg pain in the horse chestnut seed extract groups compared with the placebo groups, while another reported a statistically significant improvement compared with baseline. Leg volume was assessed in seven placebo-controlled trials. A meta-analysis of six trials that involved 502 patients suggested a decrease in leg volume when horse chestnut seed extract was compared with placebo. Results: Overall the review concluded that there was an improvement in chronic venous insufficiency with the short-term use of horse chestnut seed extract. Most of the trials found the extract more effective than placebo, and one trial indicated that taking 50 milligrams of aescin (the active ingredient in horse chestnut seed) twice daily over twelve weeks may be as effective as treatment with compression stockings. Adverse events were usually mild and infrequent. The authors concluded that more rigorous randomly controlled trials are required to confirm the efficacy of this treatment option.[3]

Another review of fourteen randomized, controlled trials found seven to be of high methodological quality, but limited by small sample sizes and short durations. These studies supported the superiority of horse chestnut seed extract over placebo, and suggest equivalence to compression stockings and to oral oxerutins (semi-synthetic derivatives of plant constituents). The authors also recommended a longer and adequately powered randomized trial comparing horse chestnut seed extract to the current common standard of care, and to further assess safety and long-term efficacy.[4]

Another review identified thirteen randomized, controlled trials of chronic venous insufficiency (1,051 patients) and three observational studies (10,725 patients). They reported that compared to placebo, horse chestnut seed extract reduced leg volume by 46.4 ml and increased the likelihood of improvement in leg pain 4.1-fold. Similarly, there was a decrease of edema and itching. Although observational studies showed significant effectiveness regarding pain, edema, and leg fatigue/heaviness, there were insufficient numbers of randomized, controlled trials done to demonstrate horse chestnut seed extract's effect on leg fatigue/heaviness or calf cramps. No severe adverse events were reported, and horse chestnut seed extract did not significantly increase mild adverse events.[5]

PRECAUTIONS AND INTERACTIONS[6] FOR HORSE CHESTNUT SEED EXTRACT

Avoid use during pregnancy and breast-feeding, if you have liver or kidney disease, or an allergy to latex.

Horse Chestnut Seed Extract and Lithium

Horse chestnut may have an effect like a diuretic and affect how the body gets rid of lithium. Increases of lithium in the body can result in serious side effects. If you are using lithium, talk with your health care provider before using this product. Your lithium dose might need to be changed.

Horse Chestnut Seed Extract and Diabetes Medication, Herbs, and Supplements

Horse chestnut might decrease blood sugar. Taking it along with diabetes medications, herbs, and supplements might cause your blood sugar to go too low. Monitor your blood sugar closely. The dose of your diabetes medication might need to be changed.

Horse Chestnut Seed Extract and Anticoagulant/Antiplatelet Medication, Herbs, and Supplements

Horse chestnut seed might slow blood clotting. Taking it along with medications, herbs, and supplements that also slow clotting might increase the chances of bruising and bleeding. Some medications that slow blood clotting include aspirin, clopidogrel (Plavix), diclofenac (Voltaren, Cataflam, others), ibuprofen (Advil, Motrin, others), naproxen (Anaprox, Naprosyn, others), dalteparin (Fragmin), enoxaparin (Lovenox), heparin, warfarin (Coumadin), and others.

CONCLUSION

There are many anecdotal observations for the use of horse chestnut seed extract topical preparations applied to varicose veins and hemorrhoids, along with other conditions, but there is a paucity of clinical trials to support topical use. More evidence is needed to rate horse chestnut for these traditionally known uses: Hemorrhoids, diarrhea, fever, cough, enlarged prostate, eczema, menstrual pain, soft tissue swelling from bone fracture and sprains, arthritis and joint pain.

Horse chestnut has not been evaluated by the FDA for safety, effectiveness, or purity. All potential risks and/or advantages of horse chestnut may not be known. Although I have not used horse chestnut in clinical practice, there is some evidence that it may be useful in relieving the pain and swelling of venous insufficiency or varicose veins of the leg.

CHAPTER 10

TEA TREE OIL FOR INFECTIONS

Jason Mackie, BSc; Cherry Tanega, BSc; Heather Boon, BScPhm, PhD;
Mel Borins, MD

In the land Down Under, where wombats burrow and joeys play, the Australian tea tree, *Melaleuca alternifolia*, grows. At maturity, melaleuca reaches a height of about twenty to twenty-five feet. The outer bark peels off, exposing a shiny white inner layer, similar to the eucalyptus tree, another member of the Myrtaceae group. When the pale green branches burst into bottlebrush blossoms of pure white, the trees look as if they've been dusted with snow, even though they grow along the humid, subtropical coast of New South Wales.

TREE OF LEGEND

According to *Australian Geographic* magazine, tea tree oil was one of the top ten Aboriginal bush medicines.[1] Indeed, aboriginal folklore suggests the tree has a long history among the people. There exists a legendary account of an aboriginal princess who took a journey through a strange forest. As she walked, she grew worried about losing her way back to her loved ones, and so she prayed to the gods of the earth for help. The gods produced seeds that scattered behind her and settled on the path where she had walked. The seeds rooted, sprouted, and reached for the light, growing into tall trees with shiny white paper bark that reflected moonlight, and that illuminated her pathway home. Over time these trees flourished, and the Bundjalung people from the coast of New South Wales came to know of their magical healing properties. They crushed the leaves and applied the paste to cuts, burns, bites, and skin ailments, and they brewed them into tea for coughs, colds, and inflammations of the throat.[2]

Historical Notes

In 1770, Captain James Cook sailed around the world, and during that journey, he explored the coasts of Australia. While anchored at a place that Captain Cook named Botany Bay, the aborigines introduced him to a hot drink made from leaves of what they called the paper bark tree. It may have been Cook who coined the term "tea tree," as a result of this drink. It is also believed that the captain gave it to his crew to prevent scurvy.

Oil of Kings and Soldiers

In 1881, George, the sixteen-year-old Duke of York and future King of England, visited Sydney, Australia. While there, he planted a tea tree in Sydney Botanic Gardens. Fifty-four years later, upon the Silver Jubilee celebration of King George V's coronation, the government of Australia sent the king a fond memento of his first visit to New South Wales. The royal gift was a glass vessel containing tea tree oil distilled from the very tree he had planted years before; the beautiful glass was mounted on a wooden base made from a portion of that same tree. One can't help but wonder what fond memories the pungent aroma elicited for the king.

In 1934, Arthur Penfold, curator of the New South Wales Technological Museum, was quoted in the Central Queensland Herald.[3] "The pleasant odor of the oil, its high germicidal efficiency, and non-poisonous properties promise a wide industrial application for it in disinfectants, germicides, and solvents, as well as in medicine and therapeutics. It has recently been discovered to be eleven to thirteen times more effective in destroying typhoid germs than carbolic acid (phenol)."

During World War II, tea tree oil was considered such an effective treatment for and preventive of so many conditions that the Australian government issued it to Australian soldiers as an essential part of their first aid kits. Since the oil was used for everything from fungal infections of the toenails to prevention of head lice, some referred to it as their head-to-toe first-aid treatment!

PROPERTIES OF TEA TREE OIL

Australian tea tree oil is a natural essential oil and natural antiseptic. The oil is steam-distilled from the *Melaleuca alternifolia* leaves. The oil has antiseptic, antibacterial, antifungal, anti-inflammatory, and antiviral properties. Tea tree oil contains over one hundred components, mostly monoterpenes, with the main active ingredient being terpinen-4-ol. It is colorless or pale yellow and has a rich distinctive odor. The minimum standard for the oil to be considered 100 percent pure, among other characteristics, requires that levels of terpinen-4-ol must be between 30 and 48 percent, and cineol needs to be below 15 percent. Basically, the higher the terpinen-4-ol levels, and the lower the cineol levels are, the better the quality rating of the oil.

TEA TREE OIL FOR ONYCHOMYCOSIS (FUNGUS INFECTION OF THE TOENAIL)

Sixty patients were treated for sixteen weeks in a randomized, double-blind, placebo-controlled study using 2 percent butenafine hydrochloride (an antifungal drug) and 5 percent tea tree oil mixed together to make a cream for the treatment of toenail onychomycosis. In the group of patients using the medicated cream, 80 percent were cured, as opposed to no one being cured in the placebo group. Four patients in the active treatment group experienced subjective mild inflammation but did not have to stop the treatment. The authors concluded that topical therapy of 2 percent butenafine hydrochloride with 5 percent tea tree oil, in combination with debridement with a nail clipper, is safe, tolerable, and significantly more effective than placebo to cure fungus infections of the toenail.[4]

Another randomized controlled trial compared the twice-daily topical application of 1 percent clotrimazole solution (an antifungal drug) to 100 percent tea tree oil for fungal nail infections. Debridement and clinical assessment were performed at zero, one, three, and six months. After six months of therapy, the two treatment groups were compared based on culture-assessed cure. The clotrimazole group showed a cure rate of 11 percent, and the tea tree oil group, 18 percent (no significant difference). After three months, about half of each group reported continued improvement or complete resolution: 55 percent of the clotrimazole group; 56 percent of the tea tree oil group (no significant difference). The researchers concluded that tea tree oil improved nail appearance and symptomatology as effectively as clotrimazole.[5] One defect of this study was that the researchers did not use a placebo group to see if either of the treatments was better than placebo. In my practice I find that topical antifungal treatments are not very effective for fungus infections of the nails.

TEA TREE OIL FOR ORAL HYGIENE

Tea tree oil kills a range of oral bacteria, suggesting that it may be of use in oral health care products and in the maintenance of oral hygiene. One study compared the antimicrobial activity of tea tree oil, garlic, and chlorhexidine gargle solutions against germs of the mouth. Thirty participants were randomly divided into 0.12 percent chlorhexidine, 2.5 percent garlic, and 0.2 percent tea tree oil. Chlorhexidine and garlic groups showed antimicrobial activity against mutans streptococci, but not against other germs of the mouth. The tea tree oil group showed antimicrobial activity against both the mutans streptococci and other oral microorganisms. The authors concluded that garlic and tea tree oil might be an alternative to chlorhexidine for oral hygiene.[6]

TEA TREE OIL FOR ORAL CANDIDIASIS (YEAST INFECTION OF THE MOUTH)

Jandourek et al. evaluated the usefulness of melaleuca (tea tree oil) oral solution in AIDS patients who had yeast infections of the mouth that were not helped with the antifungal drug fluconazole. Twelve patients were given 15 ml melaleuca oral solution four times daily to swish and expel for two to four weeks. Results: At the four-week evaluation, eight of the twelve patients showed a response (two cured, six improved), four were nonresponders, and one had deteriorated. A mycological response (decrease in fungal growth) was seen in seven out of twelve patients. The authors concluded that melaleuca oral solution appears to be effective for AIDS patients with yeast infections of the mouth that did not respond to the antifungal drug fluconazole.[7]

Another study reviewed the success of alcohol-based and alcohol-free melaleuca oral solution in patients with AIDS who had oropharyngeal candidiasis but did not respond to the antifungal drug fluconazole. Twenty-seven patients were randomized to swish and expel either alcohol-based or alcohol-free melaleuca oral solution four times daily for two to four weeks. Results: 60 percent of patients demonstrated a clinical response to both melaleuca oral solutions at the four-week evaluation. This study also seems to suggest that melaleuca oral solutions appear to be an effective alternative regimen for patients with AIDS suffering from yeast infections of the mouth that did not respond to fluconazole.[8]

TEA TREE OIL FOR ATHLETE'S FOOT

One hundred and fifty-eight patients with athlete's foot, a fungal infection between the toes, were randomized to receive a placebo or a tea tree oil solution of 25 or 50 percent strength, twice daily for four weeks. Result: A statistically significant improvement was seen in the clinical score in 68 percent of the 50-strength tea tree oil group and 72 percent of the 25-strength tea tree oil group, compared to 39 percent in the placebo group. The 25 percent tea tree oil strength was associated with fewer complications than 50 percent tea tree oil solution. Four patients applying tea tree oil developed moderate to severe dermatitis that improved quickly on stopping the medication.[9]

TEA TREE OIL FOR ACNE (MILD TO MODERATE)

Applying a 5 percent tea tree oil gel appears to be as effective as 5 percent benzoyl peroxide (Oxy-5, Benzac AC, and others) for treating acne. Tea tree oil might work more slowly than benzoyl peroxide, but seems to be less irritating to facial skin.[10]

TEA TREE OIL FOR HERPES LABIALIS (COLD SORES)

A poor quality, randomized, placebo-controlled, single-blind study evaluated topical tea tree oil in the treatment of recurrent cold sores. Double-blinding was not attempted because of the distinctive odor of the oil. The study consisted of twenty patients with self-reported histories of recurrent cold sores. Patients were randomized to receive either 6 percent tea tree oil in an aqueous gel base or placebo gel, applied five times daily. The median time to healing after treatment with tea tree oil was nine days, compared with twelve and a half days after placebo (not significantly different). The

---

CAUTION

The American Cancer Society states: Tea tree oil is toxic when swallowed. It has been reported to cause drowsiness, confusion, hallucinations, coma, unsteadiness, weakness, vomiting, diarrhea, stomach upset, blood cell abnormalities, and severe rashes. People that are allergic to other members of the myrtle family (*Myrtaceae*), such as eucalyptus, guava, clove, or allspice, may be more likely to have an allergic reaction. Those who are sensitive to pine or turpentine might also react to tea tree oil because of chemical similarities between the plants.[11]

While tea tree oil can be applied to minor cuts and scrapes, please use caution for more extensive areas of broken skin or areas affected by rashes not due to fungus. The oil may burn if it gets into the eyes, nose, mouth, or other tender areas. Some people have allergic reactions, including rashes and itching, when applying tea tree oil and it can cause contact dermatitis. For this reason, only a small amount should be applied when first using it. I would not recommend using it during pregnancy and breastfeeding. Do not take tea tree oil internally because it can cause gastrointestinal upsets and can be toxic at small doses. There have been reports of potentially fatal central nervous system depression (excessive drowsiness, sleepiness, and coma).

It is very important to keep tea tree oil out of the reach of children and pets. Because the oil breaks down into substances that can cause allergic reactions in some people, it is best to always use high quality, fresh products that have not been exposed to light, air, and heat.

---

authors concluded that tea tree oil was no more effective than placebo for treating herpes labialis.

TEA TREE OIL FOR FUTURE CANCER TREATMENT

A report released by the Australian government in July 2010 highlighted the positive role tea tree oil may play in the future in treating people with skin cancer. *In vitro* studies (done in glass dishes or tubes, versus human subject) identified that the oil has potential as an antitumor agent through necrosis (tissue death), low-level apoptosis (process of programmed cell death), and the arrest of the cancer cell cycle. They also reported tea tree oil inhibited tumor growth of subcutaneous malignant mesothelioma and of melanoma tumor models studied, and it induced tumor regression in the study mouse with a malignant mesothelioma tumor. This identification of antitumor activity is an important step in the process to identify, test, and implement effective treatments for skin cancer.[12]

CONCLUSION

Tea tree oil has been shown to possibly be useful when used for oral hygiene, yeast infections of the mouth, fungus infections of the toenail and feet, and in mild acne. It is very dangerous if swallowed internally. In my clinical practice I have found that topical antifungal drugs for athlete's foot and other prescription topical treatments for acne are more effective.

CHAPTER 11

HERBAL TREATMENT FOR BACK PAIN

Jennifer Fink, MD, and Mel Borins, MD

Back pain is one of the most common presenting problems I see in my office and one of the most frequent causes of disability, absence from work, and economic hardship. Although physicians prescribe nonsteroidal, anti-inflammatory drugs, pain medication, physiotherapy, exercise, and sometimes surgery, few of these modalities of treatment have compelling randomized, double-blind, controlled trials to show their usefulness.

Often when patients have back pain they seek out alternative forms of treatment such as acupuncture, massage, and chiropractic. Others use cranial sacral therapy, Feldenkrais Technique, the Mitzvah Technique, and the Alexander Technique, which represent other forms of therapy where research is also very scarce.

Herbs have been used by traditional societies for back pain all over the world and many patients take herbs that are given by herbalists, naturopaths, or other health care practitioners. Let's have a look at three that have been used traditionally in many different countries and have been studied in randomly assigned, controlled trials.

CAUTION: DEVIL'S CLAW (*HARPAGOPHYTUM PROCUMBENS*)

BEWARE: Many different plants share the same common name. When purchasing an herbal product or remedy, make sure to check that it has the correct botanical name. In the case of this herb, do not become confused with another devil's claw, *Proboscidea parviflora*, of the American southwest. That plant comes from the family Martyniaceae, which has completely different properties and uses.

DEVIL'S CLAW—THE HERB

Devil's claw, *Harpagophytum procumbens*, belongs to the sesame seed family: Pedaliaceae. *Harpagophytum* is taken from Greek and translates to "grapple plant," a plant that grapples, holds, or makes fast to something. The Latin descriptor *procumbens* means prostrate, which refers to the creeping characteristic of the ground-cover plant. It has a stout central taproot that grows more than five feet deep and secondary storage tubers, somewhat resembling elongated yams or sweet potatoes, which branch off horizontally and contain twice as much harpagoside—the active ingredient—as the taproot itself.[1] The leaves are large and a grayish-green color. The plant has a beautiful, trumpet-shaped blossom with a pale yellow throat opening to fluted edges rimmed in ruby pink, red, or purple. It is the spiny, woody fruits that grow from the flower and produce seeds with numerous radiating, barbed spines that inspired the names "devil's claw" and "grapple plant."

Devil's claw is native to Botswana, Zimbabwe, Namibia, and the Kalahari Desert of South Africa where it grows on open grazing lands and where poor sandy soils and overgrazing produce weak grass and herb cover. It can also be found in dry savannah or open woodland. Devil's claw seeds hitchhike on passing animals, attaching sharp hooks to their fur and hooves. Nature's clever method of distributing these seeds causes animals that tread or lie on the spines to receive an injury, leading to inflammation and infection. If the claw gets stuck in an animal's mouth or throat, it can starve, a truly hellish way to die. For this reason, many cattle farmers have tried to eradicate the plant from grazing lands.

It is difficult to cultivate devil's claw, so the majority of the secondary tubers are collected from the wild by people living in rural communities, mostly in Namibia, South Africa, and Botswana. The tubers are sold and exported for medicinal use and are an important source of income for poor Kalahari communities. On one hand, it is immensely helpful to communities to have the cash crop, but on the other, the price paid for the tubers is often so low, it encourages overharvesting.

Due to eradication practices used by cattle farmers and overharvesting by poor communities, many conservation projects and export regulations have been adopted to save the herb from extinction. The Namibian government, for example, pays a financial incentive to harvesters not to over-harvest, while other African and international programs have helped to develop techniques to propagate it outside of grazing areas, providing an alternative to wild-harvested supplies for the herbal medicine trade.

Devil's claw has recently been classified as a protected species in Botswana, Namibia, and South Africa, and permits are required both to harvest and to export it. *Harpagophytum* is also listed with CITES, the Convention on International Trade in Endangered Species of Wild Fauna and Flora, an international treaty drawn up in 1973 to protect wildlife against over-exploitation, and to prevent international trade from threatening species listed under its protection. Under EU regulations, no part of the tubers or roots can be traded within the European Union without proper licenses.[2]

Traditional Uses for Devil's Claw

People of the Kalahari have used devil's claw for centuries to treat a wide range of illnesses. The British Herbal Pharmacopoeia recognizes devil's claw as having anti-inflammatory, analgesic (pain killing), sedative, and diuretic properties (increases urine production and removes excess body fluid). It is also listed as an official treatment in the European Pharmacopoeia and is a component in many over-the-counter preparations and dietary supplements that are compiled for treating rheumatic conditions. In 2001, devil's claw accounted for 74 percent of the total number of prescriptions for rheumatism in Germany.[3]

The active ingredient extracted from the tuberous root is harpagoside, which has traditionally been used in the treatment of degenerative rheumatoid arthritis, osteoarthritis, tendonitis, kidney inflammation, and heart disease.

The Science behind Devil's Claw

A Cochrane review by Gagnier et al. looked at herbal treatments for back pain and found there is some proof that certain herbs could be useful.[4] Here is a summary of their findings:

Harpagophytum procumbens was tested at a dose of 50 mg of standardized extract harpagoside versus placebo for patients who had experienced acute episodes of chronic low-back pain for a period of more than six months. Three hundred twenty-five patients were followed in two four-week trials.[5, 6] Results: There was a significant increase in the number of pain-free patients in the 50 mg harpagoside group over placebo. The percentage with no pain or mild low-back pain increased over the four-week period whereas the percentage with unbearable or severe pain decreased. The pain subscale (subcategories of types of pain) was also significantly improved in the group that used 50 mg harpagoside. Conclusion: There is strong evidence that 50 mg harpagoside per dose of an aqueous (water-based) extract of *H. procumbens* per day reduces pain more than placebo in the short-term in patients with acute episodes of chronic low-back pain.

Another study was done with 197 patients divided into three groups in one four-week trial. They compared *H. procumbens* standardized to 100 mg harpagoside per day, versus a lower dose of 50 mg harpagoside, or a placebo. Results: The number of pain-free patients for at least five days in week four was significantly higher in the group that took 100 mg of harpagoside than the placebo or lower dose (50 mg) groups. The percentage of patients with no or mild lower back pain increased, whereas the percentage with unbearable or severe pain decreased. Conclusion: There is moderate evidence that 100 mg of harpagoside per dose of an aqueous extract of *Harpagophytum procumbens* leads to a higher number of pain-free patients for at least five days in the fourth week of treatment during acute episodes of chronic nonspecific low-back pain.

SIDE EFFECTS OF DEVIL'S CLAW

There have been a few rare occurrences of allergic reactions, such as difficulty breathing, swelling of throat, tongue, or lips, and hives. Headache, ringing in the ears, loss of appetite, and loss of taste were also listed as side effects to watch out for.[7]

WHITE WILLOW BARK (*SALIX ALBA*)—THE HERB

One of the classic children's books, *Wind in the Willows* by Kenneth Gra-
hame, is a story about animals that live along the River Thames in England. It is in this setting where the white willow tree (*Salix alba*) grows, a
peaceful scene made famous by landscape artists such as John Constable
and Claude Monet, a scene that brings to mind summer picnics and flat-
bottom punting boats amidst gentle breezes.

Wood from the European white willow, *Salix alba*, so named for
the white underside of the leaves, has been used for centuries to make
cricket bats and fruit crates as well as for decorative carvings. Willow
trees have traditionally been pollarded (branches pruned back to the
trunk) which forces new shoots to grow fast, strong, and flexible, like
reeds. These flexible shoots are the source of withies, material used for
making willow baskets. Some of the best quality artists' charcoal is also
made from willow.[8]

Medicinal Uses of White Willow Bark

Ancient civilizations have recorded the use of willow as far back as six
thousand years ago. Extracts of white willow bark were used to treat fever,
pain, and inflammation. Archaeologists have discovered clay tablets left by
Assyrians that describe use of the leaf for the same conditions. Egyptians
wrote about the curative properties of white willow prescriptions on papy-
rus leaves. Hippocrates, the ancient Greek physician, recommended that
the leaves be chewed to relieve fever and pain.[9] The active substance, salicin, is an extract of the bark and the source for salicylic acid, also known
as aspirin.

The Science behind White Willow Bark

A four-week trial[10] involving 210 patients compared a standardized dose
of 120 mg or 240 mg salicin per day, against placebo for chronic low-back
pain. There was a significant increase in the number of pain-free patients
for at least five days in week four in the treatment groups compared to
placebo. The number of patients requiring relief medication (Tramadol)

during each week decreased significantly compared to placebo. Pain scores, invalidity index (measure of disablement), and physical impairment were also significantly improved in the willow bark groups. Scores for the higher 240 mg dose were generally more favorable than the 120 mg dose in most categories. There is moderate evidence that 120 mg salicin dose of an extract of *S. alba* leads to more pain-free patients for the treatment of acute episodes of chronic nonspecific lower back pain in the short term.

Another trial[11] of 228 subjects with acute episodes of chronic nonspecific low-back pain found no differences in effectiveness comparing *S. alba* (standardized to a daily dose of 240 mg salicin) in a four-week trial, against 12.5 mg per day of Rofecoxib, a nonsteroidal anti-inflammatory (NSAID).

White willow bark can cause stomach upsets, raise blood pressure, and may even cause liver or bleeding problems. Pregnant women should not take willow bark, and if you are allergic to aspirin you should avoid using willow bark. It may also react with drugs like blood thinners, anti-inflammatory medicines, anti-hypertensives, and acetazolamide.

CAYENNE PLASTER

Cayenne, *Capsicum frutescens,* is a red chili pepper that grows wild in Central America and subtropical regions of South America. It was named after the capital of French Guiana (situated on the northeast coast of South America). The perennial shrub grows to one meter at maturity. The fruit of the capsicum plant contains a chemical called capsaicin. Capsaicin seems to reduce pain when applied to the skin.

Numerous double-blind trials have proven that topically applied capsaicin creams are helpful for a range of conditions, including nerve pain in diabetic neuropathy, post-surgical pain, muscle pain due to fibromyalgia, nerve pain after shingles (postherpetic neuralgia), osteoarthritis, and rheumatoid pain.[12] Cayenne pepper is approved by the German Commission E as a topical ointment for the relief of painful muscle spasms.

Method of Application of Cayenne Plaster

While many herbal remedies are taken orally, others are inhaled or absorbed through the skin. External applications are often by ointment, compress, poultice, or plaster. Plasters are chosen when using "hot" herbs that should not touch the skin.

Compresses, poultices, and plasters should be made fresh just before application. To make a plaster, herbal material is crushed and formed into a paste using oatmeal, bran, cornstarch, or flour as thickener, and then mixed with enough water and/or oil to form the paste. A cayenne plaster can easily be made by mixing 1 teaspoon of cayenne powder with 1 teaspoon of olive oil and 3 teaspoons of flour. A little water may be added if necessary. The paste should be spread onto a layer of clean gauze bandage, and then covered by another layer of bandage before applying to the area of pain.

Topical creams that contain between 25 and 75 percent capsaicin may also be purchased. These are applied to the affected area three or four times per day. A burning sensation may occur when the cream is applied, but should gradually decrease with each use.

How Does Cayenne Plaster Work?

Substance P is a chemical that helps our nerves to transmit pain signals from the body to the brain. Capsaicin temporarily depletes this substance so that pain signals can no longer be sent. The pain-killing effect is, therefore, temporary.

CAUTION

Cayenne is a hot pepper and an irritant that can cause redness and irritation and can burn the skin. It was even proposed for use as a chemical weapon during the American Civil War! Be sure to wash hands carefully after each use in order to prevent the plaster paste or topical cream from accidentally causing a burning sensation of the eyes, nose, or mouth. Do not apply to areas of broken skin.

The Science of Cayenne Plaster

One hundred fifty-four patients with acute episodes of chronic nonspecific low-back pain were randomly assigned to either a placebo plaster group or a capsicum plaster group for three weeks. Results: There was a significant reduction in the capsicum group in pain and total Arhus score (a back pain–specific index, including physical impairment, pain, and disability scores) compared to placebo. Physician global ratings of efficacy were considered "excellent" or "good" in 75.7 percent of the capsicum group and only 47.4 percent of the placebo group. After treatment, 13.5 percent of the capsicum group and 6.6 percent of the placebo group were completely symptom-free.[13]

In another study, 320 participants with chronic, non-specific low-back pain were randomly allocated to a placebo plaster group or a capsicum plaster group for twenty-one days. Results: The total Arhus score decreased by 33 percent in the capsicum group and by 22 percent in the placebo group. There was significant reduction in pain in the capsicum group compared to placebo. The capsicum treatment was rated as either excellent or good by investigators in 74 percent of cases compared with 36 percent for the placebo group. Compliance was reported as being very good or good in both groups.[14] This plaster is a useful alternative that can be made from ingredients and materials found in the average kitchen and first-aid kit.

CONCLUSION

There is scientific evidence that devil's claw, willow bark, and a plaster of cayenne are useful for back pain. Back pain can be the result of many different conditions. Before you focus on relieving the symptoms, consult with your physician to determine the underlying cause of the problem.

CHAPTER 12
PROBLEMS WITH HERBS

Herbs have stood the test of time, and for the most part are quite safe, but they can cause problems if used inappropriately. Just because herbs are natural does not mean they are free from side effects. Many of our modern drugs, such as digitalis, atropine, and opiate derivatives like morphine and codeine, are highly toxic if used inappropriately, and some can lead to dependency. These drugs were all developed from plants.[1] It is important that we familiarize ourselves with the risks and downsides of using herbs in order to avoid negative consequences. Now that we have discussed the use of many different herbs, let's have a look at some of the potential hazards.

STANDARDIZATION AND QUALITY CONTROL OF HERBS

Many herbs are sold as teas, foods, and food supplements. Since they are not being offered as drugs, there does not have to be any proof of the effectiveness of the herbs, and warnings about side effects are not necessarily provided. On the other hand, when a drug is prescribed the dosage and quality of the substance is more or less assured. There is at present no standardization or quality control with respect to all herbal formulations, so you need to be careful.

Let us imagine that you have visited a Traditional Chinese Medicine practitioner, received a prescription written in Chinese, and have taken it to a Chinese herbal store. You may not know what ingredients are in the prescription, and if you experience side effects, it may be difficult to determine which substance is responsible.

There have been reports that herbal preparations don't always contain what the label claims and when analyzed, the supposed active substance is not present at all.[2] Other times, serious poisoning can take place when an importer or retailer mistakes one herb for another.[3, 4, 5]

Herbs are grown under many different climatic and soil conditions that affect their potency. When the grass really is greener on the other side of the road, you can be certain it is due to the quality of the soil, the fertilizer used, or the amount of water and drainage available. When a soil is depleted of nitrogen through intense farming, or is naturally short of magnesium or selenium, for example, plants grown in that soil will also be lacking in the same minerals and trace elements. Farmers often provide salt licks for their animals to replace these minerals and trace elements.

How plants are handled is also a factor that can affect quality. When I visited the Toyama Medical and Pharmaceutical University Hospital in Japan, I saw that fresh herbs from around the world were collected, and every batch was analyzed. Great differences in the presence of the active substances were found, depending on where the substances were grown and how long the herbs were allowed to stand before they were shipped or used. In the Toyama Hospital, many of the fresh herbs are stored in a temperature-controlled storage area to ensure quality control.

TOXIC INGREDIENTS IN HERBS

Sometimes toxic ingredients, pesticides, non-declared drugs, or added chemicals contaminate herbal preparations.[6, 7, 8, 9, 10] Heavy metals like arsenic, mercury, lead, and cadmium have also been found in herbal remedies.

If you suffered from the chronic pain of arthritis you might have been tempted to try Chuifong Toukuwan, an herbal medication that claimed to relieve all your symptoms, according to the advertisement of a Hong Kong mail order company. Imagine that after taking the medication, you became very ill indeed. Thirteen people who did this developed serious side effects, including bone marrow depression, hypertension, irregular heart rhythms, and abnormal bleeding. When the pills were analyzed, they were found to contain the prescription drugs prednisone and indomethacin and the toxic heavy metal lead.[11]

Four other patients developed agranulocytosis, a condition involving a severe leukopenia (lowered white blood cell count), and life-threatening infections while taking herbal medicines for relief of arthritis and back pain. These herbal medicines were found to contain aminopyrine, a pain-killer and fever reducer that is now rarely used because of its dangerous side effects, and phenylbutazone, a powerful anti-inflammatory drug, commonly used for treating horses or dogs, but no longer sold for human use in the United States.[12]

The Canadian Drug Reaction Monitoring Program has received many reports of adverse reactions to certain Chinese herbal preparations that contained toxic heavy metals, such as arsenic, mercury, lead, and cadmium. Along with the prescription drugs mentioned above, herbal preparations also tested positive for the steroid hormone testosterone and the addictive anti-anxiety drug, diazepam.[13]

HEAVY METALS IN HERBS

All of us have small amounts of individual metals and metal compounds in our bodies. Heavy metals are in the soil, the air, the food and water we take in, and in many things we use on a daily basis. Tiny amounts of these metals will do little or no harm, and the lack of some metals would result in delayed development, illness, or even death. Iron, for example, is an essential component of red blood cells; a lack of iron can produce anemia.

Many metals are not eliminated easily from the body, and so they build up over time. We can experience metal poisoning from one exposure, or we can become chronically ill and die from repeated exposures over a long period of time. One example of this is lead poisoning in children who lived in houses where dust from lead-based paint entered their lungs and mouths. Along with several adverse symptoms in all ages, even very low levels of lead can affect mental development in young children, cause behavior and attention problems, damage kidneys, and stunt growth.

The intentional use of lead in traditional folk remedies occurs in some societies. Hmong refugees from Laos prepare an herbal formula called Pay-loo-ah, which is used to relieve fever and rashes, often in children. Unfortunately, there have been reported cases of lead poisoning[14] and arsenic and mercury contamination in Pay-loo-ah.[15]

Azarcon, which contains lead tetroxide, and Greta, which contains lead oxide, are Mexican folk remedies that have also caused toxicity.[16, 17, 18, 19] Ayurveda, the system of traditional medicine native to India, sometimes uses heavy metals in its remedies.[20, 21] Practitioners of Espiritismo, a spiritual belief system indigenous to Puerto Rico and other Caribbean islands, use mercury for good luck, protection from evil, and the envy of others. This creates a certain hazard and can easily lead to mercury poisoning.[22]

While traveling abroad, some people purchase herbal remedies and bring them back to North America. These remedies can cause problems.[23] One thirty-five-year-old man went to India and purchased Shakti and Pushap Dhanva Ras, a traditional Ayurvedic remedy for diabetes, which he brought home. He was later admitted to a Canadian hospital with a serious case of lead poisoning, caused by the remedy. The tablets not only contained high levels of lead, but mercury and arsenic as well.[24]

A similar case of lead poisoning occurred in a Korean man who bought multiple bags of dried herbs containing *hai ge fen* (clamshell powder) from a Chinese herbalist in New York. The adulterated (made impure by adding extraneous ingredients) clamshell powder contained high amounts of lead and arsenic.[25]

When safety regulations and quality controls are not practiced or sufficiently monitored in other countries, it's no wonder that western doctors are slow to accept the use of traditional medicines. It makes sense therefore to work with other countries, and to help them create reliable research facilities, adopt safety standards, and develop quality testing and ingredient controls.

TOXIC SIDE EFFECTS OF HERBS

Some reactions or side effects happen as a result of the inherent properties in the herbs. In my medical practice I have only seen problems with an herbal product on three occasions, but toxic reactions have been recorded in the medical literature.[26] For instance, cases of cyanide poisoning were reported in people who ingested the seeds, bark, or leaves of apricots, cassava beans, cherry, choke cherry, peach, plum, and other fruits.[27] Licorice, used in the treatment of gastrointestinal problems, can cause hypokalemia (a lower than normal amount of potassium in the blood), hypertension (high blood pressure), sodium and water retention, and cardiac problems.[28]

Oil from the root of the sassafras tree was traditionally used to create a favorite American soft drink and herbal tea. Yet a few drops of the oil, which contains high levels of a liver toxin named safrole, can kill an infant, and as little as a teaspoon can kill an adult. Sassafras has understandably been banned for human consumption.[29] It is also believed that sassafras is carcinogenic in animals.

There have been reported cases of serious poisoning in Hong Kong and Australia from the use of two Chinese herbal medicines: Caowu, from the root of *Aconitum kusnezoffi*, and Chuanwa, the main root of *Aconitum carmichaeli*. These herbs, used to treat rheumatism, arthritis, bruises, and fractures, contain variable amounts of toxic alkaloids. They can cause dangerously irregular heartbeats, cardiovascular collapse, and even death.[30]

Forty-eight Belgian women developed renal (kidney) failure after using Chinese herb therapy in an attempt to lose weight.[31]

Ginseng, a commonly used herb that seems to have many positive benefits, can sometimes cause hypertension, nervousness, skin rashes, and sleeplessness.[32, 33]

Perhaps you will suddenly find yourself, after reading these excerpts, suspiciously eyeing that teapot of Lapsang souchong, but don't worry; no skull and crossbones are hidden under the lid! Most teas and herbal products purchased in North America are perfectly safe when used as advised and in moderation. This book is not meant to be a scaremonger, but to encourage you to be careful when purchasing and using herbal remedies that are not regulated by the same standards as modern drugs.

Herbs as Cathartics—Purging the Bowels

Some politely refer to it as "regularity" while others call the ritual "making a deposit" or "going to the dump." No matter what term is used, having a good bowel movement on a regular basis is one of the joys that elude many people, sometimes because of poor diet and reliance on fast food. It is not surprising, therefore, that some of the most common problems I see in my medical practice stem from people using cathartics for constipation.

Many people believe that cathartics or laxatives in the form of teas or herbs are quite safe, but this is not the case. The continued use of cathartics for constipation can cause dependency, or the so-called lazy-bowel problem. Once you begin taking these herbal treatments, it may be very difficult to stop without the symptom of constipation returning.

And don't forget Sam, my patient who, like many others before him, self-medicated with laxatives to avoid going to the doctor. His decision delayed the diagnosis of a serious, but treatable disorder: colon cancer. Buckthorn, senna, dock roots, juniper berries, and even the wonder plant, *Aloe vera*, can have fairly strong irritant, cathartic effects and they will cause diarrhea if used indiscriminately. I recommend that you do not use herbal laxatives without consulting your physician.

Anticholinergic Herbs

Anticholinergics reduce muscle spasms in the intestines and are sometimes used to treat conditions such as irritable bowel syndrome. People who treat diarrhea symptoms with common herbs such as catnip, juniper, lobelia, jimson weed, wormwood, and nutmeg can suffer delirium and hallucinations.[34][35] Taking these might also produce symptoms of dry skin and mouth, flushed face, agitation, anxiety, and rapid or irregular heartbeat.

Herb Allergies

In summer when the golden blossoms of tansy ragweed appear in meadows and along the roadside, many people suffer with allergy symptoms. These are often sparked by pollen from flowers of the Compositae family, one of the largest groups of plants whose flower heads are composed of many florets. Amongst the thousands of plant varieties in this group are included asters, thistles, chrysanthemums, dandelion, sunflowers, and tansy ragweed. People with these allergies should also avoid teas made from goldenrod, marigold, yarrow, St. John's wort, and chamomile, because of the potential problem with cross-reactivity.[36][37]

Chamomile has widely been used as a remedy for minor digestive disorders, skin problems, and as a mild sedative. One source of allergic reactions is the contamination of chamomile flowers with other related but more allergenic plants, such as mayweed or dog fennel.

Herbs Dangerous During Pregnancy

Devil's claw root used for arthritis, berberis for stomach problems, dong quai for menstrual irregularities, ruta for multiple conditions, goldenseal or oil of oregano (in highly concentrated capsules) used for flu and cold infections—all should be used with extreme caution in pregnancy. Any herb that acts as a menstrual regulator (an emmenogogue) can potentially cause miscarriages or abortions.[38]

Herbs Causing Hepatitis—Inflammation of the Liver

Comfrey, a popular folk remedy in Europe and North America, is said to be useful for skin conditions, arthritis, pulmonary conditions, and even gastrointestinal conditions. It has been shown to contain pyrrolizidine alkaloids, which cause liver damage and cancer in both animals and humans.[39, 40, 41]

Jane, a fifty-year-old patient of mine, had unexplained hepatitis. When I reviewed the details of what could be causing her abnormal liver enzymes, the only unusual thing that she had been ingesting was an herb she called witch's broom. Witch's broom is not a species of plant, but an irregular growth condition that happens to a wide variety of trees and shrubs when they are invaded by certain fungi, viruses, insects, or spores. The affected tree will produce many shoots from one branch node, making what appears to be a nest or witch's broom, hence the name. Some people errantly refer to mistletoe as witch's broom. When I looked up witch's broom in my herbal books I could find no reference to it causing hepatitis, but as soon as Jane stopped using the herb, her liver tests improved.

Germander,[42] mistletoe,[43] chaparral,[44] and ragwort[45] have also been suspected of causing hepatitis. A popular Chinese herb, Chuen-Lin, commonly given to newborns in the Chinese community, doesn't cause hepatitis, but it can have a significant effect in displacing bilirubin from its serum protein binding and can cause an increase of bilirubin, producing the yellow appearance associated with jaundice. The use of this herb should be properly supervised and stopped in cases of neonatal jaundice.[46]

CONCLUSION

As I said before, people have been taking herbs for medicinal purposes for thousands of years, long before scientific trials ever existed, and in many cases achieved successful results. There are pros and cons to every substance we use, whether it is from folk, traditional, or modern Western medicine. What I have tried to make clear is that herbs can be beneficial, but they can also be dangerous. Without well-designed research trials to support the claims of healing properties, many doctors are unwilling or reticent about recommending their use.

If you decide to use herbs as an alternative to western medication, you will have a much better chance of avoiding the pitfalls if you follow the advice listed below.

1. Be cautious about taking any herbal preparations, especially if they are purchased outside of North America.

2. Do not believe unsubstantiated claims for miracle cures.

3. Get advice from a licensed health professional officially trained in the prescribing of herbs. The regulation of herbalists is very poor, so it is important to check out a practioner's qualifications before visiting him or her.

4. All remedies should be clearly labelled and all ingredients listed.

5. Pregnant patients should not take herbs unless their safety can be assured.

6. Buy herbs from a reputable source, preferably one recommended by a licensed health professional.

7. Be especially careful about buying off the Internet. Sometimes the seller will offer money-back guarantees but will then disappear after a few weeks or months.

8. Tell your doctor if you are taking herbs so that any side effects can be monitored.

9. In the United States, report any side effects to: www.fda.gov/Safety/MedWatch/HowToReport/default.htm, or in Canada to: www.healthcanada.gc.ca/medeffect.

SECTION II: ACUPUNCTURE

I never dreamed, while going through medical school and an internship, that my medical school classmate Andy Wong of all people would lead me into the world of alternative medicine. Andy had always seemed to be a conservative, down-to-earth, Western-medicine doctor.

When Bonnie and I began our first round-the-world sabbatical in 1975, we were excited to visit Andy and his wife, Luciante, in Hong Kong, where he'd taken a residency in Internal Medicine. The city was clustered on the north shore of the island, a giant, bustling doorway to Asia. Highrises, street cars, neon signs, bicycles, and throngs of people contrasted with the peaceful, rust-red sails of Chinese junks in the harbor against a background of mountains that poured their indigo blue reflection into the sea. Hawkers and market-stall holders created a cacophonic din that throbbed like an adrenaline-pumped heart, and you couldn't escape the sensation that Hong Kong's fever generated energy from every crack and corner of its silk and concrete skin.

Andy was eager to show me his acupuncture machine. Along with his Transcutaneous Electric Nerve Stimulation Machine, he had a point finder. This attachment looked somewhat like a thick pen and was used to find points on the skin that had a lower resistance to the passage of electricity than the surrounding area, and it measured a change in electrical charge. These points were consistent with acupuncture points. His enthusiasm was infectious as he explained how each person's body was represented by a sort of map on the ear, a map made up of dozens of points. Each one of these points, he said, corresponded to an area, structure, or organ of the body. When there was a weakness or problem with any part of the body, and the instrument touched the corresponding acupuncture point on the ear, it would register a difference in electric current and emit a high-pitched buzz. If anyone other than Andy had been telling me this, I probably would have thought they were crazy, but I could see my friend believed in its capability, so when he asked if I wanted to try it, I was keen to see what happened.

Andy ran the point finder tip slowly over my ear. Other than a humming sound, nothing much happened. I didn't have any health issues or weakness that I was aware of, so that made sense. When he placed the instrument on my wife Bonnie's ear, however, the point finder buzzed as soon as it touched the spot that corresponded with her kidneys. Sure enough, she had a history of kidney and bladder infections. Finally, Andy let me run the point finder over his ear. When it touched the area for his lungs, it registered a loud buzzing sound. He remarked how good the instrument was; he had suffered repeated bouts of bronchitis as a child and this is what he thought the point finder was picking up. While I found it interesting, I didn't take it too seriously. It wasn't until later that the significance of this event really hit me.

Nearly two years later, I received a letter from Luciante. Andy had gone for an X-ray to see why a persistent cough refused to go away, only to discover that he had adenocarcinoma, cancer of the lung. Andy soon died at the young age of thirty-two, my friend who had been so full of life and always shined with a passion for helping people to heal and be well. I couldn't stop thinking about the buzzing acupuncture point finder when it touched the area in the external ear corresponding to Andy's lungs. Perhaps it had identified Andy's cancer—long before his symptoms appeared and before X-rays could spot the cancer.

When our sabbatical was over, I returned to Toronto and started practicing medicine. I also took a three-day course on acupuncture with the Acupuncture Foundation of Canada under the instruction of doctors Linda Rapson and Joe Wong. The more I learned, the more I wanted to know. I continued to take training sessions every opportunity that arose, and I began using it on my patients. Particularly with some medical conditions such as tennis elbow, osteoarthritis in the knees, and neck pain, I was impressed by how consistently I was getting good results, despite my limited training. Later I went to Sri Lanka and spent time observing acupuncture there, and I also took a Traditional Chinese Medicine course in Beijing, China, through the Chinese Medical Association, which ran a course for physicians.

WHAT IS ACUPUNCTURE?

Acupuncture has been used to treat a variety of diseases, to relieve pain, and even to produce an analgesic effect for surgical procedures. Basically, acupuncture is the practice of inserting very fine needles, not much thicker than human hair, through the skin at specific points on the body in order to stimulate the body's self-healing capacities. Before discussing needles, however, one needs to grasp the basic principle of *qi*, pronounced "chee."

According to classical acupuncture theory, every living body contains pathways of energy called *qi*, the vital life force that fuels the body's organs, systems, and functions. Just as cars head down a highway or blood cells navigate the veins, the Chinese believe that currents of life energy travel through the body inside invisible channels or pathways called meridians. Two meridians are on the body's central core, or midline, and twelve paired sets of meridians run up and down the left and right sides of the body, with the flow of energy in the dorsal channel (back of the body) going in one direction and the flow of energy on the ventral channel (front of the body) traveling in the other direction, thus creating a vertical cycle, similar to that which carries blood through the body's veins and arteries from head to toe. Each meridian governs the organs after which it is named and influences the territory of the body over which it passes.

Traditional practitioners believe that when there is an imbalance caused by an excess or deficiency (of yin or yang) or a blockage of *qi* (life energy), it can result in distress or disease in the parts of the body governed by that meridian. Situated along the meridian lines are approximately four hundred points where the meridians come to the body's surface. It is on these points where lowered resistance can be measured with electronic instruments, such as Andy's point finder; it is also where therapeutic procedures are performed and diagnostic clues are obtained. This action of inserting needles is thought to reestablish the balanced flow of energy in the body, either by stimulating or suppressing the energy.

Unlike hypodermic needles that give injections through a hollow, razor-edged tube, acupuncture needles are solid and come to a very fine, tapering end. The needles are of different length and diameter depending on the area of the body that is pierced. The practitioner inserts needles at several locations along the body's meridian lines and leaves them undisturbed for usually twenty to thirty minutes. Most patients will report that they cannot feel or can just barely feel the needle's insertion, and once inserted, they feel nothing other than possibly a slight sense of warmth, ache, or vibration. However, for the treatment to be effective the practitioner stimulates the needle by twirling it or moving it gently up and down. Acupuncture analgesia happens when the patient feels soreness, numbness, heaviness, and distension following acupuncture manipulation.

HISTORY OF ACUPUNCTURE

Acupuncture was first recorded by Huang Di Nei Jing in *The Emperor's Canon of Internal Medicine,* compiled over two thousand years ago (475–221 BC). Primitive acupuncture needles dating back to around 1000 BC have been discovered in archeological finds of the Shan dynasty in China. Other similar healing practices involve the use of stones to massage over certain points on the body; these date back even further, perhaps as far as four to ten thousand years. Moxibustion, the practice of burning small plugs of the herb mugwort over acupuncture points, thus stimulating the points with heat, has also been traced back to societies that warmed specific areas of the body for therapeutic effects. Shiatsu, which is finger pressure applied to acupuncture points, and (the modern) Transcutaneous Nerve Stimulation (TENS) are all based on the same principles.

Classical acupuncture theory evolved over thousands of years and encompasses the law of five elements, the philosophy of yin and yang, pulse diagnosis, and examination of the tongue. Just as training in Western medicine demands that doctors spend many years in school followed by internship, classical acupuncture theory is complicated and requires years of study to thoroughly understand Traditional Chinese Medicine and to practice with skill.

In the late 1970s, it was apparent that the West was rising to meet and learn more about the East. Several articles began to appear in reputable scientific journals reflecting the genuine interest of Western researchers to understand if and how traditional acupuncture worked. One study reported that virtually all acupuncture points correspond to known neural structures, and another stated that it is possible to detect acupuncture points electrically with an instrument that measures skin resistance.[1, 2] A third study reported that most acupuncture points have a lower skin resistance measurement than the surrounding skin, and that the location is constant in all people. Simple dry needling of tender points (versus the use of a corticosteroid injection through a hollow needle), they concluded, can give relief to different kinds of problems. Some of these tender points correlate with trigger and acupuncture points that have been described in other conditions like fibrositis.[3]

SCIENTIFIC EXPLANATION OF ACUPUNCTURE

There are many theories about how acupuncture works. The most well known focuses on the stimulation of the body's ability to produce its own natural chemicals called endorphins. These endorphins use the same brain receptors as opioid drugs to switch on pain relief. Scientists wondered if acupuncture stimulated the release of these endorphins, thereby stimulating a natural pain-killing effect. They designed a trial to test their theory, using a drug that prevents opioid receptors from working.

The drug Naloxone is an opioid antagonist, meaning it acts to stop the effects of opioid drugs, such as morphine and heroin. In the case of a morphine overdose, the central nervous system becomes depressed so that brain signals that normally generate breathing activity stop signaling, and the person dies from respiratory failure. Naloxone was developed to prevent death by overdose. Let's say a post-surgical patient was receiving morphine for pain relief, and then suddenly stopped breathing. Naloxone would quickly be administered to counteract the depressive action of the morphine, and the patient would start breathing normally again. Unfortunately for the patient, the morphine's analgesic action would also stop working, and the patient's pain would return.

Dr. Bruce Pomeranz and Dr. Richard Cheng found that when acupuncture was used for analgesia, administering Naloxone effectively blocked the analgesic (pain-killing) action, and pain returned, implying that acupuncture analgesia is produced by stimulation of the body's endogenous opiates, or rather, endorphins. It is believed that low-frequency (2–6 Hertz) electrical acupuncture stimulates receptors that cause the release of endorphins in the spinal cord, midbrain, hypothalamus, and pituitary glands, which help in pain mediation.[4]

Another study showed that electro-acupuncture increases blood cortisol levels in horses and human beings.[5] Cortisol is the body's own anti-inflammatory. Reducing inflammation helps to reduce pain. Another possible mechanism suggests that acupuncture stimulates serotonin, GABA, and acetylcholine, which are neurotransmitters (brain chemicals) that mediate pain response.[6]

Dr. Helene Langevin, a researcher in acupuncture, believes that it is possible that the mechanical signal created by an acupuncture needle being rotated in the plane of loose connective tissue at an acupuncture point can be transduced into an electrical signal that is passed through the web of fibroblasts in the body's tissue that may correspond to the meridian system. She offers this as an explanation for the remote effects of acupuncture.[7]

A newer concept for interpreting how acupuncture works comes from Zhang and colleagues who described a collection of the activated neural and neuroactive components distributed in the skin, muscle, and connective tissues surrounding the inserted needle, and they called this area a neural acupuncture unit (NAU).[8]

This NAU is believed to contain relatively dense and concentrated neural and neuroactive components. They believe that the NAU-based local mechanisms of biochemical and biophysical reactions play an important role in acupuncture-induced analgesia.

When an acupuncture needle is inserted into a designated point and repetitively manipulated in different directions, it is assumed to cause local tissue injury and biochemical reactions, with the release of various inflammatory and immune mediators in NAUs. This acupuncture-induced tissue injury may represent a "positive" biochemical process resulting in therapeutic responses at local and systemic levels, which is due to the nerve fibers in NAUs.

Some believe that acupuncture is not only a noxious stimulus but is also mechanical and can be electrical.[9] Many inhibitory mediators, such as adenosine triphosphate (ATP), a coenzyme used as an energy carrier in the cells of all known organisms, and its metabolite adenosine, are released in response to mechanical and electrical stimulation. Acupuncture stimulation has been found to increase the extracellular concentrations of ATP and adenosine in mice's acupoint tissues, when pain relief was elicited.[10]

Other researchers also believe that acupuncture balances sympathetic and parasympathetic activity via somato-autonomic reflex. The research implies that NAU signals are transmitted by multiple peripheral and central neural pathways to different levels in the central nervous system. These signals go to the spinal cord, the brainstem, and the hypothalamus, where they are relayed to the organs of the body via autonomic nerve fibers and the neuroendocrine and neuro-immune systems. This ultimately results in a rebalance of sympathetic and parasympathetic activity thus helping to put the body into better balance.[11, 12, 13]

DOES ACUPUNCTURE WORK?

The scientific literature contains many studies that demonstrate the usefulness of acupuncture.[14, 15, 16, 17, 18] A systemic review of acupuncture for four chronic pain conditions—back and neck pain, osteoarthritis, chronic headache, and shoulder pain—looked at twenty-nine Randomly Assigned Controlled Trials (RCT) involving 17,922 patients. Acupuncture was superior to both sham and no acupuncture control for each pain condition. The authors concluded that acupuncture is effective for the treatment of chronic pain and that acupuncture is more than a placebo.[19]

Personally I have had the most success with acupuncture treating pain syndromes such as temporomandibular joint syndrome (TMJ—a disorder that may cause jaw pain, dizziness, and headaches), coccydynia (tailbone pain), headaches, plantar fasciitis (inflammation of the thick tissue on the bottom of the foot), and pain in a single joint such as the knee, shoulder, elbow, or small joints of the hands and feet. I also find it useful in the treatment of allergies, sinusitis, and for help in stopping smoking. In countries such as China and Sri Lanka acupuncture is sometimes used as anesthesia during surgery.

There is a considerable amount of research that shows acupuncture is helpful. A comprehensive systematic review (twelve studies up to 2008 involving 1,076 patients) concluded that acupuncture and moxibustion were safe and effective to treat allergic rhinitis (runny and stuffed nose caused by allergies) and may have some advantages over routine medication.[20] Another systematic review (twelve studies up to 2007) also found suggestive evidence for the effectiveness of acupuncture in persistent allergic rhinitis.[21]

Evidence of benefit has been further supported by findings from a large trial that included two randomized groups and one non-randomized group, involving 5,237 patients with allergic rhinitis. Brinkhaus and colleagues found that when acupuncture was added to routine medical care, there were statistically and clinically relevant benefits. Rhinitis Quality of Life Questionnaire (RQLQ) scores after three months of acupuncture treatment improved significantly.[22]

ACUPUNCTURE FOR DEPRESSION

There is some evidence that acupuncture can be useful for depression. After reviewing 207 clinical studies of acupuncture for depression, 113 on major depression and 76 on post-stroke depression were found. Of all those studies, twenty Randomly Controlled Trials of major depression involving 1,998 patients and fifteen studies of post-stroke depression involving 1,680 patients were considered high-quality and were included for meta-analysis. The authors found that acupuncture was as good as antidepressants alone in improving clinical response and alleviating symptom severity but not different from sham acupuncture. They did not find that adding acupuncture in addition to antidepressants could yield better outcomes than antidepressants alone. They did find that acupuncture was superior to antidepressants and wait-list controls in improving both response and symptom severity of post-stroke depression. The incidence of adverse events in acupuncture intervention was significantly lower than antidepressants.[23]

Another review also looked at the efficacy and safety of acupuncture for the treatment of depression. The authors concluded that acupuncture, including manual-, electrical-, and laser-based, is generally beneficial, well tolerated, and safe as single treatment for depression.[24]

ACUPUNCTURE FOR OTHER PROBLEMS

Most of the research for other conditions has been done in China and the review papers are written in Chinese so I cannot verify that the reviews are the gospel. However, because they are listed in Pub Med, a reliable source for acceptable journals, I am going to share some of this research by summarizing the abstracts that are written in English. These reviews looked at constipation, acne, and ulcerative colitis, a serious inflammatory disease of the large intestine.

One review looked at fifteen papers involving 1,052 patients with constipation. They concluded that the curative rate of acupuncture and moxibustion on constipation was significantly better than ordinary medication. Abdominal pain, defecation duration, and general symptom scores were statistically better than controls.[25] Another review looked at seventeen papers, including 1,613 cases, comparing the treatment of acne with acupuncture and moxibustion with routine Western medicine as control. They concluded that acupuncture and moxibustion are safe and effective treatments of acne, and are possibly better than routine Western medicine. However, they acknowledge that the studies examined were of low quality. Another review of eleven clinical studies found that the therapeutic effect of acupuncture and moxibustion on ulcerative colitis was superior to that of Western medicine with greater safety and less adverse reactions.[26]

SIDE EFFECTS OF ACUPUNCTURE

Over the thirty years that I have been doing acupuncture, the number of side effects has been exceedingly small. Two patients have had fainting episodes when I put the needles into the acupuncture points. Now I usually have patients in a lying-down position; no one has ever fainted when they were in this position. Some conditions may seem to get worse after the acupuncture treatment, but often get better after the initial aggravation. Occasionally mild pain and minimal bleeding or bruising can result at needle insertion points. I have had no incidence of infection or any other serious complication.

One must be cautious, however. Certain acupuncture points are contraindicated in pregnant women because acupuncture has been known to cause miscarriages. Also certain acupuncture points are dangerous if needled improperly. There have been reports of pneumothorax or collapsed lung after acupuncture needles were inserted too deeply into the chest cavity, causing the needle to pierce the lining of the lung. Apparently there have been thirty cases of collapsed lung presented to emergency departments in Toronto due to acupuncture needles penetrating too deep, so proper training is crucial.

There have also been reports of infections like AIDS and hepatitis B and C because the practitioner used needles that had not been properly sterilized. Most practitioners use disposable needles, and some use electrical and laser acupuncture, which avoids needles. Because there is often no regulation of practitioners, proper hygiene is sometimes overlooked. You must always be careful when choosing an acupuncturist, and select someone who uses disposable needles and allows you to see them open the sealed packages.

FINDING A QUALIFIED PRACTITIONER

While certification requirements are regulated independently by each state, currently in America, forty-three states plus the District of Columbia require the passage of the National Certification Commission for Acupuncture and Oriental Medicine (NCCAOM) examinations or NCCAOM certification as a prerequisite for licensure. Certified practitioners may be found on their website: www.nccaom.org. Also, the American Board of Medical Acupuncture lists certified, licensed practitioners: www.dabma .org/physicians.asp. In Canada, you may look up certified, licensed practitioners on the Acupuncture Foundation of Canada Institute's website: www.afcinstitute.com.

THE FUTURE OF ACUPUNCTURE

Dr. Linda Rapson, former Director of the Acupuncture Foundation of Canada Institute, said, "Someday in the future, we will be using acupuncture as a treatment of first choice in some conditions, rather than a last desperate attempt to help the patient when all else has failed."

CONCLUSION

The problem with looking at the research on acupuncture is that the outcome of the treatment is sometimes dependent on the skill of the acupuncturist, the points that are used, and the modality of acupuncture. Sometimes acupuncture may use a Traditional Chinese Medicine diagnosis and other times a Western medical diagnosis. Each diagnostic method or lens will affect which acupuncture points are stimulated.

If you have a swollen and painful knee, elbow, or finger, rather than going on a nonsteroidal anti-inflammatory drug, which has systemic side effects, or injecting that joint with cortisone, which also carries some risks, acupuncture can be useful. Sometimes even chronic joint pain can be relieved in five or six sessions. Tennis elbow, tendonitis of the shoulder, trigger finger, and TMJ dysfunction may also respond well to acupuncture.

I have had patients who complained of a frozen shoulder such as John, a fifty-five-year-old dermatologist who had a longstanding history of frozen shoulder. He was fed up with the pain and was going to get an injection of cortisone, but he decided instead to come and see me for acupuncture first. He couldn't lift or move his left shoulder at all. After a number of treatments once or twice a week for a number of weeks, he regained full use of his shoulder and was completely pain free.

Chronic back, neck, and other pain syndromes are more difficult to treat and need an experienced clinician. If you have musculoskeletal problems it is important to correct the underlying cause of the problem or the disability may return. For example, the treatment of headaches often requires the treatment of dietary, structural, and emotional aspects as well as using the needles.

For smoking cessation, acupuncture needles are put in the ears and stimulated with electricity for twenty minutes, once or twice a week for the first few weeks. Press needles can remain in the ears between office treatments. Acupuncture seems to help some smokers with the withdrawal side effects and can be used in addition to nicotine transdermal patches or any other technique.

CHAPTER 13

ACUPUNCTURE FOR OSTEOARTHRITIS OF THE KNEE

Linda Rapson, MD, and Mel Borins, MD

Osteoarthritis (OA), sometimes referred to as degenerative joint disease (DJD), is caused by the breakdown and eventual loss of cartilage between bone joints. Cartilage is protein that acts as a cushion, preventing bone from rubbing against bone. When the cartilage breaks down, joints can become inflamed, painful, and swollen. Osteoarthritis is the most common form of arthritis and usually affects people more as they age. Heredity can play a role, but causes are usually disease, injury or trauma, repetitive movement, lack of muscle tone, or just plain age.

While there is no absolute cure, the physician's goal of treatment is to reduce pain and inflammation and to improve and maintain joint function. Weight reduction, muscle-building exercise, avoidance of excessively strenuous or repetitive activities involving the joint, and diet changes are usually the first line of recommendation for patients. Treatment interventions may consist of taking nonsteroidal anti-inflammatories, pain killers, cortisone injections, or surgery, which may involve knee replacement. All of these treatments come with risks and side effects. Would acupuncture be a safer, effective treatment?

Fred is a typical example of patients who come to me with this problem. He was a forty-two-year-old businessman who had a painful and swollen left knee that was not helped by nonsteroidal anti-inflammatory drugs or physiotherapy. He had been referred to an orthopedic physician who recommended arthroscopic lavage. This surgical intervention involves making a tiny incision to insert a scope with camera, inspect the joint, fix any visible problems, and wash out the joint space with a saline solution, removing any loose debris, fluid, or blood. While lavage is a commonly used intervention, recent studies have raised questions about its effectiveness.[1]

Fred came to me as a last resort before going for surgery. I treated him once a week with electro-acupuncture. I inserted needles into the acupuncture points around his knee and at other distal points (away from the area of pain, but along the appropriate meridian lines), and I hooked up a TENS (transcutaneous electro nerve stimulation) machine to the needles. Fred received this treatment weekly for a period of ten weeks. He made a slow but complete recovery and averted the need for surgery.

While Fred's case is an excellent example of a successful outcome, one could still ask whether acupuncture caused the recovery, or would he have healed anyway in ten weeks without treatment? This is a good example of anecdotal evidence that doesn't prove anything, but combined with scientifically researched evidence, can lead one to a safer conclusion.

CLINICAL TRIALS AND ACUPUNCTURE

In the early days of scientific study on acupuncture for osteoarthritic conditions, researchers faced many challenges. Some trials recruited too few participants. Others struggled to create study method designs that provided blind and controlled conditions. Some trials were criticized for not covering a long enough period of time. When independent, randomized, double-blind, controlled trials repeatedly come out with positive results, we conclude that treatment is effective. But with all scientific research, despite the number of trials resulting in positive outcomes, there will always be one or more with negative outcomes; the nature of journalism is sometimes to focus on the one negative result, which skews public opinion about whether a treatment is effective. Good examples of this were two randomized, controlled trials with reasonable designs that showed a negative outcome for acupuncture treatment of osteoarthritis of the knee. These trials, however, included only twenty patients each, and fewer than ten acupuncture treatments were given.[2, 3]

One of the challenges in designing acupuncture trials is to create a double-blind control, where the patient, the researcher, and/or the person giving the treatment, are unaware of which group the patient is in: the experimental group (true acupuncture) or the control group (sham acupuncture or no treatment). In recent studies, sham needles have been used to try to resolve this challenge.

Acupuncture needles are cased in a hub, or hollow holder, which is used to position the needles accurately over the acupuncture point. Genuine acupuncture needles will permeate the skin when pressed, but sham needles have blunt ends that retract into the hub upon contact with skin. Research assistants who observe and collect data on pain levels and movement ability are unaware which needle is being used, but the practitioners who perform the procedure can tell the difference. What researchers needed to know was, can patients tell the difference?

One method of testing whether patients are effectively blinded by the procedure is to ask each patient after treatment if they think they received the true acupuncture, the sham acupuncture, or if they are unsure. Statistics performed upon the collected answers comparing those with treatment or sham status would reveal whether there is significant evidence of patients' ability to tell the difference between sham and real acupuncture treatment.

Another challenge, particularly in studies with people suffering from osteoarthritis of the knee, is pain. A certain number of study volunteers take medication that enables them to perform daily tasks and routines. Imagine that you rely on over-the-counter nonsteroidal anti-inflammatories to deal with your chronic knee pain. You hear about a research trial on the effectiveness of acupuncture treatment for painful knees, and they are looking for volunteers. That sounds interesting! When you call them to find out more about the trial, they say that for six months, you will have to give up NSAIDS, the one thing that gives you some relief from the painful knee. Immediately you're wondering what will happen if you are placed in the control group and get no treatment. What are the chances that you'll join the trial now? You'd have to be extremely motivated to take that risk, and most people are not.

Studies have to be designed so that they take into account any medication the participants may be taking. Once again, by collecting data about each participant and statistically analyzing individual variables against whole-group totals, researchers hope to reach a qualified conclusion about whether acupuncture treatment is effective or not. The following study emphasizes that proper clinical trials can be done to show the benefit of acupuncture.

Dr. Brian Berman from the University of Maryland completed a six-month trial of acupuncture in 570 patients with osteoarthritis of the knee.[4] All participants were age fifty or older and had significant pain in their knee the month before joining the study, but had never experienced acupuncture. They had not had knee surgery in the previous six months and had not used steroid or similar injections. Participants were randomly assigned to receive one of three treatments: 190 received acupuncture, 191 received sham acupuncture, and 189 participated in a control group that attended the Arthritis Foundation's Self-Help Course for managing their condition, a proven effective model of treatment. Patients continued to receive standard medical care from their primary physicians, including anti-inflammatory medications and opioid pain relievers.

Over twenty-six weeks, the acupuncture groups had twenty-three sessions of either true or sham acupuncture, depending on their assigned group. The real acupuncture group had two sham points used on their abdomens approximately 3 cm lateral to and slightly above the umbilicus bilaterally. This was done so that the two groups would both have similar experiences. A screen was placed so that the patients could not see the true or sham treatment on the legs but could observe the procedure on the abdomen.

Five local acupuncture points were used: GB 34, SP 9, ST 36, ST 35, and Xiyan (XL 2). Four distal points included UB 60, GB 39, SP 6, and K 3. Electrical stimulation of the needles consisted of square biphasic pulses (0.5-ms pulse width) applied at 8Hz for twenty minutes to the Xiyan points. The sham group had a mock trans-electrical stimulation unit attached to the sham needles at the knee; this unit had a blinking light and emitted a sound.

The sham technique involved tapping the skin with a guide tube and immediately affixing a needle to the skin surface with adhesive tape. The same points were used for the sham group as listed for the real acupuncture group, but with the difference that the sham group had needles inserted on the abdomen and sham performed on the legs, versus the real acupuncture group which received the reverse.

Participants were allowed to continue taking their usual medication during the trial. At the start of the trial 11 percent of participants were taking simple analgesics; 31 percent were taking non-selective NSAIDs; 28 percent were taking COX-2 selective inhibitors like Vioxx, Celebrex, Mobicox, and Bextra; and 6 percent were receiving an opioid. A careful analysis was done to ensure that medication could not have been responsible for the differences in the groups.

All participants were asked at four and twenty-six weeks whether they thought they were receiving true acupuncture, sham acupuncture, or were unsure about which one they were getting. At four weeks, 67 percent of the true acupuncture group believed they were receiving real acupuncture and 25 percent were unsure, whereas 58 percent in the sham group believed they were receiving real acupuncture, and 33 percent were unsure. Thus only 9 percent saw through the sham. By week twenty-six, more people in the true acupuncture group felt they were getting real treatment (75 percent), because they were getting better, but still only 10 percent of the individuals receiving sham treatment thought it was not real.

Assessments using WOMAC pain and function scores (Western Ontario and McMaster University Osteoarthritis Index) and Patient Global Assessments were done at baseline, four, eight, fourteen, and twenty-six weeks. The Short-form Health Survey score (SF-36) and a six-minute Walk Distance test were done at eight and twenty-six weeks. Careful attention was paid to possible adverse effects at each measurement interval.

Results: By week eight, compared with the sham and control groups, participants receiving the true acupuncture recorded a significant increase in function, and by week fourteen, a significant decrease in pain. These results, shown by declining scores on the WOMAC index, held steady through week twenty-six. Overall, those who received acupuncture had a 40 percent decrease in pain and a nearly 40 percent improvement in function compared to baseline assessments. There were no adverse effects attributable to the acupuncture or sham acupuncture.

In 2006, a systematic review and meta-analysis[5] were completed on a selection of eight randomized, controlled trials involving adults with chronic knee pain or osteoarthritis of the knee, who had received one of four treatments: adequate acupuncture, a sham treatment, another intervention, or their usual treatment care. In five combined studies involving 1,334 patients, acupuncture produced significant superior results, in both pain and function, over sham acupuncture and usual treatment care. Significant differences were also recorded after long-term follow-up. The authors of this review concluded that "acupuncture that meets criteria for adequate treatment is significantly superior to sham acupuncture and to no additional intervention in improving pain and function in patients with chronic knee pain."

CONCLUSION

While more research could always be done, it is safe to conclude that, especially for patients who are unable to take NSAIDs, acupuncture is a useful treatment for osteoarthritis of the knee.

CHAPTER 14
ACUPUNCTURE FOR NAUSEA AND VOMITING

How many of us remember family vacations when one (or worse, all) of the kids in the backseat cried out, "I'm going to be sick," and the car was in the fast lane of the highway, with little or no room to pull over? Another not-so-fond memory of many mothers is their first trimester of pregnancy, when they felt nauseous upon waking and several times throughout the day. When a pregnant woman loses her appetite for supper merely at the thought of cooking it, she wonders why it is called morning sickness.

Nausea and vomiting are common occurrences that aren't always attributed to carsickness or pregnancy. It may be indicative of food poisoning, the flu, or could be a side effect from drugs used for anesthesia or chemotherapy. Nausea can also be a sign of something more sinister, so it is important to discover the underlying cause and appropriately treat the origin of the problem. There are a number of medical conditions where symptomatic treatment is all that is required, but conventional medications do not always control nausea and vomiting, and they often have side effects. The medical community cannot forget the tragic number of children who were born with missing or severely stunted limbs after their mothers were treated with thalidomide for nausea during early pregnancy.

One alternative to taking medicine for nausea and vomiting is acupuncture. Acupuncture treatments usually require the stimulation of multiple points because symptoms are complex in nature. Understanding symptom complexes, meridians, and the insertion of the needles requires some degree of training. With nausea and vomiting, however, there is one point called P6 or Pericardium 6 that, when needled by itself, will sometimes relieve nausea and vomiting without the necessity of using multiple acupuncture points.

ACUPRESSURE SELF HELP

Some manufacturers of products for treating seasickness have designed a variety of wrist straps that utilize the P6 point. Studies have shown that acupressure wristbands offer a safe alternative to relieve nausea due to morning sickness, motion sickness/travel, chemotherapy, radiation, and anesthesia.[1, 2, 3]

To find P6, hold your right hand up, palm facing you, and bend the hand slightly forward. Under your palm, where wrist and hand meet, is at least one clearly defined, horizontal crease. Place your left thumb horizontally across the wrist, immediately below the topmost crease. The top (left side) of the thumb should be running in the same direction as the crease. Now look at where the bottom (right side) of the thumb is. Move your thumb down to run horizontally below this line. A simpler way of putting it might be to say, place your thumb, two thumbs down, beneath your wrist. Where the bottom of the second thumb lies, is where you will find P6. Using your index finger, find a vertical groove that runs between two long tendons. To make certain your index finger is in the correct groove, wiggle the little finger of your right hand; you should be able to see the left vertical tendon on your wrist move. Press the spot right in the middle; it should feel slightly different from other locations on your wrist, possibly a little tender, or just a little odd. You have now correctly identified the P6 acupuncture point.

THE SCIENCE BEHIND ACUPUNCTURE

With recent developments in technology, we can now use brain-imaging scans while the body is being stimulated, and we can chart which parts of the brain respond to that stimulation. Functional magnetic resonance imaging (fMRI) studies found that acupuncture at P6 activated parts of the cerebrum (outer brain) associated with nausea and vestibular motion sickness. These were: the left superior frontal gyrus, the anterior cingulate gyrus, and the dorsomedial nucleus of thalamus. Sham acupuncture and tactile stimulation on the skin at the same acupoint did not show activation.

The cerebellum, a tree-shaped structure situated in the hind brain (back of the skull), controls motor movement, coordination, balance, equilibrium, and muscle tone. This also showed activation under fMRI when stimulated with acupuncture at P6. The activated parts in the cerebellum were: the declive, nodulus, and uvula of vermis, quadrangular lobule, cerebellar tonsil, and superior semilunar lobule.[4]

Put simply, a visual scan of brain activity performed during acupuncture treatment confirmed that when acupoint P6 was stimulated, parts of the brain involved with motion, balance, and nausea were activated, versus sham acupuncture and tactile stimulation, which did not show activation during the fMRI scan.

ACUPUNCTURE FOR POSTOPERATIVE NAUSEA AND VOMITING

Postoperative nausea and vomiting (PONV) are common complications following surgery and anesthesia. Drug therapy to prevent PONV is not always effective. A systematic review of twenty-six trials found that there were significant reductions in the risks of nausea, vomiting, and the need for rescue antiemetics (antinausea drugs) associated with acupuncture of the P6 stimulation point compared with sham treatments.[5]

In a study of 410 women undergoing gynecological surgery there was a significant reduction of PONV in those who were given bilateral P6 acupressure (on both wrists) after surgery, as compared to sham treatment and controls.[6]

Another randomized, double-blind, sham-placebo controlled study injected 0.2 ml of glucose solution with a 1 ml tuberculin syringe vertically to a depth of 5–7 mm in the P6 acupoint before the conclusion of the surgery in 187 children between the ages of seven to sixteen. This resulted in pressure being applied to the acupoint from inside the skin. P6 injections were found to be as effective as Droperidol (antiemetic) in controlling early postoperative nausea and vomiting. The author concluded that P6-related techniques should be incorporated in the curriculum of anesthesia residency programs because the technique is quite simple to learn and is a low-cost procedure with little side effects.[7]

ACUPUNCTURE FOR NAUSEA AND VOMITING OF PREGNANCY

Two hundred thirty pregnant women who had mild to severe vomiting in early pregnancy, between weeks 6 to 12 of gestation, were randomly assigned to receive a device for nerve stimulation therapy of P6 or an otherwise identical but non-stimulating placebo device. There was a significant reduction in nausea and vomiting and more weight gain in the group who used the nerve stimulation device over P6 compared to controls.[8]

The Society of Obstetricians and Gynecologists of Canada in their Practice Guidelines have stated that P6 stimulation is a safe treatment for the relief of nausea and vomiting in pregnancy.

ACUPRESSURE FOR SEASICKNESS OR TRAVEL SICKNESS

To help with the nausea of travel, many people use wristband products such as Seabands or Psibands, which apply continuous pressure by means of a plastic stud on the P6 acupressure point between the two central tendons near the wrist. Positioning of the band is one factor that may affect the outcome. Patients anecdotally claim that these bands help them travel without nausea. Small independent studies have reported both negative and positive outcomes.[9] More randomly controlled, double-blind studies are needed before a reliable conclusion can be reached.

ACUPUNCTURE FOR NAUSEA AFTER CHEMOTHERAPY

Many patients with cancer and rheumatic diseases continue to experience nausea and vomiting when undergoing chemotherapy treatments even with preventative medications. There is evidence that stimulation of the P6 acupoint can help in relieving these symptoms.[10]

ACUPUNCTURE FOR DENTAL GAGGING

One study found that by stimulating P6 with thumb pressure, patients were more able to go through dental procedures without gagging.[11]

CONCLUSION

Acupuncture is a safe, easy to use treatment for the prevention and relief of nausea and vomiting. There is scientific evidence to support its use.

CHAPTER 15
ACUPUNCTURE FOR TENNIS ELBOW

After two long sets on the tennis court, your partner asks for one more. It's the first game of the season, and you promised yourself to make a gentle start after the long, inactive winter. Just as you go to refuse the offer, you think again. It's late Saturday morning; the sun is shedding its warmth, and the air is filled with the heady scents of spring. The longest winter you remember has finally given up its icy, blustering stance, and the only remaining traces of its fury are a few meek and melting roadside berms of wet, dirty snow. It feels great to be outdoors again. You can't resist the temptation. "Okay, one more set," you say.

You pick up your racket and twirl it, waiting for your partner to serve. He makes a killer overhand serve, trying to drive the ball home on your left side, but you're ready. You reach to make a backhand return, and suddenly, a Taser-like pain streaks from your elbow, travels down your forearm, and strikes your wrist. Your numbed hand loses its grip, the racket missiles across the court, and the ball lands on your side of the net in a pathetic, spinning roll. Dazed, you stumble over to retrieve the racket aware of a sinking feeling in your gut. Past experience tells you that this game is over and you might not be playing anymore this season. You've got tennis elbow, or rather, lateral epicondylitis.

TENNIS ELBOW—WHAT IS IT?

Lateral epicondylitis is a common condition that results from injury of the muscle tendons that attach to the bone on the outside of your elbow. Over time, these small tears called lesions happen in the tendon tissue and eventually it leads to inflammation, irritation of the nerves, and pain. The type of movement that commonly causes this injury is a repetitive twisting motion of the forearm, as happens with racket sports, and with repeated use of hand tools. Workers that experience this condition come from a number of trades: painters, builders, plumbers, electricians, keyboard operators, cooks, butchers, glassblowers, etc. When the pain occurs on the inner side of the elbow, it is commonly referred to as golfer's elbow.

The symptoms can persist for a long period of time, sometimes a year or more. The condition is often self-limiting, in that many people will rest the arm until the pain goes away, which is a recommended first treatment, along with icing, and sometimes, using nonsteroidal anti-inflammatory drugs (NSAIDs). Arm braces, stretches, and physical therapy can help, but when pain continues for more than a few months, cortisone injections or surgery may be recommended.

Since osteoarthritis of the knee often responds well to acupuncture, would it not make sense to use it for tennis elbow as well? There have been few randomized, blind-controlled studies on acupuncture treatment of lateral epicondylitis, and none of them involved high numbers of patients. Taking that into consideration, let's have a look at the research available.

THE SCIENCE BEHIND ACUPUNCTURE FOR TENNIS ELBOW

In a randomized, investigator- and patient-blinded, controlled clinical study, twenty-three patients were treated with real acupuncture, and twenty-two patients received sham acupuncture. The patients each received ten treatments, with two treatments given per week. The primary outcome variables were: maximal strength, pain intensity (using a verbal rating scale), and disability (using a questionnaire for rating disabilities of the arm, shoulder, and hand). Patients were examined one week before the start of treatment and at follow-up: two weeks and two months after the end of treatment.

At the two-week follow-up there was significantly greater improvement for all outcome parameters in the group treated with real acupuncture. At two months the function of the arm was still better in this group than in the sham acupuncture group, but the differences in pain intensity and maximal strength between the groups were no longer significant.[1]

Another randomized, examiner- and patient-blinded controlled clinical study reviewed forty-five patients. Half of the patients received acupuncture with the points being mechanically stimulated, and the other half received invasive sham acupuncture (non-acupuncture points were used) twice a week for ten sessions. The study looked at outcome measurement of pain at rest, pain on movement, pain on exertion, and frequency and duration of pain. Two weeks, two months, and one year after the end of treatment there were significant reductions in all pain variables compared to baseline in both groups. At the first follow-up, two weeks after treatment, significant group differences were registered for pain on motion and on exertion, in favor of the real acupuncture group. But at the two-month and twelve-month follow-ups, these differences in pain intensity between the groups were no longer significant. The authors concluded that, in the treatment of chronic epicondylitis, the selection of so-called real acupuncture points gives better results than invasive sham acupuncture at early follow-up.[2]

In a 2002 Cochrane review,[3] four small, randomized controlled trials were studied and reviewed, although they could not be combined in a meta-analysis due to clinical differences between trials and flaws in study designs (small populations, uncertainty about group allocation being concealed, and substantial lack of data from patients who left the study before the twelve-month follow-up). Here are their findings:

- One randomized controlled trial found that needle acupuncture results in relief of pain for significantly longer than placebo and is more likely to result in a 50 percent or greater reduction in pain after one treatment. Patients in the treatment group were treated at non-segmental distal points (homolateral leg) for elbow pain, following Chinese acupuncture rules, whereas patients in the placebo group were treated with placebo acupuncture (avoiding penetration of the skin with an acupuncture needle). Overall reduction in the pain score was 55.8 percent in the treatment group and 15 percent in the placebo group. After one treatment, nineteen out of twenty-four patients in the treatment group (79.2 percent) reported pain relief of at least 50 percent compared to only six patients out of twenty-four in the placebo group. The duration of analgesia after one treatment was 20.2 hours in the treated group and 1.4 hours in the placebo group.

- Another randomized controlled trial demonstrated needle acupuncture to be more likely to result in overall participant-reported improvement than placebo in the short term, but no significant differences were found in the longer term (after three or twelve months).

- A randomized controlled trial of laser acupuncture versus placebo demonstrated no differences between laser acupuncture and placebo with respect to overall benefit.

- A trial published in Chinese demonstrated no difference between vitamin B12 injection plus acupuncture, and vitamin B12 injection alone.

The Cochrane reviewers concluded that "there is insufficient evidence to either support or refute the use of acupuncture (either needle or laser) in the treatment of lateral elbow pain."

Finally, in 2004, a systematic review[4] was done of six studies that were considered to be of high quality (using the Jadad scale). Reviewers noted that all six studies indicated that acupuncture was effective in relieving lateral epicondyle pain. Five of the six studies found that acupuncture treatment was more effective compared to a control treatment. They concluded that there is strong evidence suggesting that acupuncture is effective in the short-term relief of lateral epicondyle pain.

CONVENTIONAL TREATMENT VERSUS ACUPUNCTURE

A Cochrane review on the use of NSAIDs for tennis elbow found evidence that topical (cream or gel) NSAIDs are significantly more effective short term for pain than placebo, and some evidence for short-term benefit from oral NSAIDs and cortisone injections (with respect to pain and function), but the benefits were not sustained over a long-term period. Significantly more gastrointestinal adverse effects were reported by those taking oral NSAIDs. The authors concluded that there remains insufficient evidence to recommend or discourage the use of oral NSAIDs.

Other systematic reviews of conventional (commonly used) treatments for this condition also found inconclusive evidence on the benefits of any treatment modalities.

What is interesting to note is that all these findings were similar to the acupuncture study findings. Short-term relief of pain caused by tennis elbow can be achieved using NSAIDs, cortisone injections, and acupuncture. But the conventional methods of treatment reported significant adverse side effects, where no adverse effects were reported with acupuncture treatment.

CONCLUSION

In my own clinical practice I have had mixed results in using acupuncture for tennis elbow, with some patients getting complete recovery after receiving only a few treatments and others not responding to acupuncture or any treatment modality such as ultrasound, physiotherapy, NSAIDs, and even cortisone injections.

With any acupuncture treatment, recovery depends on the expertise of the acupuncturist, on which acupoints are chosen (also if a Traditional Chinese or Western approach was used), whether TENS or moxibustion was used, and upon the severity of the damaged tendon condition.

Further research would be helpful to clarify just how effective acupuncture is for this common problem. I recommend eliminating the cause of the problem, doing specific exercises, and receiving acupuncture, as my first choice for the treatment of tennis elbow.

CHAPTER 16
ACUPUNCTURE FOR NECK PAIN

Don't be such a pain in the neck! Perhaps you remember saying that to your sibling, or maybe someone at school said it to you. Few people want to be accused of it, and nobody wants to have it, but most of us, at some point in our life, will experience pain in the neck. Whether the pain is acute and intense, chronic, or just plain sore, a neck that hurts is difficult if not impossible to ignore.

The average adult human head weighs between eight and twelve pounds and can be heavier. Not only is your neck responsible for supporting your head's weight all the waking hours of the day, but it makes thousands of left and right rotations of up to 60 to 80 degrees, allows chin-to-chest flexion for looking at your feet, and backward extension so you can watch eagles soar above you or change the ceiling lightbulb. It also makes 45-degree lateral bends, which means you can tilt your head halfway to your shoulder and hold the phone without using your hands. Along with the potential problems of being a flexible, weight-bearing structure, the neck is also a place where emotions such as anger, worry, fear, and stress can be stored in muscle and other tissues. (Don't get your hackles up—it hurts!) No wonder this slender bridge between brain and body gets sore.

The neck consists of a framework of seven cervical vertebrae starting with C1 (the atlas, which supports the skull) and C2 (the axis) down to C7. Collectively, the vertebrae form a protective but flexible barrier around the spinal cord, and between each vertebra are cushions called discs. Along with nerves that travel from the brain, down the spine, and through the vertebral openings, the neck contains muscles, tendons, arteries and veins, glands, and structures of the throat that allow us to breathe, speak, and swallow.

In today's world, where mechanized equipment and means of transport have replaced much of our need for movement and strength, and our work and entertainment allow us to sit motionless for hours at a time, we struggle to stay physically fit. As we age, the muscles we developed in our youth may instead begin to atrophy if we don't use them every day. Muscles help to support bony structure as well as offering some protection from trauma and injury, and when we lose muscle tone around the neck, we may be more likely to get degeneration of the joints, suffer strains, and have an injury.

Whiplash, strained muscles, osteo- or rheumatoid arthritis, pinched nerve from a herniated disc or bone spurs, and cervical spondylosis caused by chronic wear are common causes of neck pain. Any sudden onset of severe neck pain or chronic neck pain should, therefore, be seen by your doctor. After eliminating infective or other organic problems, and depending on the cause of the pain, whether from recent trauma or years of wear and tear, structural misalignment, or muscle spasm, the primary care physician may prescribe anti-inflammatory, muscle-relaxant, or pain medication; physiotherapy; a collar; or sometimes alternative therapies like chiropractic, Active Release Technique (ART), massage, cranial sacral therapy, and Feldenkrais technique. Often it takes a combination of therapies and medication to achieve good results. But what about acupuncture; does that offer a good alternative or complementary treatment?

THE SCIENCE BEHIND ACUPUNCTURE FOR NECK PAIN

Some of the first reviews published on research trials of acupuncture for neck pain were quite negative due to the low number of randomized, controlled, high-quality methodology trials. Typical judgment upon studies done at the time is shown in a 1999 review by White and Ernst[1] where they stated that "the hypothesis that acupuncture is efficacious in the treatment of neck pain is not based on the available evidence from sound clinical trials." Since then, more studies have been completed, data gathered, and further analyses and reviews published. So let's have a look and see what recent findings report.

A 2007 Meta-Analysis of Acupuncture for Neck Disorders

Reviewers considered nineteen studies using acupuncture for neck pain. Of these, only ten studies qualified for inclusion; the others were disregarded due to various design difficulties. The overall quality of the following ten studies was rated as four being considered of high quality and six as being acceptable.[2] Since there were differences in each of the studies' methodology, they have been grouped accordingly:

Acupuncture Compared to Sham

Two trials involving a total of 114 patients compared acupuncture to sham acupuncture for mechanical neck disorders. It was concluded that there is moderate evidence that acupuncture treatment is more effective for pain relief than some types of sham therapy.

Acupuncture Compared to Active Treatment (Mobilization or Massage)

Mobilization is a manual therapeutic technique, such as stretching or chiropractic, that fosters movement of the specific tissues and joints associated with the site of pain.

One study compared acupuncture to mobilization using a visual analogue score *immediately after treatment.* (In visual analogue scoring, patients draw a line on a bar between 0, meaning no pain, to 10, excruciating pain, to represent where their level of pain is at the present moment.) No differences between acupuncture and active treatment were shown.

Another study compared acupuncture to mobilization *at short-term follow-up of less than three months* (using visual analogue scores) and showed no difference between treatments.

The third study compared acupuncture to massage and showed that acupuncture was significantly better than massage at short-term follow-up.

One low-quality study looking at subjective improvement at six weeks showed that patients treated with acupuncture reported more improvement than patients treated with traction.

Acupuncture Compared to Inactive Treatment

Inactive treatment involves no therapeutic movement, but rather uses electronic (TENS) or laser acupoint stimulation. Sham treatment would have involved using fake TENS or fake laser.

Two studies looked at pain intensity *immediately after treatment*. One of these, considered less valuable due to the low number of patients, compared acupuncture to sham TENS and showed no difference between the groups. The other study compared two types of acupuncture treatments (Western and Traditional Chinese) to sham laser. There was no difference between the group using direct needling over trigger points (Western approach) and sham laser, but the group using non-local acupuncture, or rather, distal points away from the area of pain (Traditional Chinese approach), showed significant improvement over the sham laser.

Another trial of thirty-six patients showed acupuncture was more effective for pain relief than inactive treatment.

Three studies looked at pain intensity *at short-term follow-up*. Two studies comparing acupuncture to sham TENS and to sham laser did not show a difference. However, re-analysis by Vickers, using regression analysis and adjusting for baseline pain, showed that acupuncture resulted in a greater reduction in pain (9.4 points) over sham laser. One study comparing acupuncture to sham electro-acupuncture stimulation yielded positive results in favor of acupuncture at one-week follow-up, but the results were not sustained at the eight-week follow-up. Meta-analysis of these three studies found the results favored acupuncture.

Acupuncture versus Wait-List Controls

Based on the studies that also used a wait-list control group, there is evidence *at short-term follow-up* that acupuncture is more effective for pain relief than wait-list control.

The authors of this Cochrane review concluded that acupuncture was an effective treatment for neck pain but recommended a need for acupuncture trials with adequate sample size that address the long-term efficacy or effectiveness of acupuncture compared with sham acupuncture.

Acupuncture for Chronic Uncomplicated Neck Pain

In 2006, a single-blind prospective study randomly assigned 123 patients diagnosed with chronic, uncomplicated neck pain. Uncomplicated means that no other problems, such as loss of function, were presenting, only pain. The treatment with acupuncture was compared with TENS-placebo, applied over five sessions in three weeks. The primary endpoint was the change in maximum pain intensity related to motion of the neck, one week after the final treatment. There was significant improvement in pain among the acupuncture group, and the improvements in quality of life, active neck mobility, and reduced rescue medication were clinically and statistically significant. The authors felt that acupuncture presents a safety profile making it suitable for routine use in clinical practice.[3]

Acupuncture for Chronic Neck Pain

In a 2006 trial involving 14,161 patients with chronic neck pain (duration greater than six months), patients in the acupuncture group received up to fifteen acupuncture sessions over three months. Patients who did not consent to randomization (agreement to double-blind condition) received the acupuncture treatment. Of 14,161 patients 10,395 did not consent to randomization, so all of these received acupuncture treatment. Of the remaining 3,766 volunteers, 1,880 were randomized to acupuncture and 1,886 to a control of routine care alone. All subjects were allowed to receive usual medical care in addition to study treatment. Result: Treatment with acupuncture added to routine care was associated with improvements in neck pain and disability compared to treatment with routine care alone.[4]

Cost Effectiveness of Acupuncture

In another 2006 study, 3,451 patients were randomized to acupuncture or to routine care, and a cost-benefit analysis was made. As defined by the World Health Organization (WHO), international Cost-effectiveness Threshold Values are based upon interventions and programs that *maximize health for the available resources*. Acupuncture treatment was associated with significantly higher patient costs over the study duration (three months) compared to routine care, but the authors concluded that, according to international Cost-effectiveness Threshold Values, acupuncture is a cost-effective treatment strategy in patients with chronic neck pain.[5]

ANECDOTAL—A DOCTOR'S EXPERIENCE OF ACUPUNCTURE

Judy was a sixty-year-old psychotherapist who came to my office seeking help with a painful, stiff neck, along with pins and needles running down her right arm into her right hand. The disability had been progressing for many months and was not getting better. An X-ray showed she had degenerative disc disease in her cervical spine and there was evidence that a nerve, which radiated down her right arm, was maybe being pinched as it exited her cervical spine. I began doing acupuncture once a week, and in about one month, her pain, stiffness, and pins and needles were much improved. Two months later her symptoms had completely gone away.

The acupuncture seemed to have helped her problem. It is important to remember that you still need to get at the cause of the condition (improving posture, neck exercises, dealing with stress) to prevent reoccurrence.

CONCLUSION

Although the research is far from adequate, the next time somebody calls you a pain in the neck, tell them to go get acupuncture and to stop needling you.

CHAPTER 17
ACUPUNCTURE FOR HEADACHE

Have you ever looked upon the face and head of Medusa? In Greek mythology, she was one of three daughters of the gods, and her beauty gave rise to a jealous curse that left her hideously ugly, with snakes replacing her beautiful hair. Medusa's expression is fraught with pain while dozens of writhing serpents emerge from and surround her skull. Each time I see it, I am reminded of the nature of headaches. An enigma for centuries, the debilitating, chronic headache has been the subject of art, literature, and medicine since man's earliest days. Studied and lectured upon, categorized, named, and even inspiration for headache-themed blogs and self-help support groups, headaches are suffered by most people at some time in their life. Just to broach the subject and limit discussion to one chapter is a task that could leave any author, let alone a doctor, with a headache. So let us not tarry, but get on with the job. Let us look at the serpents of symptoms in poor Medusa's hair.

Headache is a common problem that manifests with a surprising variety of symptoms and guises. It can feel like pressure, as if the ears are full, or a stabbing pain behind the eye; it can be one-sided or crawl up the back of the skull. A headache can affect the face and cheekbones and get worse with movement, or it can irritate the sufferer so much that he cannot sit still and feels compelled to pace. Words to describe the pain range from squeezing, throbbing, pulsing, and pounding to a dull ache. Headaches may appear upon waking or sometimes after exercise or eating, and they might be accompanied by nausea and sensitivity to light.

Usually the main focus of treatment is to find the cause and eliminate the causal factors. It helps to determine the cause if we first categorize headaches by the range of symptoms, for one type of headache, such as migraine, may be correlated with food sensitivities, and another, such as sinus, with bacterial infection.

After identifying which type of headache the symptoms point to, your doctor will take a full history, do a general examination, blood workup, and may even do diagnostic imaging to rule out rare conditions such as aneurysm, meningitis, brain tumor, metabolic problem, hypertension, and subdural hemorrhage. Most of the time headaches have no organic component and no cause is found. Treatment will depend upon which group of symptoms you are dealing with. Doctors look for the cause on a physical, environmental, emotional, and social level.

Certain foods and improper eating habits can contribute to headaches. By keeping a detailed record of the food you eat, you can correlate it with headache patterns and frequency. Sometimes what triggers the headaches will become clear, and changing your diet and eating behavior may help to eliminate the problem. Rebound headaches can happen as a result of taking NSAIDs such as acetaminophen or ibuprofen or other pain medication on a regular basis. Whenever you stop taking the medication, a withdrawal headache can result, motivating you to take more medication and so on. Breaking this cycle may solve the problem.

Headaches are occasionally caused by environmental factors. You may be sensitive to cigarette smoke, perfumes, gas fumes, or formaldehyde. If a headache goes away when you distance yourself from the environment, but comes back when you are exposed to the environment again, identification and elimination of the pollutant may resolve the difficulty.

You might find, on the other hand, that poor posture, temporal mandibular joint dysfunction (jaw clenching), or other muscular tension brings on the headaches. Relief can sometimes be sought by alternative structural approaches such as Alexander Technique, Feldenkrais, therapeutic massage, Active Release Technique (ART), cranial sacral therapy, or biofeedback.

Sometimes headaches are caused by emotional factors. Perhaps you are under pressure from a situation in your life that needs attention, but having ignored it, your body responds with a headache. Social causes such as stress at work, marital difficulties, or family problems can be alleviated with counseling, changes in work, lifestyle, attitudes, and habits. Approaches such as Gestalt therapy, neuro-linguistic programming (NLP), hypnosis, guided imagery, cognitive behavioral therapy, or simply talking therapy can be useful. Sometimes it is necessary to combine a number of these techniques.

Often a headache is a secondary symptom and so treating the primary problem makes the headache disappear. I have seen people with chronic sinusitis who had been prescribed antibiotics over and over again. Martha is a seventy-two-year-old woman with recurrent sinusitis that was accompanied by headaches. I treated her with six sessions of acupuncture and her recurrent sinusitis was relieved along with her headache.

Acupuncture has been used for thousands of years in the treatment of headache. While I have seen some good results, I do not always have success with acupuncture treatment for patients with chronic headache. So let's have a look at the science.

CLINICAL REVIEWS OF ACUPUNCTURE FOR HEADACHES

A Cochrane review chose twenty-six randomized, controlled trials that included a total of 1,151 patients. Sixteen of these trials were conducted among patients with migraine, six among patients with tension-type headache, and four among patients with various other types of headaches. In half of the sixteen trials comparing true and sham (placebo) acupuncture for migraine and tension-type headache patients, true acupuncture was reported to be significantly superior; in four of the sixteen trials, there was a trend in favor of true acupuncture; and in two trials there was no difference between the two interventions. Ten trials comparing acupuncture with other forms of treatment yielded contradictory results. The reviewers concluded that "Overall, the existing evidence supports the value of acupuncture for the treatment of idiopathic headaches. However, the quality and amount of evidence is not fully convincing."[1]

Twenty-seven clinical trials that evaluated the efficacy of acupuncture in the treatment of primary headaches (migraine headache, tension-type headache, and mixed forms) were reviewed in the *Clinical Journal of Pain*. In the majority (twenty-three of the twenty-seven trials), it was concluded that acupuncture offered benefits in the treatment of headaches. However, because of methodological weaknesses of the trials, the authors also called for further good studies before recommendations could be made.[2]

Another review evaluated acupuncture's impact on migraine. Thirteen randomly controlled trials with a total of 1,107 participants were chosen for the study. Seven of the trials were classified as low quality, scoring two or fewer points on a methodology scale. The majority of low-scoring trials displayed positive results favoring acupuncture treatment for migraine. The remaining six studies scored greater than two on the methodology scale, rating them as being of higher quality and less likely to be biased. Two of these high-quality trials showed acupuncture to be effective. Three studies that achieved consistently high scores for reporting acupuncture and methodological quality were theoretically the most reliable studies included. These studies all had negative outcomes.[3]

ADDITIONAL CLINICAL STUDIES

In a randomized, controlled trial of 114 migraine patients, who received eight to fifteen sessions of acupuncture over twenty-four weeks, acupuncture proved to be as effective and safe as metoprolol, a drug used prophylactically to treat migraines. Of all the responders who experienced a 50 percent or more reduction of migraine attacks, 61 percent had been treated with acupuncture and 49 percent treated with metoprolol. Both physicians and patients reported fewer adverse effects in the acupuncture group. Due to missing the recruitment target (480 patients) and the high dropout numbers in the metoprolol group, the authors said the results must be interpreted with caution.[4]

In another study, seventy-four patients with chronic daily headaches were randomized into two groups. One group received medical management; the other group received medical management plus ten acupuncture treatments. After six weeks, the patients who received only medical management did not demonstrate improvement in any of the standardized measures. Patients who received medical management plus acupuncture, however, reported much less suffering from headaches at six weeks.[5]

Vickers et al. found, in a randomized, controlled trial, a notably long-lasting benefit in headache scores in migraine patients. They found that patients treated with acupuncture used less medication, made fewer visits to their doctors, and took fewer days away from work.[6]

Allais et al. in Italy compared acupuncture to flunarizine, a calcium channel blocker used in the prevention of migraine. Treatment was given weekly for two months, then monthly for the next four months. Acupuncture was as effective as flunarizine for pain relief. Acupuncture was more effective in reducing attack frequency after two and four months of treatment and in reducing severity after six months of therapy. Fewer side effects were reported with acupuncture.[7]

In 2005, fifty patients with chronic, tension-type headache were randomly allocated to treatment or placebo groups. Patients in the treatment group received low-energy laser acupuncture three times per week for ten sessions. The placebo group was treated in a similar way except that the output power of the equipment was set to zero. The acupuncture group showed significant improvement in headache intensity, median duration of attacks, and median number of days per month with headache compared to controls.[8]

Finally, in another 2005 study, 302 patients with migraine headaches were treated with acupuncture, sham acupuncture, or served as a waiting-list control. Acupuncture and sham acupuncture consisted of twelve sessions per patient over a period of eight weeks. Acupuncture was no more effective than sham acupuncture in reducing migraine headaches, but both interventions were more effective than a waiting-list control.[9]

CONCLUSION

In summary I think that the evidence for acupuncture and headaches in general is mixed. A trial of acupuncture may be indicated if you are suffering from debilitating headaches. Remember to seek medical advice to rule out serious causes of headache before searching out alternatives. Always address the underlying cause of the headache as well.

SECTION III: PHYSICAL THERAPIES

Many alternative and complementary therapies involve treatments that enter the body, such as herbs, homeopathy, vitamins or mineral supplements, and even needles, as in the case of acupuncture. But alternative medicine can be sought using other forms of treatment that work on the body from the outside. Of these, physical therapies play an important role. Increasingly more of the physical therapeutic methods are recognized and supported by insurance companies, for they can be less costly and sometimes are just as or more effective than pharmaceutical treatment.

Some physical therapies are passive on the part of the patient and may be considered relaxing and quite pleasurable, such as massage therapy. Others, such as different forms of exercise, require that the patient play a much more active role, and this may be considered pleasurable or not, depending on the measurement of the patient's couch-potato levels.

In the next few chapters, we will have a look at physical therapies that have been subjected to a modicum of scientific scrutiny by clinical trials, reviews, and meta-analysis.

CHAPTER 18
YOGA FOR BACK PAIN

Jennifer Fink, MD, and Mel Borins, MD

Back pain continues to be one of the most common reasons for physician visits. Betsy is a sixty-year-old secretary who strained her back shoveling snow. Luckily for Betsy, I could assure her that most new-onset, low-back pain settles down in time. But what I would also explain is that only about one in three injuries resolves completely over a twelve-month period. This can be difficult for patients to cope with and challenging for physicians to manage. Pain medication will relieve the pain, but it doesn't fix the injury, and it can cause even more problems ranging from adverse side effects to, in some cases, drug tolerance and addiction.

More than ever before, patients are turning to complementary and alternative medicine as part of the answer for their pain. Betsy's solution, after a few days of rest, was to join a yoga class specifically geared to people who needed gentle exercise to strengthen muscles, increase flexibility, and decrease vulnerability to accidents and injury. Despite the nagging pain in her lower back, she enjoyed getting out and being with other people. Making the commitment to join a class motivated her to practice the exercises at home as well. Considering her pain, was Betsy's choice a good one? Would yoga help to relieve the pain that had settled into her lower back?

Celebrity endorsements and a collective need to spice up the gym routine may have converted yoga into a health-conscious social fad, but what are the roles of yoga as a therapy for medical conditions, and what is the evidence? Yoga has been gaining popularity over the years and is particularly attractive in view of its non-pharmacological nature, minimal side effects, and its internationally accepted regimen for maintaining a healthy body and mind. An estimated 14.9 million Americans practice yoga, and 21 percent of them use it for treating neck and back pain.[1] Despite its greater prevalence of use over other alternative therapies, such as acupuncture and homeopathy, yoga has received less coverage in Western

120 .

medical literature, and only a few studies have been conducted using rigorous methodological approaches. We will have a look at some of those studies, but first, let's answer some basic questions.

WHAT IS YOGA?

Yoga is an ancient practice that began in India an estimated five thousand years ago. The word *yoga* is derived from the Sanskrit word *yuj*, meaning joining or union. The joining or uniting of the mind, body, and spirit is the goal of yoga. Joining, which is accomplished through the breath, requires a flexible and relaxed body and mind, and these are all achievable through the practice of yoga.

There are six major paths or types of yoga: raja (highest form of yoga), karma (selfless action yoga), bhakti (devotional yoga), jnana (knowledge yoga), kundalini (chakra yoga), and hatha (physical yoga). All paths share common elements, but some focus more on postures (asanas) and breathing exercises (pranayamas), whereas others have a greater focus on meditation, spirituality, knowledge, and chanting.

Hatha yoga is the most commonly practiced yoga in North America and Europe. It focuses on the postures and breathing techniques and is a popular practice for achieving fitness, relaxation, and health. Most of the clinical literature on yoga to date has evaluated some form of hatha yoga.

HOW DOES YOGA WORK?

The body is controlled by two systems. The first of these is the central nervous system (CNS), which includes the brain, brain stem, and neurons (nerves are brain cells that bundle and extend their axons into all parts of the body). The second system is called the peripheral nervous system (PNS), which is everything *outside* the brain, brain stem, and neurons. The PNS involves things we consciously control, such as physical movements like walking, and things we don't consciously control, like the functions of heart, lungs, and digestion. These (involuntary) functions fall under a subcategory of the PNS called the autonomic nervous system (ANS).

Autonomic functions are also divided into two systems or states of being: the parasympathetic, nicknamed "rest and digest," and the sympathetic, nicknamed "fight or flight."

When your body is controlled by the sympathetic system, you are in a stress-reaction mode. It wakes you up, increases heart rate and breathing, and pumps blood to your muscles so they can run or fight. This is important when you are in danger, but your body needs to rely on this system as an emergency survival mechanism, not a daily maintenance plan. When you are no longer under threat, your body returns to a state controlled by the parasympathetic system. Your heart rate and breathing slow down, muscles relax, and blood is free to travel to reproductive organs, the immune system, the endocrine (glands and hormones) system, and the digestive organs. Your body is now able to turn nutrients into stored energy and has time to heal damage that accumulated during its daily battles. Ideally our body needs to maintain a healthy balance between these two states.

As humans evolved into modern society, we no longer had to fight beasts of prey or hunt with arrows. Instead we became challenged with deadlines, bills to pay, driving kids to school, responding to an increasing number of attention grabbers like phone calls, texts, and e-mails, and playing warlike video games. While these demands are not life-threatening, they often fool our bodies into thinking we are under threat. When living under constant stress, the sympathetic system releases fight or flight chemicals into our body and doesn't stop doing so until we relax. Some physicians believe that these excess stress chemicals can cause inflammation, higher blood sugar, weight gain, lack of sleep, pain, and many other adverse effects.

According to a 2006 study,[2] scientists believe that the effects of yoga on health and relaxation can be explained by an alteration of autonomic function, reducing sympathetic tone (fight or flight response) and activating antagonistic neuromuscular systems (rest and digest response). This belief is consistent with the findings that heart rate, respiratory rate, and energy expenditure decrease with yoga. Basically, yoga appears to disperse the excess stress chemicals through breath and movement, and stabilizes the body's state of being, bringing it under the more relaxed and rejuvenating parasympathetic system.

Some scientists believe that when our body is under the control of the parasympathetic system, rejuvenation and strengthening of muscle tissue and tendons can happen, along with the healing of injuries and reduction of inflammation. If yoga encourages this state of being, can we presume that it will also reduce pain? Let's have a look at the science.

THE EVIDENCE ON YOGA FOR BACK PAIN

A randomized, controlled trial in 2005[3] compared the effects of Iyengar yoga therapy on chronic back pain to self-care education for a period of sixteen weeks. Iyengar is a form of hatha yoga with an emphasis on structural alignment and the use of props. Results: The yoga therapy intervention was associated with a significant reduction in self-reported disability and pain, and a reduced use of pain medication compared to the group in the educational program. These significant reductions were maintained at the three-month follow-up. One of the limitations of this study was a small sample size of only forty-four patients.

Comparing Yoga with Conventional Exercise for Treatment of Back Pain

In 2005, Sherman et al.[4] conducted a randomized, controlled trial with 101 adults to determine whether a twelve-week yoga program is more effective than conventional therapeutic exercise. The control group had no exercise regimen but read a self-care book for patients with chronic low-back pain. Results: Back-related function in the yoga group was found to be superior to reading the book and conventional exercise at twelve weeks. Pain symptoms decreased in all treatment groups during the twelve-week intervention period. However, between weeks twelve and twenty-six, only the yoga group continued to have an improvement in symptoms, whereas participants in the exercise and book groups experienced worsening symptoms.

In 2011, a further trial by Sherman et al.[5] divided 228 adults with chronic low-back pain into three groups. Ninety-two were assigned to twelve weeks of yoga classes, and ninety-one were assigned to twelve weeks of conventional stretching exercises. Although the specific exercises differed between the two classes, most of the class time was spent performing exercises designed to stretch and strengthen back and leg muscles (roughly forty-five to fifty minutes for yoga versus sixty to sixty-five minutes for stretching). The control group consisted of forty-five people who received a book about self-care of the back. Results: Compared to self-care, both yoga and stretching participants were significantly more likely to rate their back pain as better, much better, or completely gone at all follow-up times (six, twelve, and twenty-six weeks). The researchers found that physical activity involving stretching, regardless of whether it is achieved using yoga or more conventional exercises, has moderate benefits in individuals with moderately impairing low-back pain.

CONCLUSION

There is some evidence that yoga can be a beneficial therapy in low-back pain under the supervision of a qualified instructor. Yoga is safe, easy to learn, and requires very little in the way of equipment. Although exercise is a recognized treatment for back pain, there may be an added therapeutic effect with the use of yoga.

In the past number of years since yoga has become so popular, I have also seen an increase in the number of injuries from yoga. So, like any form of exercise, care must be taken to prevent injuries.

CHAPTER 19
MANIPULATION FOR BACK PAIN

In the introduction to this book, I related the story about my friend Jack who put his back out while we were living on a houseboat in Kashmir, India. The local healer who fixed Jack's back was not a chiropractic doctor, but he did apply some of the basic principles of manipulation used by today's chiropractors. Physical manipulation has been practiced for thousands of years by bone setters and other folk healers, but the formal discipline of chiropractic medicine is relatively new.

Chiropractic medicine was founded by Daniel David Palmer, who began using physical manipulation of the spine as an alternative healing practice in 1895, and he coined the term "chiropractic," which means "done by hand." Of the primary health professions in North America, chiropractic has since grown to become the third largest primary contact profession.

Palmer believed that when small dislocations or "misplacements" of the spine press upon nerves, it causes nerve interference and has the potential to damage the nerve and the tissues and structures served by that nerve. He theorized that nerve impingement results in restricted movement, and pain. Palmer coined these small dislocations vertebral subluxations, sometimes referred to as joint dysfunction. A subluxation is described as a palpable restriction of joint play (lack of motion you can feel with your hand) in a spinal joint. It is associated with surrounding muscle tightness, pain, and tenderness.

Palmer's original method of treatment was simply a matter of manipulating by twisting, levering, or applying force to the spinal vertebrae in order to take pressure off the affected nerves and to realign the spine into its correct functioning position. Manipulation involved moving the articulations (joints) beyond their usual physiological range of movement, but without passing the limit imposed on their anatomical range of movement—in other words, up to the point that the joint was originally designed to move. This manipulation is often done with a single, short, high velocity (quick), but usually low amplitude (gentle) thrust that is executed at the end of a passive movement. Taking the joint into this paraphysiological joint space results in a process called *cavitation*; this is what produces the noise (*snap* or *crunch*) associated with manipulation. This also differentiates the act of manipulation from joint mobilization. The cavitation results from gas being released from the joint's synovial fluid, which is a natural process. Research has shown that manipulation results in relaxation of the surrounding muscles, improvement in range of motion, and reduction of pain. Spinal manipulation usually is not associated with pain during the maneuver.

Chiropractors take a medical history, examine the patient structurally, palpate the spine for any irregularities in the contour of the vertebrae, and sometimes they take X-rays. Chiropractors generally believe that a vertebral subluxation takes place where there is abnormal movement in a spinal joint (stiffness), and often a structural displacement of a vertebra (palpable lump). When the vertebra is out of alignment it may press on a nerve or it may irritate the local ligaments and muscles, which causes the pain syndrome. By quickly stretching the spinal joint, possibly by shifting the vertebra back into place, the pain can be relieved. Chiropractors not only manipulate or mobilize the vertebral column, but also the peripheral joints such as the shoulder, knee, or elbow. Often today's chiropractors incorporate other physical therapies and techniques in their practice such as TENS, ultrasound, Active Release Technique for soft tissues, or application of hot and cold packs to augment the manipulations. Most important, chiropractors may also provide education about healthy posture and lifestyle habits as well as prescribe exercises to help patients self-manage their condition and prevent recurrences. At the same time, medical doctors, osteopaths, and physiotherapists may incorporate manipulation in their treatment practices.

Dr. James Cyriax, a British orthopedic surgeon who taught manipulation to physicians and physiotherapists, believed if one, two, or three manipulations don't help a problem, then there needs to be a reassessment of the proper diagnosis or manipulation will not help this condition.[1]

WHAT THE STUDIES SHOW ABOUT BACK PAIN

In the following studies, two types of pain will be mentioned: acute and chronic. Acute pain is sudden onset, often described as "sharp," and it generally settles down or goes away after a relatively short period of time. Chronic pain is pain that lasts for a long time; it may be weeks, months, or years. Some physicians call pain chronic when it lasts more than three months, while others will say it is chronic after six months or a year.

In 1990, a randomized, controlled trial of 741 patients showed chiropractic to be more effective than hospital outpatient management for the treatment of low-back pain of mechanical origin.[2]

In 2004, a practice-based observational study of 2,870 low-back-pain patients was completed. Patients received either chiropractic or medical care, with follow-up extended from two weeks to forty-eight months after treatment. Results showed better pain scores for most chiropractic patients. Most relief was achieved within three months and sustained for one year. Greatest improvement was seen in acute patients. Leg pain that radiated down to below the knee was an area that showed a particular advantage with chiropractic treatment. Researchers concluded that in an episode of lower back pain, early intervention is suggested in order to reduce intensity and number of days of pain.[3]

One UCLA study of treatments for low-back pain found that patients expressed greater levels of satisfaction with chiropractic care for low-back pain as compared to medical care.[4]

In a randomized, double-blind clinical trial, 192 patients experiencing low-back pain of two to six weeks' duration were randomly allocated to three groups with interventions applied over two weeks. Interventions were either chiropractic adjustments with placebo medicine, muscle relaxant medication with sham adjustments, or placebo medicine with sham adjustments. Only 146 patients completed the study. Results: Pain, disability, and depression decreased significantly, but lumbar flexibility did not change. Chiropractic was more beneficial than placebo in reducing pain and more beneficial than either placebo or muscle relaxants in reducing physician's global impression of severity (GIS).[5]

Because the value of medicinal and popular forms of alternative care for chronic spinal pain syndromes was uncertain, a randomized control trial for chronic spinal pain (minimum thirteen weeks) was conducted in Australia at Townsville General Hospital's spinal pain unit. Between February 1999 and October 2001, 115 patients were assigned one of three treatment modalities: medication, needle acupuncture, or spinal manipulation. For the twenty-three patients who received spinal manipulation, two twenty-minute office visits per week were given over nine weeks or until patients reported no pain or reported they had received acceptable pain relief. Follow-up was at twelve months and thirty-six months. Results: The highest proportion of early (no pain) recovery was found for manipulation (27.3 percent), followed by acupuncture (9.4 percent) and medication (5 percent). Manipulation achieved the best overall results, with improvements of 50 percent on the Oswestry Back Pain Disability Index scale, 38 percent on the Neck Disability Index, 47 percent on the Short-Form-36 Health Survey questionnaire, and 50 percent on the Visual Analogue Scale (VAS) for back pain, 38 percent for lumbar standing flexion, 20 percent for lumbar sitting flexion, 25 percent for cervical sitting flexion, and 18 percent for cervical sitting extension. However, on the VAS for neck pain, acupuncture showed a better result than manipulation (50 percent versus 42 percent). The consistency of the results provides, despite some discussed shortcomings of this study, evidence that in patients with chronic spinal pain, manipulation, if not contraindicated, results in greater short-term improvement than acupuncture or medication. However, the data do not strongly support the use of only manipulation, only acupuncture, or only nonsteroidal anti-inflammatory drugs for the treatment of chronic spinal pain. Researchers concluded that overall, patients who received spinal manipulation resulted in greater short-term and long-term improvement than acupuncture or medication.[6]

Dutch researchers did a meta-analysis of thirty-five randomized trials that compared manipulation with other treatment modalities. In eighteen of the thirty-five studies, spinal manipulation improved outcome studies. Most of the studies were of very poor quality.[7]

Edzard Ernst evaluated the effectiveness of chiropractic and massage therapy for the reduction of any type of pain. Systematic reviews of chiropractic and massage as a means of pain control were located and evaluated. Six systematic reviews were found, four of chiropractic and two of massage therapy. Promising evidence emerged from some of these reviews, but they lacked fully convincing evidence for effectiveness in controlling musculoskeletal or other pain for chiropractic or massage. Dr. Ernst believes that the notion that chiropractic or massage is effective intervention for pain control has not been demonstrated convincingly through rigorous clinical trials.[8]

A Cochrane review looked at twenty Randomly Controlled Trials with a total of 2,674 participants. The authors concluded that spinal manipulative therapy is no more effective in participants with acute low-back pain than inert interventions, sham spinal manipulation, or when added to another intervention, and it also appears to be no better than other recommended therapies. Their evaluation was limited by the small number of studies per comparison.[9]

Many countries include manipulation as a treatment for low-back pain in their national clinical guidelines, including Australia, New Zealand, the Netherlands, the United Kingdom, Europe, Canada, and the United States.[10, 11]

A systemic review of ten published clinical guidelines recommended patient education, with the short-term use of acetaminophen, nonsteroidal anti-inflammatory drugs, or spinal manipulation therapy for acute low-back pain. For chronic low-back pain, the addition of back exercises, behavioral therapy, and short-term opioid analgesics was suggested.[12]

CONTRAINDICATIONS

There are a certain number of medical conditions where I believe manipulation should not be performed:

- Bleeding disorder

- If you are on anticoagulant therapy
- Vertebral artery syndrome (loss of pain, sensitivity or paralysis to the face, difficulty swallowing, and loss of taste are just some of the symptoms typical of this rare, secondary condition)
- An abdominal aorta with extensive atherosclerosis
- A neurological lesion involving the spinal cord
- A vertebra that is weakened by osteoporosis
- The presence of an unrecognized tumor (an abnormality on an X-ray, CT scan, or MRI that has not been clearly diagnosed)
- An acute lumbar disc herniation with defined, progressive neurologic deficit, especially motor weakness
- Cauda equina syndrome (acute loss of nerve function due to compression of the bundle of nerves at the end of the spinal cord)
- Vertebral basilar insufficiency (disruption of blood supply to the back of the brain)
- Metastatic disease from cancer affecting the bone
- Infection in the joint being treated

STROKE AS A RESULT OF MANIPULATION

There has been great controversy over the relationship between neck manipulation and stroke. There are estimates that stroke can result from between 1 in 400,000 to between 3 and 6 per million manipulations.[13, 14] A comprehensive study on this issue showed that stroke in patients with neck pain is no more likely to occur within a week after the patient visits a chiropractor than if they visit a medical doctor instead.[15]

ADVERSE EFFECTS OF MANIPULATION ON HERNIATION

Is there a risk of worsening a herniated disc in the lumbar region or of causing cauda equina syndrome (CES) when using spinal manipulation?

In an attempt to provide a qualitative, systematic review of all relevant case reports, review articles, surveys, and investigations, and to estimate the risk of spinal manipulation causing a severe adverse reaction in a patient presenting with lumbar disc herniation (LDH), prospective and retrospective studies and review papers were graded according to quality, and their results and conclusions tabulated. The calculations from all the data collected for this study showed that the risk of spinal manipulation causing a clinically worsened disk herniation or CES in a patient presenting with LDH was estimated to be less than 1 in 3.7 million. This study also compared estimates of the safety of "medically accepted" treatments for LDH: nonsteroidal anti-inflammatory drugs (NSAIDs) and surgery. They concluded that the apparent safety of spinal manipulation, especially compared to safety of other treatments for LDH, should stimulate its use.[16]

CONCLUSION

Patients who present with an acute history, such as bending over to pick something up and experiencing severe back pain where something still feels out of place, can sometimes be helped with a simple manipulation.[17]

Personally I have chosen not to have spinal manipulation performed on me. However, many of my patients find chiropractic manipulation helpful for their musculoskeletal conditions, and there is scientific support for its effectiveness. Like all other health services, it is important for patients to be comfortable with the techniques that are being utilized as part of their care. Education about one's health condition and recommendations for treatment should be fully explained by one's health provider so that patients can make informed choices about the type of treatment they receive.

CHAPTER 20

MANIPULATION FOR ASTHMA

There can be few things more frightening than the inability to breathe oxygen into your lungs, or even worse, to watch your child anxiously wheeze and gasp for air, as her small chest heaves in a fight just to breathe. Asthma is a chronic disease that affects the airways serving the lungs. The condition becomes extremely uncomfortable when the mucosal lining inside the air passages swells, causing inflammation and narrowing of the passages.

Asthma symptoms can be triggered by allergens such as pet dander and dust, but toxins from secondhand cigarette smoke and forest fires may damage cells in the lungs, actually triggering asthma and other serious problems.[1, 2] Data showing that people with asthma were more likely to come from families where multiple members had the condition, than from families with no history of members having asthma, suggests there may be genetic links.[3]

STUDIES IN MANIPULATION FOR ASTHMA

There has been a suggestion that manipulation may help asthma. Let's look at some of the studies available.

Study One

Ninety-one children ages seven to sixteen, with continuing symptoms of asthma despite receiving usual medical therapy, were randomly assigned to receive either active or simulated chiropractic manipulation for four months. There had to be evidence of vertebral subluxation on palpation, as determined by a single chiropractor on screening. The subjects visited the selected chiropractor three times weekly for four weeks, followed by twice weekly for four weeks, then once a week for eight weeks. Before chiropractic intervention began, each child was tested to obtain a baseline measurement of how much breath they could expel before using a bronchodilator in the morning. This measurement was used to compare against breath expiration (peak expiratory flow) measurements taken after the children had been receiving chiropractic manipulation (or sham manipulation) for two months and again at four months. Except for the treating chiropractor and one investigator, all participants remained fully blinded to treatment assignment throughout the study. Results: There were small increases measured (7 to 12 liters per minute) in peak expiratory flow in the morning and the evening in both treatment groups, with no significant differences between the groups in the degree of change from baseline. Symptoms of asthma and use of *beta*-agonists (bronchodilator drugs) decreased, and the quality of life increased, in both groups, with no significant differences between the groups. There were no significant changes in spirometric measurements (lung volume during ventilation) or airway responsiveness (narrowing of the airway passages). In other words chiropractic manipulation did not help asthma.[4]

Study Two

In a randomized, controlled, four-week crossover trial, thirty-one adults age eighteen to forty-four with chronic asthma requiring bronchodilators or inhaled corticosteroids compared the effects of twice-weekly active chiropractic with simulated treatments. A cross-over trial involved participants being randomized to a sequence of treatments. In the first four weeks, participants received the chiropractic treatment, and at four weeks, the groups crossed over, or rather, switched sides and received four weeks of simulated or sham chiropractic treatment. Results: There were no clinically important or statistically significant differences in subjective (rated by the patient) or objective (measured by the researchers) outcomes between the groups. The ratings of symptom severity (on a visual-analogue scale) decreased by 34 percent for all the subjects, but there was no improvement in lung function.[5]

Previous trials in which there had been evidence of benefit of chiropractic treatment of asthma were inadequately controlled.

Uncontrolled Trials on Manipulation for Asthma

In the Bronfort et al. study, twenty-four asthmatic children were allocated to an active care group and twelve were allocated to a sham group. Each group was given twenty treatments over three months. Results: The active and sham group were dissimilar at baseline in terms of classification and patient-related severity. There was no attempt to make statistical comparisons between the two groups. There was no significant change in lung function, or day or night symptoms. There was improvement in quality of life scores, severity ratings, and overall self-rated improvement, which was maintained at one year. No comparisons were made between the two groups. The authors believed that these changes were unlikely to be the result of spinal manipulative therapy.[6]

In another trial, three patients being treated by conventional pharmacological means had chiropractic manipulation administered to the upper thoracic spine twice a week for a period of six weeks. Objective measurements were collected using a peak flow meter and subjective data using an asthma-specific questionnaire. All three cases resulted in increased subjective and objective measurement parameters.[7]

In a comparison study, nineteen subjects ages two to seventy years of age had improvement in mean peak expiratory flow at baseline and after two, three, five, and eight treatments, whereas eleven control (no chiropractic treatment) subjects, who were not matched for age or for respiratory status, had no change.[8]

In another uncontrolled study of fifteen subjects eight to forty-five years old, participants felt subjectively better after three, five, and seven treatments. Six patients reduced their medication and one stopped taking them entirely, reflecting a 46.67 percent decrease in the subjective need for medication while under chiropractic care, but there were no changes in the FEV1:FVC ratio (measurements of respiratory function).[9]

A systemic review of randomized clinical trials by Ernst reported in *Respiratory Medicine* found three trials that were considered to be of excellent methodological quality and all used sham manipulation as a control. None of the studies showed that real manipulation was more effective than sham manipulation in improving lung function or subjective symptoms.

The author concluded that manipulation was not an effective treatment for asthma.[10]

CONCLUSION

Although there are uncontrolled trials that show spinal manipulation may be helpful for the symptomatic relief of asthma, the randomized assigned controlled trials did not show any difference between sham and manipulation. But it's important to note that both showed improvement over no treatment at all.

There are many possible reasons why sham treatments may provide equally good results as manipulation. Patient education, family support, and the daily use of asthma diaries used in these studies may have been very important. Teaching parents and children how to recognize and rate their asthma symptoms and how to perform peak flow measurements, assess readings, and to use beta2-agonists appropriately increased participants' knowledge and their sense of control. When asthma patients write about stressful life events, it seems to increase pulmonary lung function. It's also possible that the visit to the chiropractor and receiving caring physical contact (even when manipulation was not done) plays an important role in their subjective experience of symptoms.

CHAPTER 21
MASSAGE THERAPY

Massage therapy has been practiced since the beginning of recorded time. There are many different schools of massage including Swedish, Thai, Traditional Chinese Medicine, Shiatsu, and offshoots of massage like cranial sacral therapy.[1] Therapeutic massage has been designed specifically for animals such as horses, dogs, pigs, elephants, dolphins, and even walrus. Perhaps because I'm a doctor and teacher and spend much of my time caring for others, I give massage a high rating on my personal Feel Good Factor scale. I really enjoy the magic of a therapeutic, thumb-deep body massage.

Have you ever sat at your desk and realized your shoulders were throbbing or stood at a grocery counter and your back began to ache? Wouldn't it have been wonderful to stop whatever you were doing and have someone rub that tension away? Just for a moment, try a little experiment of your own. Close your eyes and take a stroll through the various parts of your body. See if you can find a place of tension. Have you found it? Good. Now, close your eyes again and take a minute or two to imagine someone pouring drops of warm oil on the tense area, and rubbing the oil in with deep, firm strokes that are smooth and warm. Did your body relax at just the thought of that touch?

The largest organ of the body is the skin, and it contains a surprising number and variety of receptors. These nerve receptors collect essential information and send it directly to our brain, telling it about temperature, movement, pressure, and many other things important to our comfort, health, development, and survival.

Visits to massage therapists are increasing. A 1998 national US survey of patients who reported back or neck pain in the last twelve months revealed that 37 percent had seen a conventional medicine provider, whereas 54 percent had used complementary therapies to treat their condition. Fourteen percent had visited a massage therapist, and of those, 65 percent had found massage "very helpful" as opposed to only 27 percent who rated conventional medicine providers as "very helpful."[2]

Anyone who has experienced therapeutic massage knows it feels good, but is there any scientific proof that massage is helpful for medical conditions?

THE SCIENCE BEHIND MASSAGE THERAPY

Researcher Tiffany Field, believing that massage therapy generally facilitates growth and relieves pain, conducted a series of massage therapy trials that focused on a variety of conditions that might benefit from therapeutic massage techniques using deep-tissue manipulation designed to stimulate pressure receptors. In her published review of these trials,[3] she also included data from the literature of other studies that met the criteria of adequate sample size and random assignment to control, treatment, or attention control groups. Her studies included both children and adults. Unless otherwise specified, adults received eight thirty-minute sessions over four weeks (two per week) that were given by a professional therapist or trained partner, and children were treated by their parents every night over thirty days for fifteen minutes. The following results were recorded from her review:

- When parents were taught to massage their infants it seemed that parents had less anxiety and reduced stress.

- Pregnant woman who were massaged versus receiving relaxation therapy reported lowered anxiety and depression, less pain, and fewer obstetrical and postnatal complications.

- When significant others were taught to massage their pregnant partners during childbirth, the massaged women had lower anxiety and depression, less need for medication, less postpartum depression, and fewer days in hospital compared to women who received standard breathing coaching.

- Preterm infants who were given a fifteen-minute massage (three times a day for ten days) while still in the incubator gained 47 percent more weight than control group infants and performed better on infant development scores. Similar results were found in cocaine-exposed babies, HIV-exposed babies, and in full-term infants.

- Pain and anxiety were reduced in burn patients undergoing debridement (removal of dead tissue).

- Postoperative patients' perception of pain was significantly reduced.

- In chronic pain conditions of juvenile rheumatoid arthritis, fibromyalgia, migraine, and low-back pain, patients experienced decreased anxiety and pain, less stiffness and fatigue, and less depression.

- Patients with spinal-cord injury and multiple sclerosis reported improvements in mood compared to controls.

- Medical school faculty and staff who received fifteen-minute chair massages during their lunch breaks reported heightened awareness and showed decreased alpha brain wave activity and improved scores on a math computation task.

Field also reviewed studies that showed massage was helpful in post-traumatic stress disorder, ADHD, autism, depression, eating disorders, and chronic fatigue syndrome. Parents were taught to massage their diabetic and asthmatic children daily at bedtime for twenty minutes for one month. Diabetics noted improvements in glucose control, and asthmatics had fewer attacks and significantly improved pulmonary function tests. Field noted decreases in cortisol and catecholamine levels, and she postulated increased parasympathetic activity as an underlying mechanism for changes. Many of the studies quoted had many methodological weaknesses and need to be replicated.

A meta-analysis of massage therapy research looked at thirty-seven studies involving 1,802 subjects under random assignment. After a single massage, a statistically significant reduction of anxiety, blood pressure, and heart rate was recorded. This is consistent with the theory that massage may promote a parasympathetic response. After a course of treatment there was a statistically significant reduction in pain, anxiety, and depression.[4]

One randomly assigned control trial evaluated 122 ICU patients who received massage, massage with 1 percent lavender (*Lavendula vera*) oil, or rest periods. Those patients who received the massage with lavender oil reported a greater improvement in mood. The study was very brief and there were many methodological weaknesses.[5]

Another randomly assigned, controlled trial examined seventy-two hospitalized children and adolescents, half suffering from an adjustment disorder and half with depression. They either received a thirty-minute back massage daily for five days or watched a relaxing video. Those who received the massage had significantly lower depression scores after massage compared with pretreatment values. However, with such a small sample size and short treatment period, the data was insufficient to judge the value of massage for depression.[6]

MASSAGE THERAPY FOR BACK PAIN

Back pain is one of the most common reasons people visit a massage therapist. Subjects with subacute low-back pain were randomly assigned to one of four groups: comprehensive massage therapy, soft-tissue manipulation only, remedial exercise with posture education only, or a placebo of sham laser therapy. Each subject received six treatments within approximately one month. The patients were evaluated at baseline, after treatment, and at a one-month follow-up. The comprehensive massage therapy group had improved function, less-intense pain, and a decrease in the quality of pain. At one-month follow-up, 63 percent of subjects in the comprehensive massage therapy group reported no pain, as compared with 27 percent of the soft-tissue manipulation group, 14 percent of the remedial exercise group, and 0 percent of the sham laser therapy group.[7]

A review of six studies for the treatment of chronic low back pain using Swedish or Thai massage found that both Swedish and Thai massage relieve chronic low back pain by enhancing physical functions, providing pain relief, improving disability and range of motion, improving psychological functions, reducing anxiety, and improving mood.[8]

A Cochrane Collaboration review looked at thirteen randomly assigned studies and concluded that massage might be beneficial for patients with subacute and chronic low-back pain, especially when combined with exercises and education.[9]

Another systemic review looked at nine systemic reviews for the treatment of non-specific low-back pain. The authors concluded that massage may be an effective treatment option when compared to placebo for non-specific low-back pain especially in the short-term.[10]

A panel looked at evidence-based clinical practice guidelines on therapeutic massage for low-back pain and concluded that massage interventions are effective to provide short-term improvement of sub-acute and chronic LBP symptoms and decrease disability at immediate post treatment and short-term relief when massage therapy is combined with therapeutic exercise and education.[11]

MASSAGE THERAPY FOR HEADACHE AND NECK PAIN

Twenty-six migraine sufferers were randomly assigned to a wait-list control group or had two thirty-minute massages per week for five consecutive weeks. The massage therapy patients had fewer distress symptoms, less pain, more headache-free days, fewer sleep disturbances, and an increase in serotonin levels.[12]

A systemic review and meta-analysis of fifteen RCTs showed that massage therapy experienced better immediate effects on pain relief compared with inactive therapies.[13] A Cochrane view was unable to make recommendations with respect to effectiveness for neck pain because of the poor quality of the studies but did say that massage as a stand-alone treatment was found to provide immediate or short-term effectiveness for pain and tenderness.[14]

MASSAGE THERAPY FOR AUTISM

In the *Journal of Clinical Psychiatry*, a review team evaluated six studies that involved the use of massage therapy for children with autism. All of the study results indicated massage may be effective for children with autism. The conclusion of the authors was that limited evidence exists for the effectiveness of massage as a symptomatic treatment of autism. They felt that there was a high risk of bias in many of the studies because there were often no controls. Therefore they felt that firm conclusions cannot be drawn. It is no surprise that they suggest more rigorous randomized clinical trials.[15]

MASSAGE THERAPY FOR DEPRESSION, CANCER, AND FIBROMYALGIA

Seventeen RCTs were of moderate quality and showed that massage therapy had a positive effect on depressed people.[16]

A systemic review of ten trials suggested that massage therapy might relieve anxiety in patients with cancer in the short-term and may have beneficial effects on physical symptoms of cancer such as pain and nausea.[17]

Nine randomized controlled trials involving 404 patients showed that massage therapy with duration ≥ 5 weeks had beneficial immediate effects on improving pain, anxiety, and depression in patients with fibromyalgia.[18]

CONCLUSION

Massage therapy seems to be useful for many medical problems. However, to date most of the research done is of very low quality and there are many different types of massage and a wide range in the quality of massage therapists' skills. The best way to find a massage therapist is most likely through referral by someone who has had successful outcomes or through your primary care physician. Perhaps in the future, massage therapy could be more integrated into routine community care. Certainly more high-quality reproducible research needs to be funded.

CHAPTER 22
EXERCISE FOR DEPRESSION

Until her retirement at age seventy, Marian was a librarian, one of those people who seemed to live a conventional, ordinary life. Ordinary that is, until you asked her about her experiences during World War II. At that point her eyes would glisten and she'd talk about her wartime work as a code-breaker and later, a counter-espionage spy. Every day this tiny, bird-like woman had ridden her bicycle down the winding country lanes of Devon, to secret headquarters where she decoded enemy transmissions. She had a knack for entering a room with such an unobtrusive presence that she was easily overlooked and often ignored. Marian, adept with the intricacies of code-breaking, had mastered several languages and was familiar with European culture and habits that would give away a person's true origin. Her combined skills made her a perfect choice for a spy. On three occasions she went to France specifically to gather information about enemy movement and bring it back to England. Not only did Marian risk her life several times and survive to tell the tale, but she remained physically fit with an active, sharp mind into her late nineties. Never the sort to sit around and watch life pass her by, she wasn't someone you'd normally expect to slip so quickly into clinical depression. But that's exactly what happened in her mid-eighties.

Marian and her dog Pip walked into the village every day, a three-mile journey. They would stop to chat with shopkeepers and friends, buy food for the day, and then walk home again. Marian's neighbor had offered to drive her into town, but Pip hated cars and suffered with travel sickness, so Marian always refused the offer. One day, the neighbor observed Marian walking toward town, but this time she was alone. When questioned, Marian explained that Pip had died. This time she accepted the ride, and for the next few months, the women journeyed together every day by car. Marian began to complain about a lack of appetite, chronic aches and pains, and poor sleep. She couldn't concentrate on anything, not even a good book. She just couldn't lift the melancholy she'd felt since Pip's death. Get another dog, friends suggested, but Marian didn't want to adopt an animal that she probably wouldn't outlive. It didn't seem fair to the dog, she replied. Six months after Pip's passing, Marian had lost so much weight and seemed so unwell, the neighbor became very concerned. She took Marian to the doctor who diagnosed mild to moderate clinical depression and prescribed SSRI antidepressants. When Marian read the list of possible side effects, she refused to take the medication.

Frustrated and worried, Marian's neighbor finally said, "I'm taking you out tomorrow. Don't ask me where we're going; it's a surprise." The next day, the neighbor drove Marian to the county shelter where they were introduced to an older dog desperate for a good home. Despite being perfectly healthy and well mannered, no one had wanted to adopt the dog because they didn't want an animal that might not live more than a couple of years. The women took the dog out for a brisk walk, and Marian was soon laughing for the first time in weeks. It felt good to be out in the fresh air again, she said. When they got back, the woman who ran the shelter said, "If he isn't adopted by Friday, he will be euthanized. We just don't have enough room." Marian's grip on the leash tightened and she wrapped her arm around the dog's shoulder. "There'll be no need for that. I'm taking this one home." The next day, Marian walked to town with her new friend beside her. Her neighbor stopped as usual and offered to drive both Marian and the dog, but Marian refused the ride, saying her dog needed the exercise. Within days, people were coming up to Marian saying how well she looked. It must be the companionship, they said. Marian agreed, but she suspected that walking three miles a day also made a big difference. "I didn't realize how much I missed the physical movement. Even when I'm reluctant to go for the walk, by the time we get home, I'm full of energy. I feel stronger, I'm sleeping better, have my appetite back, and I don't suffer from the aches and pains anymore. The best medicine for me is my dog and his daily walk." The next time Marian visited her doctor, he was delighted to hear her depressive symptoms were gone. The solution to her depression had been as simple as a canine fitness coach.

Jack's depression reflected a completely different background and scenario. Eldest child of an alcoholic single mother, by the age of eight Jack was left routinely to care for his younger siblings and often had to steal to get food for them. At twenty years of age, drugs and alcohol had become Jack's main coping mechanism for dealing with his depression. By the time he reached thirty, the substances no longer worked for him, and desperate to stop the emotional pain, he tried to take his own life with an overdose. The hospital that saved him placed him into a long-term treatment program where he received counseling, group therapy, and antidepressant medication. At four months into the program, Jack relapsed and nearly killed himself again. When he got out of the hospital the second time, Jack's counselor urged him to take up some kind of physical fitness activity. She observed that clients who regularly exercised to the point of sweating and being out of breath had fewer anxiety attacks, better overall mood, and less urge to use the drug of their choice. Jack took up running and a few weeks later joined a kickboxing club. This time, his recovery lasted. When Jack completed his first year of clean sobriety, he thanked his counselor for her suggestion.

Depression is one of the most common problems we treat in clinical practice. Unlike mood fluctuations that result from hormone cycles or situational melancholy, when depression sets in with long-lasting, moderate to severe intensity, it becomes a serious health condition. The person suffers physical, cognitive, psychological, and emotional symptoms that can prevent day-to-day functioning. According to data gathered in 2012 by the World Health Organization, more than 350 million people of all ages across the globe suffer from depression, and the numbers are rising. Especially when it is long-lasting and presents with moderate or severe intensity, depression is a serious health condition. The affected person suffers greatly and functions poorly at work, at school, in social environments, and in the family.[1]

Even though drug therapy and psychotherapy are effective at alleviating symptoms, much depression remains undiagnosed and inadequately treated. Many patients, as in the case of Marian, refuse to take medication. Oftentimes better results are produced when psychotherapy, medication, and other treatment modalities are combined. An exercise routine has proven to be a beneficial treatment addition in many ways.

HOW EXERCISE WORKS FOR DEPRESSION

Exercise may have an effect on mood by releasing the body's own pain-killing and euphoria-producing chemicals (endorphins) and other neurotransmitters that send electrical and chemical signals to the brain, affecting sleep, appetite, alertness, and level of energy. Often exercise is done in groups or with a trainer, and the social contact may be a critical element for improving mood. If exercise is done outdoors, or away from the person's home, the very act of getting out and doing something positive may be therapeutic. Exercise can also act as a diversion for negative thinking and helps to take the patient out of the hopeless, withdrawn, "dark" state of mind.

WHAT IS THE EVIDENCE?

A meta-analysis of eighty studies (regardless of their methodological quality) revealed that exercise decreased depression scores significantly when compared to controls who did not exercise. The antidepressant effect occurred with all types of regular exercise, independent of sex or age, and overall mood increased with the duration of therapy.[2]

A Cochrane review of thirty-seven trials compared exercise to no treatment or another form of treatment. The authors concluded that exercise is moderately more effective than a control intervention for reducing symptoms of depression. When they analyzed the trials, those studies that were of the highest quality showed that the impact of exercise was less on relieving the symptoms of depression. Exercise was no more effective than psychological or pharmacological therapies for depression.[3]

Another meta-analysis looked at seventy-two potentially relevant studies. Of these, only fourteen studies fulfilled the inclusion criteria for their analysis. Unfortunately, the fourteen studies had important methodological weaknesses: Only three trials adequately concealed randomization to groups; intention-to-treat analysis (where none of the patients are excluded and all patients are analyzed according to randomization) was undertaken in only two of the trials; and assessment of outcome was blinded in only one. Results: When the exercise treatment groups were compared with no treatment, exercise significantly reduced symptoms of depression. The size of the effect was significantly greater in trials that had shorter follow-up times. The authors concluded, however, that they could not determine from these poorly designed trials the effectiveness of exercise in reducing symptoms of depression. They stated that there was a lack of good-quality research available with data gathered from clinical populations that included adequate patient follow-up.[4]

Martinsen and Stephens identified eight experimental exercise-intervention trials in clinically depressed patients. They found that exercise was associated with reductions in depression scores in all of the studies.[5]

One hundred fifty-six adult volunteers with major depressive disorder were randomly assigned to one of three groups: aerobic exercise, sertra-line therapy (a SSRI antidepressant prescription drug), or a combination of exercise and sertraline over a four-month period. At the completion of the four months, patients in all three groups exhibited significant improvement; the proportion of participants whose depression went into remission was comparable across the three treatment conditions. After ten months, however, remitted subjects in the exercise group had significantly lower depression relapse rates than subjects in the medication group. Exercising on one's own during the follow-up period was associated with a reduced probability of depression diagnosis at the end of that period. These findings suggest that perhaps in the long term, exercise as a therapy may have a better chance of reducing or eliminating depression symptoms, and the people who motivate themselves to continue with an exercise practice are more likely to get respite from depressive symptoms.[6]

It is often difficult to treat elderly patients who are depressed. Regular physical exercise in the elderly is associated with decreased depressive scores. In one study those moderately depressed elderly subjects who were randomly allocated to walking exercises showed a significant decrease in depression compared to controls at six weeks.[7]

Another study examined thirty-two elderly depressed patients in a twenty-week, randomized, controlled trial, with follow-up at twenty-six months. Exercisers engaged in ten weeks of supervised weight-lifting exercise followed by ten weeks of unsupervised exercise, whereas controls attended lectures for ten weeks. Depression was significantly reduced at both twenty weeks and twenty-six months for the patients who exercised, versus the controls who showed no significant change. At the twenty-six-month follow-up, 33 percent of the exercisers were still regularly weight lifting, versus 0 percent of controls.[8]

Many people in northern climates suffer from seasonal affective disorder. A randomized controlled trial on 120 indoor employees in southern Finland was done. The subjects were allocated to supervised fitness training under bright (2,500–4,000 lx) or ordinary (400–600 lx) light conditions in a gym, two to three times per week for eight weeks, or supervised relaxation training once a week over the same period as active placebo. Fitness training under bright light resulted in greater relief from atypical depressive symptoms, and more vitality than in ordinary room light.[9]

CONCLUSION

There is enough evidence to suggest adding exercise to psychotherapy and drug treatment will help with depression. I highly recommend the book *Spark: The Revolutionary New Science of Exercise and the Brain* if you are interested in the topic.[10] I have found that when patients exercise under supervision such as with a fitness coach or in an exercise class, and have to go out to exercise, the results seem to be better. Depressed patients often find it difficult to adhere to an exercise prescription when feeling apathetic and unmotivated. Committing to a class or regular appointments with a fitness coach helps to provide the impetus they need to get up and go. Even a "work-out buddy" can promote and motivate!

SECTION IV: PSYCHOLOGICAL THERAPIES

When Sigmund Freud, the founder of psychoanalysis, used "talking therapy" to understand and treat patients, it was just the beginning of modern physicians' recognition that resolving conflicts of the mind was a necessary step toward healing the psyche, and often, the body. Early psychologists believed that any kind of trauma or inner conflict (particularly those experienced in infancy and childhood) can result in a psychological injury that then manifests as emotional or developmental problems later in life. Until the initial conflict is resolved, a person may continue to suffer from some level of psychological discomfort, stunting of emotional growth, and even a state of physical disease. Freud's theories and work inspired others to further develop approaches to psychotherapy and establish treatments and interventions based on resolving past trauma and inner conflict.

Until recently, little was known about the exact physiological role that the brain plays in physical, emotional, and mental health. In the last two decades, especially with the use of brain imaging, leaps and bounds have been made in our understanding of how the brain works at cellular and global levels and how we can utilize this knowledge to help us heal. Learning which structures of the brain are involved with memory, learning, sensory perception, language, stress, and emotions, and how they all interconnect and influence each other, are some of the developments that modern medicine has been able to use to great advantage, especially when dealing with trauma to the brain, whether that trauma was physical, psychological, or both.

What we now know is that everything we experience registers in specific regions of the brain and then, through electrical and chemical signals, travels to and affects many other regions. For example, as you prepare to cross a road, the sight of a car coming towards you will register first upon the nerves situated at the back of the eyeball. The message is then sent to the back of the brain—the occipital region (vision), to the frontal cortex (decision making), to the cerebellum (a structure at the rear base of the brain that controls spatial awareness and gross motor movement), and to several other structures in the left and right hemispheres of the cerebral cortex (outer brain). This conference call between brain regions enables us to absorb, perceive, organize, understand, respond to, and resolve whatever stimulus is happening around us.

The nature of our survival is to learn from, understand, and effectively resolve what we experience. When we don't accomplish nature's goal, our brains are designed to repeat the memory (or the behavior) until we reach that understanding and resolution. For example, observe a baby who, with a fluffy ball hanging above him, waves his arms and legs and accidentally makes contact. He stops, entranced with the ball's bouncing swing. Waving his arms and legs again, he soon makes another contact and the ball reacts again. The baby may keep repeating his physical behavior until he understands that he has control over his legs, and when he kicks the ball, he can make the ball dance!

THERAPY FOR POST-TRAUMATIC STRESS INJURY

We hear a lot today about post-traumatic stress disorder (PTSD) in people who cannot return to their normal responsibilities and enjoyment of life as a result of trauma they have experienced, whether they are soldiers returning from war, or people who suffered abuse, tragedy, or a harrowing accident. This is nothing new; only the term we use to identify the condition has changed over the years. In World War I, for example, the term *shell shock* was coined, referring to soldiers who returned from battles in the trenches where months of constant attack by enemy fire and extreme hardship in living conditions had caused them to suffer psychological, as well as physical, injury.

When a person goes through a highly traumatic experience, the brain is flooded with stress chemicals that can, in effect, encapsulate that experience, and hard-wire the experience in the brain. When the person is in a similar environmental, situational, or emotional situation, the brain will crack open the capsule. Physical, mental, and emotional reactions attached to the original trauma flood over the person, often accompanied by a replay of the traumatic scene over and over. This memory is so disturbing, that each time it repeats, the person will physically and emotionally suffer great distress.

In the case of a soldier who witnesses her buddies being blown up by a suicide bomber, or a boy who is severely beaten by gang members while fearing for his life, the revisited scene will affect them with a fear-based, autonomic fight-or-flight physiological response as if it is actually happening. This is one of the major signs of PTSD. Other common symptoms of the disorder are mood swings and depression, loss of short- and/or long-term memory, inability to concentrate, disturbance and irregularity of sleep patterns, physical pain for no apparent reason, panic attacks, loss of self-confidence, feelings of isolation and hopelessness, difficulty with being in public places, and coping with stressful circumstances. Often people with these symptoms will seek prescription medication and then self-medicate with drugs and alcohol, which can easily turn into substance abuse and addiction, and in far too many cases, can even lead to acts of suicide. Whether a person suffered the trauma as an adult or as a child, unless and until it has been identified, acknowledged, and resolved, they may suffer psychological discomfort or disorder and physical conditions or disease. Rather than treat these patients solely with pharmaceuticals to reduce symptoms and regulate mood, we are now aware that psychological treatments can be effective in dealing with the source of the physiological distress. In other words, by treating the heart and mind, the body can respond and heal the disease.

In the next chapters, we will look at three psychological approaches and the scientific research surrounding them.

CHAPTER 23

EYE MOVEMENT DESENSITIZING & REPROCESSING (EMDR) FOR PTSD

EMDR is a relatively new therapy for post-traumatic stress disorder. It is believed that by stimulating both hemispheres of the brain (with eye movement), and connecting old traumatic memories (through visualization of the trauma followed by free association) within a secure and safe environment, people may open the walls that encapsulated the trauma and bring it to some form of resolution. By re-experiencing and processing the old memory under new (safe) conditions, it desensitizes the person at a deep level and gives them an alternative physiological experience that leads to a reduction or elimination of distressful symptoms. Therapists who use this modality claim good results with shorter durations of treatment compared to other approaches.

In EMDR therapy, a patient is asked to think of a place where they feel safe, comfortable, and have a positive sense of self. This becomes a place where they can mentally retreat at any time during or after the intervention. The patient is then asked to visualize the negative memories and emotions of a traumatic event that has been triggering symptoms. These events would have been identified with the therapist in a previous session. Negative images are then brought to the foreground for fifteen to twenty seconds, while at the same time the patient's eyes follow an object that the therapist moves horizontally or vertically. As the patient reflects on the images and emotions, they verbalize other associations they experience during the eye movements. The therapist stops at regular intervals and asks the patient to identify physical and emotional responses and to score their level of discomfort (on a scale of

1 to 10 with 10 being highly disturbed). The procedure is repeated until traumatic memories and emotions are no longer eliciting symptoms and the patient reports their level of disturbance as being in the neighborhood of 0 to 1.

Apparently the eye movements are just one of many useful types of stimulation, and only one component of this complex, integrated treatment. The evidence in support of EMDR is encouraging for this inexpensive, simple therapy. Further research is warranted in larger samples with longer periods of follow-up.

THE SCIENCE BEHIND EMDR

In 2000, Shepherd, Stein, and Milne published a review of sixteen randomized, controlled trials that compared EMDR with alternative psychotherapy treatments, with variants of EMDR, and with delayed treatment groups. Studies were generally small with the mean number of patients at thirty-five, and there was variable quality in methodology. Only five studies reported blinding of outcome assessors to treatment allocation, and in some cases, there was a high loss to follow-up. All but one trial found EMDR to be effective at reducing symptoms up to three months after treatment. Two studies suggested that EMDR is as effective as exposure therapies, and three claim greater effectiveness with EMDR in comparison to relaxation training. While examining specific treatment components, two studies found that treatment with eyes moving was more effective than eyes fixed, while three studies found the two procedures (using eye movement or not using eye movement) to be of equal effectiveness.[1]

A review published in 1999 looked at four rigorously controlled studies of EMDR and reported that 84 to 100 percent of single-trauma victims no longer maintained the post-traumatic stress disorder diagnosis after the equivalent of three ninety-minute sessions.[2]

Another review compared EMDR with a cognitive behavioral therapy variant (trauma treatment protocol, TTP) in the treatment of PTSD, via a controlled clinical study using therapists trained in both procedures.

Researchers' findings showed TTP was both statistically and clinically more effective in reducing pathology related to PTSD, and this superiority was maintained and, in fact, became more evident by three-month follow-up.[3]

A meta-analysis of thirty-four studies examined EMDR with a variety of populations and measures. Process and outcome measures were examined separately. EMDR showed a significant effect when compared with no treatment and with therapies not using exposure to anxiety-provoking stimuli. Post-treatment comparisons also showed an effect with EMDR. There was no significant difference found, however, when EMDR was compared with other exposure techniques.[4]

In a 2011 study conducted in Australia, researchers investigated the effectiveness of eye movement, which is used during EMDR treatment while patients are reprocessing distressfully negative memories. Sixty-two nonclinical participants with negative autobiographical memories were randomly assigned to one of three groups. One group received EMDR treatment without eye movement; the other two groups received treatment that included eye movements of varied or fixed rates of speed. Subjective scores of distress and vividness of memory were recorded at pre-treatment, post-treatment, and at a one-week follow-up. Results: Both groups with eye movement led to greater reductions in distress than the group with no eye movement. The fixed rate of eye movement showed the most significant reductions in distress. Physiological scores based on heart rate, heart rate variability, skin conductance, respiration, and orientation responses all showed significant, positive changes versus the group using no eye movement. Researchers stated their findings indicate that the eye movement component in EMDR is beneficial, and is coupled with distinct physiological changes that may aid in processing negative memories.[5]

In 2007, Bisson and Andrew included thirty-three studies of trauma-focused interventions in a review of randomized controlled trials that followed the guidelines of the Cochrane Collaboration. The authors stated that in the treatment of PTSD there was evidence for EMDR and TFCBT (another trauma-focused individual treatment) being superior to stress management and they were more effective than other therapies.[6]

CONCLUSION

The United States Department of Veterans Affairs and Department of Defense, in their (2010) *Clinical Practice Guideline for Management of Post-Traumatic Stress*, make a strong recommendation that "patients diagnosed with PTSD should be offered one of the evidence-based, trauma-focused psychotherapeutic interventions that include components of exposure and/or cognitive restructuring, or stress inoculation training." EMDR was listed under the "A" category (highest recommendation) for treatment interventions.

CHAPTER 24
MINDFULNESS-BASED STRESS REDUCTION (MBSR)

Mindfulness-based stress reduction (MBSR)[1] is a therapy program that was founded by Jon Kabat-Zinn in 1979 in the Department of Behavioral Medicine at the University of Massachusetts Medical Center. Patients were taught to develop non-judgmental, moment-to-moment awareness of thoughts, feelings, and body sensations through a number of mind-body practices. Many subsequent programs have been modeled on this one, and a number of research studies have shown the approach useful for many divergent conditions.

If you have ever played golf, you might wonder why I even dare to mention the sport in the same chapter that discusses stress reduction. People who attempt to hit the little white ball over hundreds of yards of obstacle-infused fairways, bunkers, water hazards, and putting greens, and try to land it in a hole smaller than the width of their palm, know that golf can be anything but stress-reducing. When the fairway is straight, smooth, and wide as a highway, and the green is sitting there like a pot of gold at the end of the rainbow, why oh why, golfers ask themselves, did they hit the ball into the trees or lose it in the tall grass? Even professional golfers, who drive the ball with practiced form, skill, and distance, can be seen shaking their heads in self-accusatory dismay when the shot they planned doesn't pan out. It's hard not to feel like a failure when your ball lands only twelve inches from the hole, hesitates, rolls in the other direction as if pulled by a magnet, and drops with a soul-destroying plop into the pond. On the other hand, when the ball complies with your wishes, it's tempting to pat yourself on the back and assume you have mastered the game. Oh, you are so clever! Your newly inflated ego and desire to do it again are certain to ruin the next shot. You wanted it too much. Once again, disappointment inspires negative self-judgment and sends you to the dunce corner.

It wasn't until my friend took golf lessons with a sports psychologist that she learned a form of mindfulness practice. "Before I hit the ball," she said, "I visualize where I want it to go; then I relax, breathe, trust my swing, and allow myself to observe what my body is doing at each step of the way. After I hit, regardless of whether the result is fantastic or drastic, the only response I allow myself to say or think is 'that's interesting.' By avoiding self-critical or self-lauding reactions, I eliminate expectation and disappointment, which enables me to be curious about the result and learn from it instead."

My friend claims her golf game has improved, but more important, she feels relaxed and happy throughout the eighteen-hole course, and she no longer berates herself when she gets unexpected results. Instead she is more aware of what her body did to produce those results, and she learns from each experience of hitting the ball. When she consciously practices the same mindful principles in her daily life, she says it reduces stress, improves her general outlook, and enriches everything she does, whether she is working, doing daily chores, or partaking in leisure activities.

MINDFULNESS MEDITATION

Meditation is the intentional self-regulation of attention from moment to moment. Mindfulness is a non-judgmental and non-reactive way of paying attention in the present moment to what is happening within us and around us whether we are meditating or doing something active. It has its roots in Buddhism and yogic traditions. Rather than restricting attention to one focus point, as in Transcendental Meditation, this approach emphasizes detached observation of a constantly changing field of focus points. At first, patients learn to concentrate on one focus point such as the successive inflow and outflow of breaths; then they are trained, over a number of sessions, to expand their field of attention to include all physical and mental events such as body sensations, thoughts, memories, emotions, perceptions, intuitions, and fantasies.

In awareness meditation practice, no event is considered a distraction but simply another object of observation. No mental event is accorded any relative or absolute value or importance in terms of its content (such as the place where the golf ball lands). All thoughts are just noted as they arise and are not judged. The implication is that, when we pay attention without judgment, we see things more clearly and develop a greater understanding of why things are the way they are. The intention is to approach each moment with more calmness, clarity, and wisdom. The patient is taught to respond consciously rather than react automatically to events. Patients learn how to be more mindful of what is occurring in the body, to be less judging, and more accepting of themselves and life's challenges, and to be more compassionate and kind with themselves and others.

WHAT IS THE MINDFULNESS-BASED STRESS REDUCTION (MBSR) PROGRAM?

Usually the program runs for eight to ten weeks in a small group setting. Patients attend once a week for two hours, and usually there is a six-hour intensive meditation retreat held in the sixth week of the program. There is one hour of homework per day, six days a week, to learn and practice the techniques of mindfulness (logging self-observation, readings, and meditation).

Patients are often given audio recordings to help with daily practice. Mindfulness meditation practice includes:

- Doing a "body sweep" or "scan" while being noncritically aware of posture, movement, resistance, spatial orientation, and using periodic suggestions of relaxation and breath awareness;
- Mindfulness of breath, thoughts, emotions, and other perceptions;
- Hatha yoga involving simple stretches and postures;
- Doing eating, walking, and standing mindfulness meditation exercises;
- Reading informative material regarding physiology and coping with stress.

The intention of the program is to teach patients simple techniques that they can continue to practice and utilize in their daily lives after the program is over.

MBSR FOR PAIN

Fifty-one chronic pain patients who had not improved with traditional medical care participated in a ten-week program. Sixty-five percent of patients showed a significant (greater than 33 percent) reduction in pain scores, and half of these patients showed a greater than 50 percent pain-reduction result. There were also significant decreases in medical symptoms reported and reductions in mood disturbances and psychiatric symptomatology.[2]

A similar study also found decreases in drug use for pain-related symptoms and an increase in self-esteem.[3]

MBSR FOR STRESS

Twenty-eight individuals who participated in an eight-week stress-reduction program based on training in mindfulness meditation had significantly greater reductions in overall psychological distress symptoms, an increase in a sense of control in their lives, and higher scores on a measure of spiritual experiences when compared with controls.[4]

Two studies done on medical students showed the program significantly improved the way students handled stress. They had decreased anxiety and depression, increased scores on overall empathy levels, and increased scores on a measure of spiritual experiences after the program.[5]

Fifty-nine adults in an eight-week program showed significant decreases from baseline in: daily hassles (24 percent), psychological distress (44 percent), and medical symptoms (46 percent). These results were maintained at the three-month follow-up compared to control subjects.[6]

MBSR FOR CANCER

Eighty-nine patients with a wide variety of cancer diagnoses, stages of illness, and educational background entered a seven-week mindfulness program of one and a half hours per week. They reported decreasing mood disturbance and stress symptoms for up to six months.[7]

Fifty-nine patients with breast or prostate cancer, after an eight-week MBSR program, showed enhanced quality of life and decreased stress. There were also changes in cancer-related cytokine production (toxic to cells, causing damage to cell structure or growth), and other changes consistent with a shift in immunity towards a more normal state of health profile.[8]

MBSR FOR ANXIETY AND DEPRESSION

A number of studies have shown improvement in depression and anxiety as well as physical symptoms after an MBSR intervention. Mindfulness-based cognitive therapy also reduced the risk of relapse in those patients with a history of three or more previous episodes of depression.

A systemic review and meta-analysis of 47 trials with 3,515 participants demonstrated that mindfulness meditation programs improved anxiety and depression.[9]

MBSR FOR PSORIASIS, ALTERED IMMUNE FUNCTION, AND BRAIN INJURY

Thirty-seven patients with psoriasis, who were about to undergo ultraviolet phototherapy (UVB) or photochemotherapy (PUVA), were randomly assigned to either a mindfulness meditation-based stress reduction intervention, guided by audiotaped instructions during light treatments, or a control condition that consisted of light treatments alone with no taped instructions. Results: Those using the brief audio intervention showed a significant increase in the resolution rate of their psoriatic lesions.[10]

Patients who participated in an MBSR program and afterwards received an influenza vaccine had greater increase in antibody titres compared to wait-list controls. Measurement of their electrical brain activity showed significant increases of activity in the left-side anterior brain, a pattern that is associated with positive mood.[11]

Ten participants with traumatic brain injuries who attended a twelve-week mindfulness-based therapy had improved quality of life scores when other treatments offered no help.[12]

MBSR COMPARED TO RELAXATION TECHNIQUE

In 2007 researchers compared the efficacy of two well-known interventions for psychological distress and anxiety. Eighty-three university students with symptoms of distress were assigned to one of three groups: mindfulness meditation, somatic relaxation techniques, or a no-treatment control. After a brief training session in the mindfulness (MBRS) or relaxation technique, students practiced the intervention treatment over a thirty-day period. Throughout the trial, measurements were taken for positive state of mind and for distractive and ruminative thoughts. Results: Brief training and practice of either mindfulness meditation or somatic relaxation techniques significantly reduced distress and improved mood over the no-treatment control group. Researchers also found that those who learned mindfulness techniques had a larger stress-reduction effect and, unlike the relaxation group, showed a significant decrease in distractive and ruminative thoughts.[13]

MBSR STUDY REVIEWS USING META-ANALYSIS

After combining results of thirty-nine previous studies involving 1,140 patients, researchers concluded that mindfulness therapy was effective for relieving anxiety and improving mood. The treatment seemed to help ease the mental stress of people recovering from cancer and other serious illnesses, but it had the strongest benefits for people diagnosed with mood disorders, including generalized anxiety disorder and recurring depression.[14]

While mindfulness-based stress reduction (MBSR) has been shown to have a significant positive effect on persons suffering from distress due to mental and physical disorders, one group of researchers performed a review and meta-analysis of ten randomized controlled trials that looked at the efficacy of MBSR in healthy people. Results: A nonspecific beneficial effect was shown on stress levels compared to control, both for reducing stress and enhancing spirituality values, including measured increases in empathy and self-compassion. Researchers concluded there is a need for more high-quality trials.[15]

CONCLUSION

Although many of the studies on MBSR had no matched or comparable controls designed into their study, it seems fairly apparent that most people with a variety of conditions can benefit from attending mindfulness-based stress reduction classes. The challenge for them is maintaining motivation to complete the program, do the homework, and continue with the exercises after the program is over. This form of alternative practice is best suited to those who are willing to become actively involved in their own care. Many of my patients have taken MBSR courses and have noticed dramatic improvement in their health. I highly recommend this effective program for improving well-being.

CHAPTER 25

LAUGHTER IS THE JEST MEDICINE

Humor is a powerful tool to improve communication and put people at ease. Victor Borge, the famous comedian, once said, "Laughter is the shortest distance between two people."[1]

Not only is laughter therapeutic, but it can be a way of uniting and uplifting us as human beings. Laughter has been described as a release of tension mediated through the autonomic nervous system.[2] A good belly laugh will relieve pain,[3, 4] boost immunity,[5, 6] and rest the brain.[7]

Humor, when used in a sensitive, caring manner, builds rapport and breaks down barriers of communication. It has even been referred to as the bulletproof vest against the ravages of negative emotions. When you can laugh at a problem, the problem ceases to exist in its original form and becomes more manageable and less threatening. Dr. Joel Goodman, director of the HUMOR Project and pioneer in the area of the therapeutic effects of laughter says, "Laughter can take you from moping, to coping, to hoping."[8]

I remember watching a YouTube video that quickly went viral on the Internet. In it, a female passenger standing inside a commuter train began to laugh. The more she laughed, the more strangers around her noticed. First they smiled, and then, chuckled. The woman's laughter continued to grow and became so infectious that soon most of the people in her end of the train car were laughing too. When the train pulled into the station, a man entered the car and the passengers who stayed on board shared another round of belly-shaking mirth. At first the man looked bemused, and then a little worried. Was something wrong with these people? Maybe his fly was undone. Glancing down, he eliminated that possibility. He moved to the farthest end of the train car, which caused the jolly passengers to break into a fresh round of hilarity. I found it impossible to watch the video without laughing myself. The most intriguing thing to observe was how quickly complete strangers had become united in a sort of laughter conspiracy, as if they were old friends and acquaintances. With the exception of the passenger who started laughing in the first place, none of the gigglers had any idea what they were laughing about. And *that* was really funny![9]

LAUGHTER AS A WEAPON

Unfortunately, humor can also be used to ridicule, degrade, and ostracize people. Derogatory laughter is used in many societies as a method of control; it maintains the status quo of the privileged "in group." These derogatory jokes cause the object of the humor to feel shame, fear, and hurt. Be assured, they are abusive. They are usually about gender, nationality, religion, or ethnic background. People who use ridicule as a form of humor try to increase their own self-esteem by negating those who they perceive as different. It is a way of accentuating differences, stigmatizing, and discriminating against groups or individuals. When you see a person trying to inflate their ego on the backs of others, one good response is: *You don't have to snuff out their candle in order for yours to burn more brightly.*

Children first begin to learn this kind of humor from watching and listening to parents and other adult models. When we teach children to laugh at others who are different, we are setting up barriers and teaching them prejudice. Many studies have shown that children begin to learn prejudice as early as three years old and show acts of discrimination by the time they are five.[10] What we could be teaching children with our own behavior-modeling is that laughter at the expense of other people's feelings is not only degrading, but it helps to create rifts between individuals and nations. This kind of humor also leads to bullying—a serious problem that can end not in laughter, but in acts of suicide or homicide.

Think back over some of the most embarrassing moments in your life. What was so distressing? One of a child's greatest fears is to be laughed at or ridiculed, and this concern carries over into adult life. Many children and adults will avoid interacting with others, entering social situations, or standing up in front of audiences because they fear making fools of themselves or that people might laugh at them. Often with these people, a parent may have repeatedly embarrassed them in public when they were a child.

Sandra, a twenty-seven-year-old nurse, was in a Gestalt therapy group of mine. After many weeks I noticed that she had not participated at all. When I confronted her, she said that she had three older brothers who constantly laughed at her and poked fun at everything she said and did. She grew up very self-conscious and became afraid to talk in public. Not only had this challenged her at school, but it also held her back in many social situations.

Sometimes there are people in our life who put a damper on our humor or our ability to play and have fun. A thirty-three-year-old physiotherapist named Monika was in that same Gestalt therapy group. She wanted to improve her ability to play with her four-year-old son. She felt extremely inhibited and was unable to engage in spontaneous play with him. She grew up in Holland after the war, and her father was a strict, serious man. He suffered greatly during the war and believed life was not for fun. If Monika smiled or laughed he would send her to her room, and sometimes, he even slapped her. She learned that it was not okay to have fun or play. This impacted her ability to play with her son.

As part of her therapy, Monika did an empty-chair technique, which is used in psychodrama and Gestalt. I asked her to imagine that her father was seated in the empty chair and encouraged her to talk to him, expressing all the anger and resentment she had felt toward him during her early years. She screamed and yelled and pounded the floor. After the session was over Monika felt different. She said she felt much lighter and freer and she began to dance around the room. When she came back the next week she reported that, for the first time since he was born, she was able to get down on the floor and play with her son.

A patient of mine who survived the Nazi death camps told me that his sense of humor is what helped him stay alive. He was the only surviving member of his family and he had lost his home and all of his possessions. No matter how terrible things were, there was always a part of him that could see the humor or the absurdity of a situation. They could never take his smile away. As long as he could laugh he felt human. Laughter is a way of "thumbing one's nose" at the inescapable and incomprehensible vagaries of existence and declaring "I choose to rise above this. I choose to meet life head on—excited about the varied possibilities in each day." Laughter is freedom.[11]

You don't have to be Tina Fey or Jerry Seinfeld to bring humor into your life. The first thing that is necessary is a willingness to acknowledge how important laughter and play can be especially when we are sick. George Bernard Shaw said, "Life does not cease being funny when people die, any more than it ceases to be serious when people laugh."[12] When people take anything too seriously they put blinders on, which cause them to miss the important aspects of what is going on around them. They develop "tunnel vision," which limits and distorts their perception of reality.[13]

Tunnel vision can be disastrous for any leader. Historically, jesters or "fools" were valued by the crown because they served criticism disguised as humor. Wit was often the only way a ruling monarch could listen to negative news, consequences of his decrees, or the public's opinion of and reaction to his rule. The entertainment and mirth inspired by his jester's witty comments made deflating, but important, lessons bearable. While a jester who went too far with his critique might be whipped or banished from court, a clever fool could earn the king's special favor, even when delivering news that no one else would have dared to give. In 1340, Philippe VI's jester was asked to bring the devastating news to the French king that the whole of his royal fleet had been destroyed in a battle with the British. Knowing his delivery would affect how the news was received, the wise jester, after relating the unhappy details, said of the English sailors that "they don't even have the guts to jump into the water like our brave French."[14]

Researchers interested in how humor affects learning found that the use of humor by teachers increased student attention; reduced test anxiety; improved critical thinking, literacy skills, and concept learning; and promoted positive classroom climate.[15] Humor stimulates learning. When something is learned with humor it is learned well.

Humor is not necessarily joke-telling; it is a sense of delight and exuberance that life is funny. Alison Crane, a nurse who teaches how to bring laughter into health care settings, says, "You don't have to be a stand-up comic to get your patients to relax, but just have a cheerful, spirited approach and be willing to respond to their humor."[16] Carl Simonton, author of *Getting Well Again*,[17] said that play is essential for health, not elective. He found that play is one of the first things to go when patients get cancer.

The pursuit of happiness is one of the basic precepts of the Declaration of Independence and the men who wrote it were not blind to the importance of a happy countenance. John F. Kennedy was purported to have said, "There are three things which are real: God, human folly, and laughter. The first two are beyond comprehension. So we must do what we can with the third."[18]

There is so much humor in our day-to-day life that when you begin to look at the frailty of the human condition, you can see the funny side in all predicaments. Jeanne Robertson, a comedienne and inspirational speaker for over forty years, looks for the funny things that happen between her and her friends and family every day. Referring to her husband as LB, which is short for "Left Brain," she tells hilariously funny stories about their escapades that everyone can relate to because they're based on the simple things of life, like shopping, camping, and traveling. In the midst of story-telling, Jeanne reminds the audience that we should learn to accept what we can't change, look for the funny side of things, and keep smiling.

Humor can be a way of raising consciousness and getting closer to each other, regardless of language barriers. Years ago the comedian Danny Kaye used humor to communicate across all racial, religious, and cultural communities. His cross-cultural humor didn't need language because his skits centered on the human condition and they were understood across the world. One scene I will never forget was filmed for the *Danny Kaye Show* in 1962. It earned so many laughs from fans that in 1976 NBC included it in their 50th anniversary special. In this particular skit, Danny took Lucille Ball to a Japanese restaurant where they tried to act with their best, culturally sensitive manners. Without a word of dialogue, they played out one of the funniest scenes I have ever watched. Recently I found it on YouTube and laughed just as hard.

CONCLUSION

Frederich Froebel said, "Play is the highest expression of human development in childhood for it, alone, is the free expression of what's in a child's soul."[19] All of those clichés are true: Remember, catch someone laughing and join in. You don't have to be happy to laugh; you are happy because you laugh. What happens to a duck that flies upside down? He's apt to quack up. Laugh and the world laughs with you. Always remember that a smile is your umbrella. It's sugar-free, fat-free, salt-free, and tax-free! When you look in the mirror, if you think you need a facelift, try smiling. Suddenly you will look ten years younger. Your smile is available 24/7, and you don't need a prescription. He who laughs, lasts. There's no assembly required, and you don't need to buy batteries. Smiles are environmentally friendly, and best of all, they are contagious!

Dr. Mel Borins's Laugh Prescription

1. Never make irreversible negative statements about your ability to be funny.
2. Learn one new joke a day, write it down, and practice telling it.
3. Take a two-week break from sadness, violence, and fear. Read, listen, and watch only funny books, movies, and TV shows.
4, If you find someone laughing and it's not putting someone else down or degrading, join in and laugh.
5. Wear a funny article of clothing for tense days.
6. Have a joke area in your home with favorite funny books, CDs, videos, joke collections, funny sayings, etc.
7. Create joy in the workplace—have joke contests, theme days, silly dress-up, or a bulletin board of jokes.
8. When you are sick, that's the time to start paying attention to laughter and play.
9. Stop telling everyone to stop being so silly. Be silly too.
10. Laugh for no reason daily.

SECTION V:
HOMEOPATHIC MEDICINE

Imagine suddenly being thrust upon a throne that you never wanted, one that you inherited only because your brother abdicated from his royal duty as King of England. Now visualize yourself standing at Westminster Palace, in front of thousands who have come to see their king. In a few minutes you will broadcast live a speech that is meant to reassure and encourage the nation. But you suffer from a serious, lifelong disability. Every time you open your mouth to speak it is sheer agony, for you can't get the words out, and when you do, you will stutter disgracefully. These were the circumstances of Queen Elizabeth's father, George VI, beautifully portrayed in the 2010 award-winning film, *The King's Speech*.

What many people don't know is that along with the speech therapy portrayed in the film, King George was also receiving homeopathic treatment. Years later, when the king was so appreciative of another homeopathic treatment that healed a nerve injury, he named his prize-winning racehorse after the remedy: Hypericum. He also granted a royal title to the homeopathic hospital in London, naming it the Royal London Homeopathic Hospital.[1]

Members of the British Royal Family have used homeopathic medicine ever since Queen Adelaide (1792–1849), wife of King William IV, publicly voiced her interest in this "new medicine." Suffering a serious malady that court physicians had not been successful in treating, the queen called for the services of Dr. Johann Stapf, one of the oldest colleagues of Dr. Samuel Hahnemann, father of homeopathy, hoping he might be able to relieve her of the condition. The queen became a great supporter of homeopathy after the treatment cured her.[2] It is said that Queen Elizabeth travels with a box of eleven homeopathic remedies to cure any of her problems.

The United Kingdom now has five homeopathic hospitals integrated into the National Health System, and many British medical practitioners use homeopathy. In 1996 the European Parliament asked the European Commission to examine whether homeopathy is helpful. The commission's Homeopathic Research Group concluded their review with a recommendation that homeopathy be integrated into medical practice. In January 1998 the French Conseil National de l'Ordre des Medecins called for official recognition of homeopathy and inclusion in the undergraduate medical curriculum.

The use of homeopathy in North America has increased more than fivefold since 1990, most of it in the over-the-counter, self-treatment market. Twenty years ago the practice of homeopathy was hardly visible in North America, but now there are schools of homeopathy and remedies are being stocked at health food stores, pharmacies, and even grocery stores.

Several years ago a friend of mine had a dog that suffered from a chronic, itchy skin syndrome called folliculitis. Their vet had been treating it with diet changes, hydrocortisone creams, medicated shampoos, and steroid injections, but while some treatments helped for a short period of time, nothing had cured the problem. The poor animal couldn't stop scratching, and when he did, hair follicles became inflamed and exacerbated the problem. My friend, a skeptic toward alternative medicine, was so desperate to help her dog that when she read about homeopathy being used to treat itchy skin conditions in people, she found a homeopathic practitioner and asked if he could help her dog. He agreed to try and asked her a long list of questions about the dog's personality, eating habits, preferences, and medical history. Finally he gave her a remedy to put in the dog's water. There was no possibility of a placebo effect since the dog could not possibly understand what he was taking or the intended results. Within two days, the dog's itching stopped, and with the exception of one minor episode that she quickly treated with another homeopathic dose, my friend's dog has had no further problems with his skin.

HOMEOPATHY AND THE LAW OF SIMILARS

The "law of similars," originally described by Hippocrates and followed by many ancient physicians, is not a law of nature, but a theory. It states that there is a parallel action between the toxic power of a natural substance and its therapeutic action. In other words, like cures like, or rather, the same thing that causes symptoms of a disease in healthy people will cure the disease in those who are ill. Hippocrates saw that white hellebore, which causes cholera-like diarrhea, could also be used successfully to treat cholera.

Dr. Hahnemann, the father of homeopathy, was a German physician in 1790. After ingesting some cinchona bark (quinine), purported by a Scottish physician to effectively treat malaria, he experienced the same symptoms (fever, shivering, and joint pain) as those suffered by people with malaria. Hahnemann found that when he used very small or infinitesimal doses of the substance, the remedy could be used to treat the disease. Excited with this discovery, Hahnemann began gathering many known plants, animals, and biological substances. He tested them on himself, his family, colleagues, and volunteers, and he recorded the symptoms that resulted. These symptoms were called *provings*. He believed that remedies retained their biological activity if they were serially diluted and shaken between each dilution. A concentrated solution was made: one part of the solution was diluted with 100 parts water to make a 1C dilution. Then one part of that solution was further diluted and shaken with 100 parts water to make 2C dilution. Successive dilutions made a 6C, 30C, or 200C dilution.

In allopathic medicine doctors attempt to oppose, suppress, or cover over symptoms; whereas, in homeopathic medicine, remedies are matched *to* the symptoms. For example, we know that when we peel onions, it causes tearing of the eyes and a profuse runny nose. If a patient presented to his homeopathic doctor with allergy symptoms similar to those experienced when peeling onions, he might be given a diluted remedy of *Allium cepa* (onion). Similarly, if a patient had sunburn and she was red as a beet, dry as a bone, and confused or delirious, then she might be given belladonna in a highly diluted form because ingesting the concentrated belladonna would cause those same symptoms.

HOW HOMEOPATHIC MEDICINES ARE PREPARED

Most homeopathic medications are made from fresh plant, mineral, metal, animal, or biological sources. Tinctures are produced and diluted to varying degrees and then shaken to transfer energized particles from the material into the solution. One part of the original concentrated solution is diluted with nine or ninety-nine parts of water or alcohol. This dilution is then shaken and then further diluted with nine or ninety nine parts of water or alcohol. This diluted solution is then given a potency rating: the 1 in 9 parts solution is called a 1X dilution, and the 1 in 99 parts is considered a 1C dilution. This is again diluted with nine or ninety-nine parts of water or alcohol and vigorously shaken and it then becomes a 2X or 2C dilution. At each stage this solution is further diluted and further shaken, and the more diluted it becomes, apparently the more potent it becomes. The most commonly used dilutions are 6C, 30C, and 200C, with the 200C being the most dilute and considered the most deep acting. Medications are administered in the smallest dosage believed necessary to be effective.

Sometimes the solution is dispensed in little bottles and taken as drops, or the solution is absorbed into powder or pellets the size of a small ball-bearing made from milk sugar (lactose). The patient will take the homeopathic drops in a glass of water or dissolve the small tablets under their tongue. The more dilute the substance becomes, the less of that substance is present in the dilution, so there is little chance of serious side effects in taking homeopathic remedies. The belief is that, as the substance is diluted, energy from the substance—a form of subatomic energy—remains, and that large amounts of energy can be released from very small amounts of matter.

You can imagine, as the solution is diluted further and further, eventually there are no molecules left. How highly dilute solutions work is a mystery, and this has led many doctors to dismiss the whole thing as nothing more than placebo. To further confound things, there are many styles of homeopathic practice. Some classical homeopaths use only one remedy at a time matched to the totality of a patient's symptoms. Homeotherapeutics might use combinations of multiple remedies for certain disease states. These combination remedies can be bought over the counter and are promoted for those do-it-yourself patients who want to reach for an easy fix.

Before making your mind up, let's have a look at the scientific research.

HOMEOPATHY AND NEGATIVE TRIALS

Homeopathy has not been shown to be useful for headaches, migraines,[3] and chronic asthma.[4] Arnica, a popular remedy for trauma and bruising, was not shown to be useful in a review of eight trials.[5] Ernest Ernst, a researcher in the area of complementary medicine, wrote a systematic review of other systematic reviews[6] and believes that there is no evidence that homeopathy is better than placebo. Many physicians believe that several of the positive studies suffer from major drawbacks, and there are claims that there has not been duplication of the successful research.

HOMEOPATHY AND POSITIVE TRIALS

Homeopathy was shown to be useful in randomly assigned, double-blind controlled trials in postoperative ileus (bowel obstruction),[7] in the treatment of influenza-like syndromes,[8] vertigo,[9] acute otitis media (middle ear infection),[10] and for the use of homeopathic remedy *Galphimia glauca* in pollinosis (hay fever).[11]

Jennifer Jacobs et al. reported in *Pediatrics* a statistically significant decrease in duration of diarrhea in the homeopathic treatment group of their trial as compared to the control.[12] Later she pooled the data of three combined studies and found a consistent effect-size difference of 0.66 days.

Taylor et al. reported in the *British Medical Journal* that patients with perennial allergic rhinitis who were given a homeopathic remedy matched to their principal allergen did better than placebo.[13] Furthermore, when patients with hay fever were given a homeopathic preparation of mixed grass pollen, they had better symptom improvement than placebo.[14]

A double-blind, placebo-controlled trial from Harvard found that patients with mild traumatic brain injury who were treated with homeopathy did better than placebo.[15]

Leptospirosis is an infectious disease common in the tropics where the incidence peaks in rainy seasons. The symptoms of this disease are variable and dangerous. Meningitis, pneumonia, hepatitis, nephritis, and other potential complications make the illness difficult to diagnose and treat. Vaccination is an effective option but of reduced effectiveness in emergency situations. In three provinces in Cuba, a homeoprophylactic formulation was prepared from dilutions of four circulating strains of leptospirosis. This formulation was administered orally to 2.3 million persons at high risk in an epidemic in a region affected by natural disasters. After the homeoprophylactic intervention a significant decrease of the disease incidence was observed in the intervention regions. No such changes or results were observed in comparable regions of Cuba that did not get the homeopathic treatments. In the intervention region the incidence of leptospirosis fell below the historic median. This observation was independent of rainfall. The homeoprophylactic approach was associated with a large reduction of disease incidence and control of the epidemic. The authors suggest the use of homeopathy as a feasible tool for epidemic control. Of course they also recommend further research.[16]

Fifty patients with chronic obstructive lung disease who were in an intensive care unit and were breathing spontaneously with continuous positive airway pressure were given a homeopathic dose of potassium dichromate 30C or placebo. The group given the homeopathic remedy twice a day had less tracheal secretions, their breathing tube could be taken out earlier, and their length of stay in the intensive care unit was shorter than the placebo group.[17]

META-ANALYSIS OF HOMEOPATHY

Kleijnen et al. in the *British Medical Journal* (1991) assessed the methodology quality of 107 controlled trials in ninety-six published reports. The results of the meta-analysis showed a positive trend regardless of the quality of the trial or the variety of homeopathy used. Overall, of the 105 trials with interpretable results, 81 trials indicated positive results; whereas, in 24 trials, no positive effects of homeopathy were found. The conclusion of the authors was that there is a legitimate case for further evaluation of homeopathy.[18]

Klaus Linde et al. examined eighty-nine randomly assigned, double-blind, placebo-controlled studies. They found that the positive results were not due to placebo.[19] He later reported on thirty-two trials and found that, in nineteen placebo-controlled trials, individualized homeopathy was significantly more effective than placebo, but when the analysis was restricted to the methodologically best trials, no significant effect was seen.[20]

Another meta-analysis of 118 randomized trials stated there is some evidence that homeopathic treatments are more effective than placebo; however the evidence is low because of low methodological quality of the trials.[21]

Blinded, multi-center research carried out at four centers showed that high dilutions of histamine (10neg thirtieth to 10neg thirty-eighth), similar to homeopathic dilutions, inhibited the degranulation of basophils by acting on H2 receptors. This demonstrated that dilute solutions can perform similar to concentrated substances.[22]

Homeopathy is fairly safe and rarely causes serious side effects. In almost all of the studies the adverse effects were rarely greater than placebo. The remedies themselves are often very inexpensive, but a visit to a homeopath can be costly. The biggest concern is that patients will delay the diagnosis, or treatment, of a treatable medical condition in favor of homeopathy. Some physicians combine homeopathic remedies with modern drugs. It is important to get advice from a licensed health professional that has been officially trained in homeopathy.

One area of worry is in the whole area of immunizations. Some people believe that they can immunize their children with homeopathic medicines and that this will give adequate protection against measles, rubella, polio, and pertussis. There is no proof whatsoever that homeopathic medicine can immunize people against anything, and I strongly recommend that children and adults receive proper immunization, which I believe is safe.

HOMEOPATHIC HEALTH TECHNOLOGY ASSESSMENT

The 2006 Health Technology Assessment (HTA) report on homeopathy was commissioned by Swiss Health Authorities, the Federal Social

Insurance Office (FSIO), within the context of an overall evaluation of Complementary and Alternative Medicines (CAMs). The report was to help the Swiss government to decide if homeopathy should be covered by government sponsored health insurance. It was written by a team of German-speaking academics and edited by G. Bornhöft and F. Matthiessen of Witten/Herdecke University in Germany.

An HTA is an established scientific procedure which, in contrast to the meta-analyses and systematic reviews specified by the Cochrane Collaboration Standards, examines not only the efficacy of a particular intervention, but especially also its "real-world" effectiveness, its appropriateness, safety, and economy. They include material that is normally not taken into consideration, such as observational studies, good case series, and longitudinal cohort studies. This report, amounting to three hundred pages, exhaustively reviews the scientific literature in homeopathy. It summarizes twenty-two reviews, twenty of which show positive results for homeopathy. Four of these showed strong evidence that homeopathy, as a system of medicine, is effective. It also finds strong supporting evidence for the homeopathic treatment of allergies and upper-respiratory-tract infections. In summary, the report concludes there is sufficient evidence for the preclinical effectiveness and the clinical efficacy of homeopathy and for its safety and economy compared with conventional treatment.[23]

Homeopathy is practiced in many countries around the world, and is most popular in Germany, India, Pakistan, France, and Britain. A number of schools are teaching homeopathy to mainly medical doctors. In India there are some hundred thousand practitioners of homeopathy, and one quarter of them are MDs.[24] Many people buy a book, read up about the constellation of their symptoms, and then choose a remedy themselves. Other people may receive homeopathic remedies from a naturopath or other health practitioner who has had some training in the dispensing of medicines. A properly trained homeopath goes through a rigorous training program very similar to medical school, however, in many states there is no recognition or licensing of doctors of homeopathy and the practice is unregulated.

Since the philosophy is totally contrary to modern medical training, most physicians are skeptical and hesitant about trying homeopathic remedies. Perhaps this will change with research of the future and this therapeutic modality will someday be part of a physician's armamentarium.

CHAPTER 26

HOMEOPATHIC OSCILLOCOCCINUM FOR TREATMENT OF FLU

Oscillococcinum is a patented homoeopathic preparation manufactured from wild duck heart and liver, which are said to be reservoirs of influenza viruses. An extract of the liver and heart is prepared, shaken in a test tube, and then poured off. A hydroalcoholic solution is then added to the test tube to dilute the drops remaining on the sides of the glass. This is again shaken and poured off and the process repeated a total of two hundred times. The resulting medicine is so dilute that a typical dose does not contain even a single molecule of the active ingredient. It is commercially available over the counter at health food stores and some pharmacists in North America and is a very popular remedy in France.

RESEARCH ON OSCILLOCOCCINUM

Ferley et al.[1] gave 237 patients Oscillococcinum while 241 received a placebo. Patients recorded their rectal temperature twice a day and the presence or absence of five cardinal symptoms (headache, stiffness, lumbar and articular pain, and shivers) along with cough, runny nose, and fatigue. Recovery was defined as a rectal temperature less than 37.5 degrees C and complete resolution of the five cardinal symptoms. The proportion of cases who recovered within forty-eight hours of treatment was greater among the active drug group than among the placebo group (17.1 percent against 10.3 percent).

A Cochrane review[2] looked at six studies using Oscillococcinum for influenza. Two studies were prophylaxis (prevention) trials involving 327 young to middle-aged adults in Russia, and four were treatment trials with 1,196 teenagers and adults in France and Germany. The standard of trial reporting was considered poor and methodological aspects had unclear risk of bias. While there was no significant difference shown to support the use of Oscillococcinum as preventative treatment, two treatment trials supported its use in symptom relief with a symptom reduction of 7.7 percent more than placebo. The authors concluded that there are insufficient good-quality studies and non-compelling evidence to make any conclusions about Oscillococcinum in the prevention or treatment of influenza and influenza-like symptoms. Further research is warranted but requires large sample sizes.

CONCLUSION

Oscillococcinum is an inexpensive, easy-to-take, and safe remedy. While the poor quality of trials has made it difficult for science to make qualified conclusions, through my own anecdotal experience and from the experience of my patients, I take Oscillococcinum at the first sign of flu symptoms. Jonas et al.[3] suggested that until homeopathy is better understood, physicians should be open-minded about its value and maintain communication with patients who use it. The case of Oscillococcinum is an excellent example of why it is so important to encourage government and companies to fund and put more effort into producing unbiased, independent research with large numbers of volunteers, good design methods, and replication of trials in multiple places.

SECTION VI: NATURAL HEALTH PRODUCTS

It is hard to go anywhere today without seeing another advertisement for some life-enhancing, miracle-working vitamin, mineral, hormone, or other so-called natural health substance. This one will stop weight gain; that one will make you live longer while still enjoying sex. These products are neither food nor drug, but supplements, which means they do not fall under the same regulations for safety, efficacy, or quality. On the label of each supplemental product you will find a disclaimer stating that the product and claims about its benefits have not been evaluated by the Food and Drug Administration, and that the product is not intended to diagnose, cure, or prevent any disease. Notice the missing word here is "treat." Shoppers may treat themselves with anything they choose.

While some supplemental products are new to the market and based on either dubious claims or valid scientific research, others have been around for generations. You may be a member of the baby boomer generation who remembers when the children's multivitamin that we kept forgetting to take was suddenly reformulated in delicious fruit flavors and colored like candy. Suddenly mothers across the nation stopped having to remind their children to "take your vitamins, dear." Instead it became a matter of making sure the kids didn't try to eat too many!

Due to many changes in society and how we live today, important aspects of our diet may be missing. With indoor jobs, lack of physical activity, easy availability of fast food, and many other changes in how we live, such as where we get our food from and what we eat, essential vitamins and minerals that we used to ingest or absorb no longer make their way into our bodies in adequate amounts. Also, as we age, many people's systems become less efficient at breaking down and metabolizing these substances.

As with all health-oriented products, it is important to buy from reputable manufacturers and dealers, for there is no guarantee with supplements that what is stated on the label is what is inside the bottle. Many products have been tested and given seals of approval by consumer organizations, such as the Good Housekeeping Seal of Approval or the Consumer Lab Awards.

In the next few chapters we will have a look at the science for some of the more common supplemental products that have been touted as being beneficial for a variety of health conditions. Because of the nature of these studies, you may find some of these chapters a little challenging to digest. If that is the case, I recommend reading the introductory sections and then skimming farther down, paying attention to the summaries and conclusions. For those of you with physics, biology, and chemistry backgrounds, you will, I hope, appreciate the more detailed information given in the research sections.

CHAPTER 27

VITAMIN D—THE SUNSHINE SUPPLEMENT

The sun is our primary source of vitamin D, a family of vitamins that are vital for bone development and healing. The active form of vitamin D is a hormone called calcitrol, and our bodies use this to absorb the calcium we ingest. To create vitamin D, we must expose our skin to sunlight. Because the atmospheric ozone layer is considerably thinner than it once was, sun exposure comes with increasing risks of skin cancer, and dermatologists strongly advise against any unprotected exposure to the sun. At the same time, many experts say that we need a minimum of 1,000 International Units (IU) of vitamin D every day to remain healthy. Our body creates ten times that amount in thirty minutes when fully exposed to sunlight.

Humans make at least 10,000 units of vitamin D within thirty minutes of full body exposure to the sun.[1] But people often cover exposed parts of their bodies with sunscreen, as recommended by dermatologists, and so they don't always get the exposure they need. In addition, during winter in northern climates, people cannot get the vitamin D exposure they require no matter how long they stay outside.

A number of research studies have suggested that your mortality risk increases the lower your levels of vitamin D.[2, 3, 4] Supplementing elderly people living independently or in institutional care with vitamin D3 seemed to decrease mortality.[5]

VITAMIN D DEFICIENCY

Despite the fact that vitamin D is easy to produce, vitamin D deficiency is much more common than people realize. When I began testing patients in my general practice, a surprising number of people were deficient in this essential vitamin. Although North Americans probably have one of the highest vitamin D intakes in the world, from fortified foods and supplements, a seasonal insufficiency of vitamin D has been reported in adults, adolescents, and children.[6–16] Severe deficiency can lead to rickets, osteoporosis, and other health problems. To help combat deficiency, many jurisdictions, including Canada, put a supplement (usually vitamin D3) into milk.

Vitamin D is particularly important for women who are breastfeeding, the recommended method of infant feeding, because it provides infants with necessary nutrients and immune factors. A study of breastfed infants in Iowa found that vitamin D deficiency, including severe deficiency, was common in breastfeeding infants, even though most breastfed infants are able to synthesize additional vitamin D through routine sunlight exposure. Due to that deficiency, it is recommended that all breastfed infants receive vitamin D supplements.[17]

In 2008, the American Pediatric Association increased its recommended daily allowance for children from 200 IU to 400 IU per day until the age of one. In the absence of exposure to sunlight, many experts say that a minimum of 1,000 IU per day is required for optimum health.

NATURAL VITAMIN D SOURCES

Because of restricted exposure to sun, most people do not receive enough vitamin D. Few foods, other than fatty fish, liver, and egg yolks, are high in the vitamin, so most people need to consider taking a vitamin D supplement either directly or by consuming fortified foods.

Food	IU per serving	% Daily Allowance
Cod liver oil, 1 Tbsp.	1,360	340
Sockeye salmon, 3 oz.	447	112
Mackerel, 3 oz.	388	97
Canned tuna, 3 oz. (drained)	154	39
Liver (beef), 3 oz.	49	12
Yolk of 1 large egg	41	10

Source: Office of Dietary Supplements, U.S. National Institutes of Health. http://ods.od.nih.gov/factsheets/vitamind

VITAMIN D AND DIABETES

There are several reasons why children should be given vitamin D supplements from birth, not the least of which is the vitamin's role in bone development. More recently, it has become clear that the vitamin may also reduce the risk of Type 1 diabetes.

In northern Finland, researchers gave questionnaires to expecting mothers and followed up with them one year later. Of the 10,366 children included in their study, 81 were diagnosed with diabetes. Children who regularly received a recommended daily vitamin D supplement were 80 percent less likely to develop Type 1 diabetes.[18]

While our understanding of diabetes is still developing, Type 1 diabetes is thought to be caused when insulin-producing cells are broken down by the autoimmune system. The causes may be genetic, perhaps a mitochondrial disorder, or they may be environmental. A case-controlled study of 820 patients and 2,335 control subjects in Europe found that vitamin D supplements given to stave off rickets were also preventing the onset of diabetes. The researchers had similar findings in centers from Eastern Europe to Northern Ireland, so no localized environmental factors are likely to have influenced the results. They concluded that vitamin D deficiency in childhood could increase the risk of developing diabetes.[19]

As seen on the table of natural vitamin D sources, cod liver oil is an easy way to get the vitamin, and many of you may recall receiving a daily dose of one teaspoon of cod liver oil as children. Cod liver oil clearly was a good idea, but not just for schoolchildren. Use of vitamin D supplements during the first year of life and maternal use of cod liver oil or vitamin D supplements during pregnancy were associated with a lower incidence of childhood-onset Type 1 diabetes.[20] Another study also showed that by taking cod liver oil or other vitamin D supplements during pregnancy, mothers could lower their children's risk of developing Type 1 diabetes.[21]

VITAMIN D AND FALLS

Just as vitamin D is important for children, so it is for adults, particularly older adults. A review of randomized, double-blind, placebo-controlled trials looked at data from five studies involving 1,237 participants. For ambulatory or institutionalized people who are generally healthy, vitamin D supplements reduced the risk of falls by 20 percent.[22]

In another study, forty-eight elderly women were given 1,000 IU of ergocalciferol (a form of vitamin D2) per day, while another forty-eight received a placebo. All the women were vitamin D deficient at the study's outset. After tracking the study participants for two years, the researchers found that the group given supplements not only had higher vitamin D levels in their blood serum, but they also had 59 percent fewer falls. Given the risk of serious injuries from falls (like hip fracture) such a reduction certainly makes it worth taking a vitamin D supplement. Increases in the relative number and size of type II muscle fibers and improved muscle strength in the vitamin D–treated group were also noted. Hip fractures occurred in four of the forty-eight placebo group members and none in the forty-eight members of the vitamin D2 group during the two-year study period. The researchers concluded that vitamin D may increase muscle strength by improving atrophy of type II muscle fibers, which may in turn lead to decreased falls and hip fractures.[23]

One long-term study found that taking cholecalciferol for two years had a huge positive effect on elderly women in residential care even if they were vitamin D deficient to begin with. While there was no significant effect on men, elderly ambulatory women suffered 46 percent fewer falls after taking supplements. The results were particularly significant for less-active women; their fall rate decreased by 65 percent.[24]

In Australia, 22 percent of women in low-level care and 45 percent of those in high-level care were deemed vitamin D deficient. Even after accounting for all variables, the researchers found that fall risk went down 20 percent when vitamin D levels were doubled, and they concluded that vitamin D levels are a predictor of falls.[25]

In fact, the vitamin is so significant that, of 400 consecutive patients attending a falls clinic and screened for the vitamin, 72 percent were found to be deficient. The researchers suggested that, absent any toxic effects, it would be pragmatic to give a vitamin D supplement to everyone attending a falls clinic.[26]

A systemic review and a Cochrane review both concluded that treating older patients with vitamin D prevented falls.[27, 28]

VITAMIN D AND FRACTURES

When falls do occur, vitamin D again proves to be useful. Another meta-analysis of hip fractures looked at the results of studies involving more than 18,000 people and concluded that taking 700 to 800 IU of vitamin D or cholecalciferol (a form of vitamin D3) reduced the risk of hip and non-vertebral fractures. It also concluded that 400 IU a day is not enough to prevent fractures.[29]

Since vitamin D supplements are directly tied to fewer falls and hip fractures, it is important to regularly monitor your vitamin D levels or take an adequate dose of vitamin D especially when you are getting no sun exposure.

VITAMIN D AND CHRONIC PAIN

There are a number of studies linking chronic pain with low levels of vitamin D. In Switzerland thirty-three female asylum-seekers from other countries who were complaining of chronic pain were evaluated. Of these women, 90 percent were diagnosed with somatization-related diagnoses, which are described as a long history of many physical complaints that start before the age of thirty. Seventy percent of the women wore a partial or complete veil and gloves. The patients received either two doses of 300,000 IU intramuscular cholecalciferol as well as 800 IU of cholecalciferol with 1,000 mg of calcium orally, or the oral treatment only. Results showed that 66.7 percent of the women responded completely to treatment; the remaining patients were considered to be non-responders. After treatment was initiated, the responders' symptoms disappeared completely after 2.84 months.[30]

Another study looked at 150 patients who presented consecutively, between February 2000 and June 2002, with persistent, nonspecific musculoskeletal pain to the Community University Health Care Center, a university-affiliated inner city primary care clinic in Minneapolis, Minnesota. Of the African American, East African, Hispanic, and American Indian patients, 100 percent had deficient levels of vitamin D. Of the total number of patients, 93 percent (140 out of 150) had deficient levels of vitamin D. The authors concluded that all patients with persistent, nonspecific musculoskeletal pain are at high risk for the consequences of unrecognized and untreated severe hypovitaminosis D. This risk extends to those considered at low risk for vitamin D deficiency: non-elderly, nonhousebound, or non-immigrant persons of either sex. Non-immigrant women of childbearing age with such pain appear to be at greatest risk for misdiagnosis or delayed diagnosis. Because osteomalacia is a known cause of persistent, nonspecific musculoskeletal pain, screening all outpatients with such pain for hypovitaminosis D should be standard practice in clinical care.[31]

RECOMMENDATIONS FOR VITAMIN D

Because the risk of toxicity from vitamin D3 is low, supplements are generally a good idea, particularly for breastfed infants, pregnant women, housebound, and elderly patients. Doctors should be measuring 25-hydroxyvitamin D [25(OH)D] levels routinely in housebound and institutionalized patients and supplementing them with vitamin D. Take a minimum of 1,000 IU of vitamin D3 per day and remember to take it with food. Ask your physician for his or her advice about taking more, especially if you are at risk for chronic pain, falls, and osteoporosis. Be sure that you do not have hyperparathyroidism before you take high levels of vitamin D.

The Endocrine Society issued guidelines in 2011 recommending that adults at risk for vitamin deficiency take 1,500 to 2,000 IU/day of vitamin D.

CONCLUSION

Vitamin D contributes to bone development, and can prevent falls and fractures, particularly for elderly women, but may also help to prevent the onset of Type I diabetes and help with chronic pain syndromes when there is a deficiency. There is also some evidence that your risk of dying may be inversely related to your level of vitamin D. Vitamin D deficiency is more common than we may think, especially in those who have little or no exposure to sunlight or have darker skin pigment. Many of my patients are vitamin D deficient. The risk of toxicity is low with cholecalciferol or vitamin D3. So it is smart to check for vitamin D deficiency and, if present, take vitamin D3.

CHAPTER 28

VITAMINS & LUTEIN FOR AGE-RELATED MACULAR DEGENERATION

If you are younger than sixty, when the first signs of age-related macular degeneration often begin to appear, you may think this chapter is of no relevance to you. But just for a moment, imagine you have been told that in twenty years or less you will not be able to drive, read a book, or clearly see the faces of your children and grandchildren. What if there is something you can take now to prevent it? Wouldn't you want to know what this wonderful product was?

WHAT IS AGE-RELATED MACULAR DEGENERATION (AMD)?

Macular degeneration is one of the leading causes of poor vision in North America. While getting older does not always result in poor vision, approximately 170,000 new cases are diagnosed every year in the United States. Many people are not diagnosed until their poor eyesight causes them to see a doctor. The condition is not painful, and it happens over a period of time. Firstly, let's consider the anatomy of the eye. The human eyeball is an amazing orb filled with a transparent gel called vitreous humor. The membrane surrounding this gel is the retina, which lines the sides and back wall of the eyeball. The retina contains rod- and cone-shaped receptors that respond to light waves and send signals along the optic nerve. Encasing the retina are two more layers: first the choroid, a vascular layer of connective tissue that provides oxygen and nourishment through the blood vessels to the retina. Finally, the outer layer, commonly called the white of the eye, is the sclera.

When light enters the front of the eye through the pupil, it penetrates the cornea, lens, and vitreous humor until it strikes the retinal membrane directly at the back of the eye. Here lies a pale yellow, oval-shaped region of the retina called the macula. This tiny structure, only two cells in thickness, has, at its center, an area called the fovea (like the bull's eye zone on a dartboard). Because the largest concentration of photoreceptors is situated there, when light strikes the receptors on the macula, we score! Sharp, clear central vision results. Peripheral vision, on the other hand, happens when light stimulates photoreceptors outside the bull's eye zone of the macula. Because the population of receptors in this area is much less dense, peripheral vision is fuzzier and less color sensitive. Its job is more about picking up shape and movement in the peripheral field than it is about seeing color variance or fine details. We still score, but not as much.

To illustrate how the difference in receptors affects your sight, let's try a little experiment. Look straight ahead for a moment and, without moving your eyes, find an object in your peripheral field of vision. As an example, you might notice a lamp with a white shade. If you then turned your head to look directly at the lamp, you'd see much more detail, such as the ribbed texture of the lampshade material, and you'd realize that the material is not white, but pale beige. Your peripheral sight worked; it just wasn't capable of giving you accurate color and sharply detailed images.

Without bull's eye vision, driving, watching TV, reading, seeing and interpreting facial expressions, and doing things that require central vision—often the activities that enhance and make life meaningful—are difficult or impossible to do. Macular degeneration tends to affect one cell at a time, while the healthy cells continue sending messages to your brain. Macular degeneration often affects both eyes, but the second one may not become involved for many years. For this reason, the awareness of visual degeneration usually creeps up on a person, often without them noticing until a great deal of damage has happened. A regular eye checkup is vitally important, for it may be the eye doctor who is first to recognize the condition.

SYMPTOMS AND DIAGNOSIS OF AMD

- Straight lines, such as telephone poles or lines on a page, appear distorted or wavy.

- Blurry shadows or white-out appear in central field of vision
- Color perception changes or diminishes

When the eye doctor shines a bright light in your eye, he can see the retinal membrane, blood vessels, optic nerve, fovea, and macula. If there is any macular damage, tiny yellowish spots of lipid (fat) deposits called drusen will be visible. In the early stages of age-related macular degeneration (AMD), there are a few small drusen. As AMD progresses, the drusen become more plentiful and then larger, blocking the vision of the affected eye.

Eye tests for this condition may involve looking (with one eye at a time) at a dot that is at the center of a pattern of lines called the Amsler grid. People with AMD will see some distortion on the grid, with parts of lines missing or appearing wavy. A snapshot image of the macula, called optical coherence tomography, may also be taken. Another test, called a fluorescein angiogram, involves dye being injected into a vein in the arm so that pictures of the retinal blood vessels can be taken.

WET OR DRY AMD

There are two types of AMD. Approximately 90 percent of macular degeneration cases are the dry form, where loss of central vision progresses slowly with mild to moderate damage of macular cells, and only rarely, with severe damage. The more severe form of AMD is called the wet form. These degenerative changes may involve fluid or abnormal vessel growth under the macula, which can then cause bleeding and scarring, seriously harming the vision. Only 10 percent of AMD patients have the wet form, and of these, 90 percent experience a severe loss of central vision.

CAUSES OF AMD

While AMD may have hereditary factors, no one specific cause has been identified, other than age and, possibly, head trauma injury.

Annual eye examinations are extremely important, especially after age fifty when many conditions common in older people (heart disease, diabetes, glaucoma, etc.) appear with increasing frequency.

Smoking, high blood pressure, high cholesterol, and obesity have been associated with a higher incidence of AMD. Quitting smoking and resolving other health issues may reduce chances of getting AMD or severity of already-developing AMD.

THE SCIENCE BEHIND TREATING AMD

Although there is some controversy whether vitamins and minerals should be used to treat dry AMD, there is some good evidence to support their use and this is summarized below:

Study One

Ninety patients with age-related macular degeneration were divided into three groups in a randomized, double-blind, placebo-controlled trial. Daily, over twelve months, patients in Group 1 received 10 mg lutein; Group 2 received a broad-spectrum supplement consisting of 10 mg lutein, antioxidants, vitamins, and minerals; and Group 3, a placebo of maltodextrin. Patients in Groups 1 and 2 experienced notable benefits including increase in the mean eye macular pigment optical density of approximately 0.09 log units from baseline, and the Snellen equivalent visual acuity improved by 5.4 letters for Group 1 and by 3.5 letters for Group 2. In addition both groups had an improvement in contrast sensitivity, and there was a net subjective improvement in Amsler grid tests in Group 1 concerning glare. Placebo Group 3 had no improvements.[1]

Study Two

Another follow-up study tracked 77,562 women (Nurses' Health Study) and 40,866 men who were at least fifty years of age (Health Professionals Follow-up Study). All participants had no evidence of AMD or cancer at the beginning of the study. The women were followed for up to eighteen years and the men for up to twelve years. Fruit and vegetable intakes were assessed with a validated semi-quantitative, food-frequency questionnaire (up to five times for women and up to three times for men) during the follow-up. Results: The higher the daily fruit intake, the lower the chance was of developing neovascular AMD. Participants who consumed three or more servings per day of fruits had a significantly less risk of developing AMD compared with those who consumed less than 1.5 servings per day. The results were similar in women and men. Intakes of vegetables, antioxidant vitamins, or carotenoids were not strongly related to either early or neovascular AMD.[2]

Study Three

Thirteen trials, which randomized 6150 people with signs of age-related macular degeneration, are included in this review.[3] The majority of people (3640) were randomized in one trial that found a modest beneficial effect of antioxidant and zinc supplementation on progression to advanced age-related macular degeneration. People who were supplemented with antioxidants and zinc were less likely to lose fifteen or more letters of visual acuity (equivalent to a doubling of the visual angle). This effect was seen more strongly in people with moderate to severe disease. There were few events in people with early signs of the disease. The trial evaluated many safety outcomes, of which hospitalization for genitourinary problems was more common in people taking zinc, and yellowing of skin was more common in people taking antioxidant micronutrients. The other trials in this review were small and the results were inconsistent.

Study Four

In a large Age-Related Eye Disease Study (AREDS), sponsored by the US Federal Government National Eye Institute, 3,640 participants aged fifty-five to eighty years were randomized to four groups. Group 1 received antioxidants (vitamin C, vitamin E, and beta-carotene); Group 2 received minerals (zinc and copper); Group 3 received a combination of antioxidants and minerals; and Group 4 received placebo. Each group contained patients at four different stages of AMD including the following levels: no AMD, early AMD, intermediate AMD, and advanced AMD. Participants were followed for an average of 6.3 years. Result: A significant reduction in the development of advanced AMD was shown in Groups 2 and 3 (taking minerals alone or the antioxidants plus minerals). Those at high risk of developing advanced AMD actually lowered their risk by about

25 percent when treated with mega dosages of the antioxidants and zinc combination.[4] About 7.5 percent of participants assigned to the zinc treatments—compared with 5 percent who did not have zinc in their assigned treatment—had urinary tract problems that required hospitalization. Yellowing of the skin, a well-known side effect of large doses of beta-carotene, was reported slightly more often by participants taking antioxidants. The AREDS formulation did not have an effect on the rate of prostate cancer in men participating in the study.

Study Five

The Ophthalmology Department at the University of Alberta studied the use of dietary supplements in their patients with AMD to determine if recommended doses from the AREDS study (as above) were being achieved. Of the 108 patients surveyed, eighty-five (79 percent) were taking dietary supplements, and seventy-three (68 percent) were taking at least one AREDS ingredient, but the mean dosages of antioxidants and zinc were all below those recommended in the age-related eye disease study. None of their patients met the recommended dosages for all four ingredients. Conclusion: Patients with AMD may not be receiving the dosages of beta-carotene, vitamins C and E, and zinc and copper recommended in the AREDS study. Until new formulations of high-dose antioxidant and mineral supplements are made available, it is important for patients to meet the recommended dosages by combining individual available supplements.[5]

Other Research Findings

There is some evidence that suggests that omega-3 from fish oils or flax seed oils is beneficial at reducing the risk of progress in macular degeneration. Lutein and zeaxanthine are also felt to have a protective effect and may be beneficial.

AREDS RECOMMENDED DOSE

The specific daily amounts of antioxidants and zinc used by the study researchers were:

- 500 mg vitamin C
- 400 IU vitamin E
- 15 mg beta-carotene (often labeled as equivalent to 25,000 IU of vitamin A)
- 80 mg zinc as zinc oxide
- 2 mg copper as cupric oxide

Copper was added to the AREDS formulation containing zinc to prevent copper deficiency anemia, a condition associated with high levels of zinc intake.

CAUTION

Smokers need to take a modified version of the above AREDS formula supplement without added beta-carotene due to a possible increased risk of lung cancer in smokers who take beta-carotene supplements. A Cochrane review[6] examining whether antioxidants reduce mortality has actually found the opposite to be true. Beta-carotene and vitamin E seem to increase mortality. Although there have not been any major adverse effects shown in the AREDS studies, the concerns seem to be mostly about the synthetic form of vitamin E used in cardiovascular disease and prostate cancer research. There is even some concern that vitamin E may increase the risk of prostate cancer and colorectal adenoma.

CONCLUSION

Previous studies have suggested that people who have diets rich in green leafy vegetables have a lower risk of developing AMD. Please understand that the AREDS vitamins and minerals, omega-3, and carotenoids are *not* a cure for AMD. They will not restore vision already lost from the disease, but they may delay the onset of advanced AMD. For people who are at high risk for developing advanced AMD, following the recommended dosage from the AREDS study may help them to keep their vision.

There is no known treatment that can prevent the development of AMD. The study did not show that the AREDS formulation prevented people from developing early signs of AMD. No recommendation has been made for taking the AREDS formulation to prevent early AMD.

These high levels of vitamins and minerals are difficult to achieve from dict alone. In addition, the levels of antioxidants and zinc are considerably higher than the amounts in any daily multivitamin. A multivitamin contains many important vitamins not found in the AREDS formulation. For example, people with osteoporosis need to be particularly concerned about taking vitamin D, which is not in the AREDS formulation. In the Age-Related Eye Disease Study, two-thirds of the study participants took multivitamins along with the AREDS formulation. Before taking these high levels of vitamins and minerals, you should talk with your doctor about the risk of developing advanced AMD and whether taking the AREDS formulation is right for you.

CHAPTER 29

VITAMIN E FOR NON-ALCOHOLIC FATTY LIVER DISEASE

Today, as many as 20 percent of Americans who drink little or no alcohol have accumulated fatty deposits in their liver. This condition is called non-alcoholic fatty liver disease (NAFLD). For many people, no symptoms or complications will occur, but left unchecked, increasing fatty deposits may eventually enlarge the organ, and it could develop into non-alcoholic steatohepatitis (NASH).

WHAT IS NON-ALCOHOLIC STEATOHEPATITIS (NASH)

Up to 5 percent of Americans develop NASH, an inflammation of the fatty liver that causes damage to cells and scar tissue formation (fibrosis). When enough scarring occurs, the liver, no longer soft and pliable, shrinks and then hardens, eventually becoming unable to work. That stage of disease is called cirrhosis of the liver, a serious, permanent condition. Many patients with cirrhosis may live without symptoms of their disease for many years before dying of some competing cause. Cirrhosis is not necessarily fatal, nor does it necessarily cause symptoms. It's only when liver failure develops as a result of cirrhosis that patients experience symptoms.

Because NASH is mostly symptomless in the early stages, the condition is often referred to as a silent disease. While fatigue may be noticeable at any time, patients usually won't develop symptoms, such as weight loss and weakness, until the more advanced stages of NASH or when cirrhosis develops. Often NASH isn't discovered until routine health-monitoring blood tests reveal higher than normal levels of liver metabolizing enzymes alanine aminotransferase (ALT) and aspartate aminotransferase (AST). Abnormal readings can happen as a result of medications, viral hepatitis, or excessive use of alcohol, so further blood tests could be done to eliminate other causes, and ultrasound or other imaging may be ordered to look for fatty deposits in the liver. Finally, NASH can be confirmed by doing a liver biopsy.

OUTLOOK FOR NASH

NASH may progress quickly or slowly over many years; it can also stop developing or reverse without therapeutic intervention. Once serious scarring occurs, however, the condition is non-reversible and very little can be done to stop progression of the disease. According to the United States National Institute of Health, NASH is the third major cause of cirrhosis in America after hepatitis C and alcoholic liver disease. Most disturbing is that the rate of people affected by this condition is steadily increasing and is associated with obesity, the rate of which has doubled in adults and tripled in children over the last ten years.[1]

CAUSE OF NASH

The cause of NASH has not been fully determined. It happens mostly in middle-aged, overweight or obese adults, but it also occurs in normal-weight adults and can happen in children. Association has been noted with diabetes and pre-diabetes, and with elevated blood lipids (fats), and high cholesterol. However, many patients with these conditions do not have NASH, and some NASH patients have healthy weight, blood lipids, and cholesterol readings. Factors that have been identified as possibly having some causative effects are: insulin resistance; release of toxic inflammatory proteins by cytokines (fat cells); and oxidative stress (deterioration) inside liver cells.

TREATMENT FOR NASH

The most important thing to do if you have a fatty liver and are overweight is to lose weight gradually. It is also helpful to avoid unnecessary medications, alcohol, and herbs or supplements known to affect the liver.

Following these recommendations (particularly in the early stage of the disease) may help to slow or even halt progression.

RESEARCH ON VITAMIN E FOR NASH

The antioxidant vitamin E has been shown to inhibit transforming growth factor (TGF)-beta, which is one of the toxic inflammatory proteins involved with liver degeneration. In animal experiments, vitamin E has been shown to protect against liver damage induced by oxidative stress.

Blood tests showing elevated liver enzymes ALT and AST are a sign of liver abnormalities. So when enzymes decrease, it is a sign that the liver may be repairing itself. One randomized, controlled trial showed vitamin E lowered the level of ALT (aminotransferase) measured in the blood of patients suffering from viral hepatitis C.[2]

FOUR TRIAL RESULTS SHOWING VITAMIN E IS USEFUL FOR NASH

Trial 1

Forty-eight patients with elevated liver enzymes (ALT and AST) were randomly assigned to one of three treatment groups. For two years, Group 1 received daily vitamin E (400 IU) plus ursodeoxycholic acid (UDCA; 12–15 mg per kg); Group 2 received UDCA with placebo; and Group 3 received only placebo. Liver biopsies were taken at the beginning and end of the two-year trial period. Patients' body mass index readings remained unchanged during the study. Forty patients completed the whole two-year trial. Results:

- Placebo/Placebo Group—no improvement in ALT or AST liver enzymes or in biopsy tissue.

- UDCA/Placebo Group—only ALT levels improved; no improvement in AST or liver biopsy tissue.

- Vitamin E/UDCA Group—A significant decrease in both ALT and AST liver enzymes was shown. Under the microscope, the activity index of biopsied tissue was improved significantly, mostly as a reduction in fatty cells. The fibrosis also improved.

Conclusion: The combination of Vitamin E with UDCA not only improves the laboratory values (blood enzyme levels), but also the hepatic (inflammation and fat cells) histology.[3]

Trial 2

Twenty non-diabetic, non-cirrhotic subjects with NASH in a randomized prospective trial were given either vitamin E alone (400 IU/day) or vitamin E (400 IU/day) and pioglitazone (30 mg/day). Treatment with vitamin E only produced a significant decrease in fatty changes in the liver. Combination therapy produced a significant decrease in steatosis (fat accumulation), cytologic ballooning (enlarged cells), Mallory's hyaline (reddish filaments found in impaired liver cells), and pericellular fibrosis (chicken-wire appearance of damaged liver cells) showing the liver was improving at a cellular level.[4]

Trial 3

Forty-five patients in a prospective, double-blind, randomized, placebo-controlled trial received either antioxidant vitamins E and C (1,000 IU and 1,000 mg, respectively) or placebo daily for six months, based on their initial biopsied diagnosis of NASH. Additionally, all patients were given standard weight-loss counseling and encouraged to follow a low-fat diet (less than 30 g fat per day). Vitamin treatment resulted in a statistically significant improvement in fibrosis score. No improvement in necroinflammatory activity or ALT was seen with this combination of drug therapy.[5] Since there was improvement of fibrosis in the antioxidant group, the authors concluded that vitamin E and C may be helpful.[6]

Trial 4

Eleven obese children with NASH were given 400 to 1,200 IU of vitamin E daily in an open-label, non-placebo-controlled trial for four to ten months. Their body mass index (BMI) readings did not change significantly during treatment. Blood tests at beginning and end of trials showed a normalization of serum aminotransferase (ALT and AST) and a decrease in alkaline phosphates (ALP—enzymatic symptom of liver damage) levels during treatment. Two children discontinued treatment, and there was elevation of aminotransferase within two months.

THREE TRIAL RESULTS SHOWING VITAMIN E OFFERS NO BENEFIT FOR NASH

Trial 1

Sixteen patients with biopsy-proven NASH were given a Step 1 American Heart Association diet, plus aerobic exercise with or without 800 IU of vitamin E daily. Biochemical assessment of liver function, lipid profiles, and body mass index significantly improved during the first six weeks of therapy and remained stable during the following six weeks. Plasma hyaluronic acid (HA) concentrations and interleukin 6 decreased in parallel with weight loss. Lifestyle modifications (low-fat diet and exercise) were associated with improvement in liver enzymes, cholesterol, and plasma HA levels in patients with NASH, whereas the level of vitamin E supplementation used in this short-term pilot study provided no apparent added benefit.[7]

Trial 2

In an open-label, randomized trial, fifty-five non-diabetic NAFLD patients were given metformin (2 g/day) for twelve months. The control cases were given either vitamin E (800 IU/day) or were treated by a prescriptive, weight-reducing diet. Aminotransferase levels improved in all groups, in association with weight loss. Metformin treatment was better than a prescriptive diet or vitamin E in the therapy of NAFLD patients receiving nutritional counseling.[8]

Trial 3

The MRC/BHF Heart Protection Study and the Women's Angiographic Vitamin and Estrogen Study found that vitamin E did not improve cardiovascular risk for cardiovascular events. In the HOPE and HOPE-TOO trial, vitamin E had been associated with a higher risk of heart failure. A meta-analysis of vitamin E studies found that doses greater than 400 IU were associated with an increase of all-cause mortality. In most of these studies, a synthetic form of vitamin E, dl-alpha-tocopherol, was used as opposed to gamma-tocopherol, the naturally sourced vitamin E. Many researchers believe that the reason vitamin E in these studies was of no benefit was because a synthetic form was used. This may explain why vitamin E from food is more effective than the synthetic form used in previous positive-epidemiological heart protection studies.

CONCLUSION

Regarding the efficacy of vitamin E for NASH, as often happens, research trials differ in their conclusions. This may be due to the quality of the trial design, number and choice of participants, and the use of synthetic (versus natural source) vitamin E. Also the best assessment for degree of impairment is a liver biopsy, and few of the studies used this marker as an assessment for improvement. There has been research expressing concerns about the safety of vitamin E. If you do consider using vitamin E, I would recommend using gamma-tocopherol only and in doses no greater than 400 IU per day. Choose a natural source of vitamin E (labelled as gamma-tocopherol, *not* dl-gamma tocopherol or dl-alpha tocopherol, the synthetic versions). Many physicians feel that there is no reliable evidence for or against vitamin E, and in the absence of evidence of benefit, vitamin E should not be promoted as helping with NAFLD.

It is a good idea to discuss this treatment with your primary care physician in order to make a collaborative and informed decision.

CHAPTER 30
COENZYME Q10 FOR HEALTH

Coenzyme Q10 is a naturally occurring, fat-soluble, antioxidant enzyme manufactured in the body and is found in fish oils, nuts, meat, and vegetables. It was first identified in heart tissue, where it plays a crucial role in energy production and supporting cardiovascular health.

Coenzyme Q10 is an essential element of the mitochondrial electron transport chain. Its main function is the production of adenosine triphosphate. It may also act as an antioxidant preventing lipid peroxidation and is an indirect stabilizer of calcium channels to decrease calcium overload. It also goes under the name of vitamin Q10, CoQ, and ubiquinone. It has become a common ingredient in many vitamin-mineral preparations and its use as a single agent is growing.

COENZYME Q10 FOR MITOCHONDRIAL DEFICIENCY CYTOPATHIES

Although I have never seen a patient with a mitochondrial deficiency disorder, there are a number of studies that show Coenzyme Q10 improved cardiac conduction defects in patients with Kearns-Sayre syndrome, which is an uncommon mitochondrial deficiency disorder. Muscle weakness and fatigue were improved in patients with chronic muscular dystrophies and neurogenic atrophies. There are also trials showing its possible benefit in patients with rare mitochondrial encephalomyopathies.

COENZYME Q10 FOR HEART FAILURE

A randomized, double-blind, placebo-controlled three-month trial of CoQ10 therapy in thirty-five patients with heart failure showed significant improvements in symptoms and a trend towards improvements in exercise time.[1] There are a number of trials that had small sample sizes but showed significant improvement in heart function. In a double-blind, randomized, controlled trial of thirty-nine patients with heart failure, half were given 50 mg of CoQ10 three times a day and the other half placebo. There was a significant improvement in heart function and an increase in exercise tolerance in the Coenzyme Q10 compared to controls.[2] Thirty-eight children with enlarged hearts because of cardiomyopathy (heart muscle disease) were given Coenzyme Q10 or placebo and after six months the children on Coenzyme Q10 showed significant improvement in heart function and heart failure compared to the control group.[3] Although other trials also found improvement in dyspnea and edema, most of the trials were of small number and inadequate methodology.

COENZYME Q10 FOR HYPERTENSION

Forty-six men and thirty-seven women with isolated systolic hypertension were given 60 mg of Coenzyme Q10 twice daily in a randomized, double-blind, placebo-controlled twelve-week trial. The mean reduction in systolic blood pressure of the CoQ10-treated group was 17.8 +/- 7.3mm Hg (mean +/- SEM).[4] Rosenfeldt and his colleagues in Australia reviewed twelve published trials of CoQ10 in hypertension and showed a mean decrease in systolic blood pressure of 17mm Hg and up to 10mm Hg drop in diastolic blood pressure without significant side effects.[5] Even though the studies were small and there were many confounding variables, CoQ10 may prove to have a role as an adjunct to conventional agents in the treatment of hypertension.

COENZYME Q10 FOR CARDIAC SURGERY AND HEART ATTACKS

Patients undergoing elective cardiac surgery were randomized to receive 300 mg per day of oral Coenzyme Q10 or placebo for two weeks preoperatively. Biopsies of pectinate trabeculae from the right atrial appendages of the heart were taken, and mitochondria were isolated and studied. Trabeculae were subjected to thirty minutes of hypoxia, and contractile recovery was measured. Sixty-two patients who received Coenzyme Q10 had significant increased Coenzyme Q10 levels in serum, atrial trabeculae, and isolated mitochondria compared with placebo levels. Mitochondrial respiration (adenosine diphosphate/oxygen ratio) was more efficient and mitochondrial malondialdehyde content was lower with Coenzyme Q10 than with placebo. After thirty minutes of hypoxia in vitro, pectinate trabeculae isolated from patients receiving Coenzyme Q10 exhibited a greater recovery of developed force compared with placebo.[6]

Thirty-two patients with end-stage heart failure awaiting heart transplantation were randomly allocated to receive either 60 mg U/day of CoQ10 or placebo for three months. All patients continued their regular medication regimen. The twenty-seven patients who completed the study showed significant improvement in the six-minute walk test with a decrease in shortness of breath, New York Heart Association (NYHA) classification, nocturia, and fatigue. No significant changes were noted after three months of treatment in echocardiography parameters or ANF and TNF blood levels.[7]

Seventy-three patients in a randomized, double-blind, controlled trial were given 120 mg of Coenzyme Q10 per day over one year after an acute myocardial infarction. Total cardiac events (24.6 vs. 45.0 percent) including non-fatal infarction (13.7 vs. 25.3 percent) and cardiac deaths were significantly lower in the Coenzyme Q10 group compared to the control group. Adverse effect of treatments showed that fatigue (40.8 vs. 6.8 percent) was more common in the control group than Coenzyme Q10 group.[8]

COENZYME Q10 FOR DIABETES

Although a number of trials showed Coenzyme Q10 had no effect on glycemic control, in one study seventy-four patients with uncomplicated Type 2 diabetes and dyslipidemia were involved in a randomized, double-blind, placebo-controlled trial. Patients were randomly assigned to receive an oral dose of 100 mg CoQ twice daily, 200 mg fenofibrate each morning, both, or neither for twelve weeks. Fenofibrate did not alter blood pressure, or HbA1c levels. There was a three-fold increase in plasma CoQ concentration as a result of CoQ supplementation. Coenzyme Q10 significantly decreased systolic (-6.1+/-2.6 mmHg) and diastolic (-2.9+/-1.4 mmHg, P=0.048) blood pressure and HbA1c (-0.37+/-0.17 percent).[9]

COENZYME Q10 FOR MIGRAINE

CoQ10 (3 x 100 mg/day) was used in forty-two migraine patients in a double-blind, randomized, placebo-controlled trial. CoQ10 was superior to placebo for attack frequency, headache days, and days with nausea in the third treatment month and well tolerated; 50 percent responder rate for attack frequency was 14.4 percent for placebo and 47.6 percent for CoQ10 (number-needed-to-treat: 3). The researchers concluded that CoQ10 is efficacious and well tolerated.[10]

COENZYME Q10 FOR PARKINSON'S DISEASE

A Cochrane review of four randomized, double-blind, placebo-controlled trials with a total of 452 patients examined the effects of Coenzyme Q10 on Parkinson's disease. Overall, there were improvements in activities of daily living, Unified Parkinson Disease Rating Scale (UPDRS) and Schwab and England Activities of Daily Living Scale for Coenzyme Q10 at 1,200 mg/day for sixteen months versus placebo. In safety outcomes, only the risk ratios of pharyngitis and diarrhea are mildly elevated between Coenzyme Q10 therapy and placebo and there were no differences in the number of withdrawals due to adverse effects.[11]

SIDE EFFECTS OF COENZYME Q10

On average side effects and drug interactions were rare and less than 1 percent of patients reported gastrointestinal symptoms like nausea, diarrhea, heartburn, appetite suppression, and epigastric discomfort. There are also reports of insomnia, headaches, dizziness, and skin reactions. There are no good long-term studies to show the effects of this supplement over long periods of time. Although many health care professionals are using

Coenzyme Q10 extensively, many physicians are waiting for larger confirmatory trials to prove its efficacy.

CONCLUSION

A number of my patients have had a reduction of migraine attacks from taking Coenzyme Q10. It may also be good for heart failure, as an add-on to hypertension therapy and for cardiac surgery.

CHAPTER 31
FOLIC ACID FOR DEPRESSION

Sixty years ago, children commonly heard their mothers say, "Eat your green vegetables; it will make you strong!" And the once-a-week liver and onions, unloved by so many children, were not only considered good for them, but also less expensive than steak or roast, an excellent way to stretch the family food budget. Mothers weren't wrong in their advice. If you are a mother now, you may remember that during pregnancy, your physician recommended taking multivitamins every day, especially those containing folic acid, one of the B complex. Seniors have often heard their physicians urging them to get enough folate through healthy diet and daily supplements. Alcoholics who have gone through treatment and recovery centers may remember the advice to "take B vitamins every day."

WHY IS FOLIC ACID SO IMPORTANT?

Folic acid and B12 are essential for building healthy blood cells; a deficiency can cause certain types of anemia. Folates act as important methyl donors in DNA synthesis and amino acid metabolism and they are vital for the functioning of the nervous system at all ages. Developmental delay in neonates, infants, children, and adolescents, and inborn errors of folate transport and metabolism are associated with folate deficiency in the womb and while growing up. Other problems associated with a lack of this essential vitamin (including those with adults and seniors) are cognitive deterioration, motor and gait abnormalities, behavioral or psychiatric symptoms, and seizures. Many adults with megaloblastic anemia due to folate deficiency have neuropsychiatric disorders, with depression being the most common.[1]

Homocysteine is an amino acid that is made by the breakdown of protein. There has been an association of high homocysteine and heart disease. Folate and other B vitamins are needed in the methylation of homocysteine, which is necessary for its conversion to S-adenosylmethi-onine (SAM). SAMe has been shown to influence serotonin metabolism and has been used in the treatment of depression.[2] So if folate is low then homocysteine is not metabolized and this can have negative consequences.

The best sources of folate include liver, kidney, yeast, and deep-green, leafy vegetables such as spinach, kale, parsley, and watercress. Since 1998, in the United States and Canada, flour has been fortified with folic acid, and the prevalence of folate deficiency has decreased.

Fifty to ninety-five percent of folate may be destroyed by prolonged cooking or by high heat. Although poor diet is probably a factor in some cases, sometimes the cause of folate deficiency may be due to drugs (anti-epileptic, methotrexate), chronic illness, increased stressors and demands, or malabsorption of food and supplements. One reason for the apparently high incidence of folate deficiency in elderly people is that folate concentrations in blood serum and cerebrospinal fluid fall, while plasma homo-cysteine level rises with age, perhaps contributing to the ageing process.

FOLIC ACID IN THE TREATMENT OF DEPRESSION

A number of studies have described the association of folate deficiency in depression, revealing that the association is more common than previously realized. Lower serum folate concentrations were also associated with greater severity of depression. Subjects with dysthymia alone (chronic low mood) had lower red blood cell levels (RBC-levels) of folate than patients who were never depressed, even though their serum levels did not differ. There is also evidence that low folate is a factor contributing to depression in chronic alcoholism.

Bottiglieri et al. identified a biological subgroup of patients with depression, raised plasma homocysteine concentration, folate deficiency, and impaired monoamine neurotransmitter metabolism.[3]

In his summary article, E. H. Reynolds reviewed a number of controlled clinical trials of folate therapy given in addition to standard psycho-tropic medication, and all trials reported positive outcomes.[4]

In an open study of thirty-eight folate-deficient elderly subjects with depression, lethargy, and memory impairment, folinic acid given at 50 mg per week for 120 days significantly improved visuomotor performance, visuospatial memory, logical reasoning, associative memory, and activities of daily living.[5]

In a double-blind, placebo-controlled trial, depressive patients treated with lithium, who also took 200 µg of folic acid for one year, significantly improved their depression scores.[6]

Similarly, the addition of 500 µg of folic acid to 20 mg of fluoxetine for ten weeks significantly improved the antidepressant response, especially in women. Homocysteine, a naturally occurring amino acid found in the blood, has been associated with heart disease when the levels are too high. In this trial, homocysteine levels decreased significantly in the women of the folic acid group. In the men, however, there was no significant difference in homocysteine levels during treatment and no significant difference in therapeutic response between men receiving folic acid or placebo. It was thought that this was the result of too low a dose of folic acid being given.[7]

In another double-blind, placebo-controlled trial 15 mg of methylfolate was added to standard psychotropic medication. Researchers reported significant and increasing clinical and social recovery of depressed patients and schizophrenic patients who were folate-deficient over a six-month period.[8]

An eight-week open study showed that 15 to 30 mg daily of folinic acid enhanced the effect of SSRI antidepressant medication in treatment-resistant depression.[9]

LEVEL OF FOLATE AFFECTS TREATMENT OUTCOMES

Alec Coppen and Christina Bolander-Gouaille reviewed the impact of low vitamin B12 and folic acid status in blood serum in relation to depression and treatment outcomes.[10] Here is a summary of what they found:

A study of 101 depressed inpatients treated with different antidepression drugs showed that the therapeutic effect was inferior if serum folate was low.

A study of severely depressed outpatients showed that the patients who responded to treatment with desmethylimipramine had significantly better folate status than non-responders. There was also an inverse association between RBC folate count in blood serum and severity of depression. Another association was seen with increasing age and disease appearance.

Therapy resistance to fluoxetine was significantly increased in patients with low serum folate and there was a higher relapse rate in patients treated with fluoxetine who had lower folate levels.

The therapeutic effect of both a selective serotonin reuptake inhibitor (SSRI) (sertraline) and a tricyclic antidepressant (nortriptyline) was shown to be dependent on baseline RBC folate, even though all folate levels were in the normal range. Higher folate status in geriatric depression predicted better outcome and the association was strongest for sertraline.

A placebo-controlled double-blind study of forty-one patients with major acute depression or schizophrenia, and whose blood serum folate levels were below normal, showed that daily supplementation with 15 mg of methylfolate for six months, in addition to standard psychotropic treatment, enhanced the therapeutic effect in both diagnoses; the positive effect also increased with time.

SIDE EFFECTS OF FOLIC ACID

High doses of more than 5 mg folic acid per day have caused muscle restlessness, jerking, and occasional seizures, but at 1 mg/day side effects have been rare. Folic acid should be used with caution in patients who are deficient in B12, because high levels of folic acid may worsen the neurological consequences of a vitamin B12 deficiency. Some research showed that epileptic seizures may be increased with folic acid use, and it is known that folic acid lowers phenytoin (seizure medication) levels. There is some controversy about the possibility that supplementation with folic acid may increase the risk of certain cancers. This debate is ongoing.

CONCLUSION

Folic acid deficiency is fairly rare these days. It can be low in people taking medications like methotrexate and anti-epilepsy drugs, or it can also be lacking in people with inflammatory bowel disease or chronic alcoholism. It is extremely important for women who intend to become pregnant to take folic acid to prevent neural tube defects in their children. Be cautious in taking folate if you have a vitamin B12 deficiency as well.

If you are suffering from depression or increasing memory loss, I would strongly recommend asking your physician to do a blood test to check your blood levels for vitamin B12 and RBC folate. I believe folic acid at appropriate doses is a safe vitamin to take when you get depressed. Talk it over with your doctor to make sure it is appropriate for you to take it.

CHAPTER 32

OMEGA-3 FATTY ACIDS

Omega-3 fatty acids are a form of polyunsaturated fat that the body cannot make on its own and must be obtained from food. There are two types of fat that are essential: omega-3 and omega-6 fatty acids. Docosahexaenoic acid (DHA) and eicosopentanoic acid (EPA) are both long-chain omega-3 fatty acids that are major structural fats of the brain. Dopamine and serotonin receptors that facilitate neurotransmitters in brain health are composed mainly of omega-3 fatty acids. Mackerel, tuna, salmon, sturgeon, mullet, bluefish, anchovy, sardines, herring, and trout are fish that are rich in omega-3 fatty acids. There is about 1 gram of omega-3 fatty acids in about 3.5 ounces of fish.

An omega-6 fatty acid, arachidonic acid (ARA), is also important for brain development in babies and is found in meat, eggs, and milk. Omega-3 is anti-inflammatory and omega-6 is inflammatory. Generally, our Western diets contain too much omega-6 fat and we need to increase omega-3s. The Mediterranean diet, which has become quite respectable lately, is high in omega-3s.

OMEGA-3 FATTY ACIDS FOR ARRHYTHMIA (IRREGULAR HEARTBEATS)

Electric impulses cause the muscle tissue of the heart to contract, and it is this contraction that makes the heart beat and the blood circulate. When something goes wrong with these electric impulses, whether they skip, speed up, or slow down too much, the heart reacts. It flutters, flip-flops, or races through beats that are too shallow to contract muscle cells. This irregularity of heartbeat is called arrhythmia. Arrhythmias are fairly common and not necessarily a problem. When tachycardia (heart rate too fast) symptoms are present, a person may feel like their heart is fluttering. They may become breathless, dizzy, light-headed, suddenly weak, or even faint. A slow heartbeat may also produce no symptoms, but if the heart rate is too low, a person may have difficulty concentrating, mental confusion, shortness of breath, difficulty exercising, or the dizzy, faint-headed symptoms mentioned before. If the heart slows down too much a person can lose consciousness. Atrial fibrillation (AF) is a potentially serious heart rhythm that can cause a clot to form in the heart chamber and can lead to a stroke.

Long-chain fatty acids from fish are thought to reduce the risk of sudden death from ventricular arrhythmias (tachycardia and fibrillation). There have been some studies to assess the effectiveness of treating with fish oil supplements. In animal studies, fish oil, a source of eicosapentaenoic and/or docosahexaenoic acids (EPA/DHA), appeared to have beneficial effects on two heartbeat abnormalities: ventricular tachycardia (VT), a dangerous heart rhythm abnormality, and ventricular fibrillation (VF) that were ischemia-induced (damage from restriction of blood supply to tissues). In a meta-analysis of thirteen studies using rat models, fish oil showed a significant protective effect for both ischemia- and reperfusion-induced arrhythmias by reducing the incidence of VT and VF. Supplementation with alpha-linolenic acid (precursor of EPA and DHA) did not show a significant difference.[1]

There is controversy whether omega-3 fatty acids have a positive impact on arrhythmias. In one study of 203 patients scheduled for on-pump cardiac surgery, half were randomized to placebo and half to supplementation with n-3 polyunsaturated fatty acids (2 g/day) (eicosapentaenoic acid:docosahexaenoic acid ratio 1:2), vitamin C (1 g/day), and vitamin E (400 IU/day). The addition of omega-3 fatty acids and vitamins C and E reduced postoperative atrial fibrillation, increased antioxidant potential, and attenuated oxidative stress and inflammation.[2]

One meta-analysis that included 2,687 patients concluded that preoperative supplementation of n-3 polyunsaturated fatty acids significantly prevents the occurrence of postoperative atrial fibrillation in patients undergoing cardiac surgery, particularly in coronary artery bypass surgery.[3]

However, two other meta-analyses did not show a protective benefit. One meta-analysis included 16 out of 124 trials including 4,677 patients.

Eight studies (1,990 patients) evaluated n-3 PUFA effects on AF recurrence among patients with reverted AF and eight trials (2,687 patients) on postoperative AF. The conclusion was that n-3 PUFAs did not reduce recurrent or postoperative AF.[4]

The second meta-analysis involved a total of 32,919 patients in nine trials; 16,465 patients received omega-3 PUFA and 16,454 received placebo. When comparing omega-3 PUFA to placebo, they concluded that taking omega-3 does not affect the risk of sudden cardiac death or ventricular arrhythmias.[5]

Although there is some evidence in humans that omega-3 acid infusion reduces the beginning of ventricular tachycardia among patients with a recent episode of sustained ventricular arrhythmia and an implantable cardioverter defibrillator (ICD), fish oil supplementation did not reduce the risk of VT or VF and may actually aggravate irregular heart rhythms in some patients.[6] In the SOFA trial, omega-3 fatty acids did not reduce arrhythmias in patients with implanted defibrillators.[7] If you have an implantable ICD device, do not take omega-3 fatty acids.

OMEGA-3 FATTY ACIDS FOR CORONARY ARTERY DISEASE PREVENTION

Coronary artery disease, the most common type of heart disease, is present when arteries (carrying blood to the heart) become hardened and narrowed, due to accumulation of plaque and cholesterol (atherosclerosis), and blood cannot sufficiently feed the heart muscle with oxygen. Eventually, the weakened heart muscle becomes vulnerable to heart failure and arrhythmia, and patients can suffer angina (pain) and heart attack.

Yzebe and Lievre did a meta-analysis of ten randomized, control trials with 14,727 patients. Data showed that the daily intake of omega-3 fatty acids for a mean duration of thirty-seven months decreased all causes of mortality by 16 percent and the incidence of death due to heart attack by 24 percent. However, because of the suboptimal quality of the studies included in the meta-analysis and the absence of data in patients receiving statins, the authors suggest that these results do not justify adding fish oils systematically to the heavy pharmaceutical assortment already recommended in coronary heart disease patients.[8]

Harper and Jacobson also looked at trials comparing the impact of omega-3 polyunsaturated fatty acids, including EPA, DHA, and ALA. They concluded there was a reduction in total mortality and sudden death without a clinically significant reduction in nonfatal heart attacks. The six trials with ALA supplements or with an ALA-enriched diet were of poorer design and smaller size than the fish oil trials, and so their findings were less impactful. The researchers concluded there is a role for fish oil (EPA/DHA) or fish in preventing a second heart attack because recent clinical trial data have demonstrated a significant reduction in total mortality, coronary heart disease death, and sudden death.[9]

Several large randomized control trials have shown fish oils to be associated with a decreased risk of cardiovascular events.[10, 11, 12]

However, in a large general-practice cohort of 12,513 patients with multiple cardiovascular risk factors who were given 1 g daily with n-3 fatty acids, there was no reduction of cardiovascular mortality and morbidity compared to placebo.[13]

OMEGA-3 FATTY ACIDS FOR RESTENOSIS (SECONDARY CORONARY ARTERY DISEASE)

Angioplasty is a common treatment for unblocking an artery. A small catheter is inserted into an artery in the groin or arm and fed up through the artery, past the blockage in the heart. A small wire is then fed through this catheter to the end, where it is threaded to the artery. Another smaller catheter is slipped over the wire and slid up the larger catheter, then threaded at the end to the same artery. At the end of this inner catheter is a little balloon device, which is then inflated. As the balloon grows, it pushes against the blockage, stretching the artery walls open, allowing the much needed blood supply to flow freely again. During some angioplasties, a stent is then inserted. This wire mesh stent looks like a miniature tube of chain link fencing, and it holds the shape of the weakened artery wall, keeping it open. While the intervention offers good results, leaving patients feeling much better than before, there are a certain number of patients whose arteries narrow and block up again after the angioplasty and stenting. This recurrence is called restenosis.

Balk, Lichtenstien et al. conducted a systematic review of the clinical literature on the effect of omega-3 fatty acids on measures of vascular structure and function. They found that overall, although there were variability and differences among the studies, there may be a trend toward a net reduction of coronary artery restenosis with fish oil supplementation.

They also suggested that the data available seemed to say that fish oil consumption may improve exercise capacity among patients with coronary artery disease, although the effect may be small and that fish oil may possibly beneficially affect cardiac atherosclerosis; however, the data are inconclusive about carotid atherosclerosis.[14]

Yet another meta-analysis of cohort studies of over 200,000 patients combined with a twelve- to thirteen-year follow-up indicated a significant reduction in CHD mortality for those consuming two to four servings of fish per week (23 percent) and greater than five per week (38 percent).[15]

A Cochrane review looked at forty-eight randomized, controlled trials and forty-one cohort analyses and concluded that it is not clear that either dietary or supplemental omega-3 fats alter total mortality, combined cardiovascular events, or cancers in people with, or at high risk of, cardiovascular disease or in the general population. They stated there is no clear evidence that omega-3 fats differ in effectiveness, whether from fish or plant sources, dietary or supplemental sources, dose, or presence of placebo. They also said there is no evidence to say we should advise people to stop taking rich sources of omega-3 fats, but further high-quality trials are needed to confirm suggestions of a protective effect of omega-3 fats on cardiovascular health.[16]

Another meta-analysis looked at 360 articles and selected 11 well-done, randomized, double-blind, placebo-controlled trials involving 15,348 patients with a history of heart disease. Patients in these studies were given omega-3 fatty acid supplements of at least 1 g/day, and for at least one year. They found a statistically significant protective effect for cardiac death, sudden death, and myocardial infarction. The authors concluded that long-term effect of high-dose omega-3 fatty acid supplementation may be beneficial for the onset of cardiac death, sudden death, and myocardial infarction among patients with a history of cardiovascular disease.[17]

Recommendations from the Canadian Cardiovascular Society suggest that n-3 polyunsaturated fatty acid therapy at a dose of 1 g daily should be considered for reduction of morbidity and cardiovascular mortality in patients with mild to severe heart failure.[18]

OMEGA-3 FATTY ACIDS FOR HYPERTRIGLICERIDEMIA (HIGH TRIGLYCERIDES)

Lovers of Mary Poppins and the supercalifragilisticexpialidocious word may enjoy getting their tongues around this diagnosis, but they won't enjoy having this problem. When the levels of triglycerides found in your blood serum test are too high, it means that you have too much fat in your blood, which puts you at risk for heart disease.

Ten studies reported long-chain omega-3 fatty acids to be effective in the treatment of hypertriglyceridemia. The average decrease in triglycerides was 29 percent, total cholesterol 11.6 percent, very low density lipoprotein (VLDL) 30.2 percent, and low-density lipoprotein (LDL) 32.5 percent. One study found LDLs to increase by 25 percent. Reviewers concluded that although there is reasonably strong evidence supporting the use of omega-3 fatty acids in the secondary prevention of hypertriglyceridemia, until there are larger numbers of high methodological quality trials they did not recommend that practitioners treat hypertriglyceridemia patients with omega-3 supplementation.[19]

OMEGA-3 FATTY ACIDS FOR STROKE

Ecologic/cross-sectional and case-control studies have generally shown an inverse association between consumption of fish and fish oils and stroke risk. Inverse means that when one goes up, the other goes down. In this case, the more fish and fish oils people consumed, the less likely they were to suffer from stroke. Results from five long-term studies have been less consistent, with one showing no association, one showing a possible inverse association, and three demonstrating a significant inverse association. The Nurses' Health Study showed a non-significant, lower relative risk of total stroke among women who regularly ate fish than among those who did not. A significant decrease in the risk of thrombotic (due to blood clot) stroke was observed among women who ate fish at least two times per week compared with women who ate fish less than once a month. These data support the hypothesis that consumption of fish several times per week reduces the risk of thrombotic stroke and does not increase the risk of hemorrhagic (leaking blood vessel) stroke.[20]

OMEGA-3 FATTY ACIDS FOR DEMENTIA

There is conflicting evidence with respect to dementia and omega-3. Although one study found no association for fish or omega-3 on cognitive function with normal aging, four studies seem to suggest a trend in favor of omega-3 fatty acids (fish and total omega-3 consumption) toward reducing risk of dementia and improving cognitive function. However, the available data are insufficient to draw strong conclusions about the effects of omega-3 fatty acids on cognitive function in normal aging or on the incidence or treatment of dementia.[21]

OMEGA-3 FATTY ACIDS FOR INFANT DEVELOPMENT

There is evidence that infant formulas containing DHA provide improved performance on the Mental Development Index in full-term infants and better mental development in preterm infants. One study demonstrated significantly better visual maturation of term infants fed long-chain fatty acids including DHA compared to control formula for a twelve-month period. A meta-analysis of five randomized controlled trials involving term infants and three trials involving preterm infants found that, in term infants, ALA supplementation was associated with increased weight and length at twelve months, which was recorded at least four months after the end of dietary intervention. There was a transient improvement in the retinal function of preterm infants fed ALA-supplemented diets compared with controls.[22]

EPA AND DEPRESSION

Several epidemiological studies suggest as rate of seafood consumption goes up the rate of mood disorders goes down. Biological marker studies indicate there are deficits in omega-3 fatty acids in some people with depressive disorders. Several treatment studies indicate therapeutic benefits from omega-3 supplementation.[23]

A meta-analysis of fifteen trials involving 916 participants assessed the effect of supplements with EPA ≥ 60 percent with dose range from 200 to 2,200 mg EPA in excess of DHA. This meta-analysis showed benefit on standardized mean depression scores. However, supplements with EPA <60 percent did not have the same benefit. They suggest that DHA is not helpful in depression.[24]

Another meta-analysis looked at the use of omega-3 fatty acids for the treatment of bipolar depression. The meta-analytic findings provided strong evidence that bipolar depressive symptoms may be improved by adjunctive use of omega-3. The evidence, however, does not support its adjunctive use in attenuating the mania aspects of bipolar disease.[25]

Although some studies have found mixed results as to whether taking omega-3 fatty acids can help depression symptoms, several studies have found that people who took omega-3 fatty acids in addition to prescription antidepressants had a greater improvement in symptoms than those who took antidepressants alone.[26]

Sixty outpatients who were suffering from a major depressive disorder were randomly allocated to receive daily either 1,000 mg EPA or 20 mg fluoxetine, or their combination, for eight weeks. EPA and fluoxetine had equal therapeutic effects in major depressive disorder. EPA + fluoxetine combination was superior to either of them alone.[27]

CONCERNS ABOUT OMEGA-3 FATTY ACIDS

Taking high doses may keep blood from clotting and may increase the chance of bleeding. High doses of fish oil might also reduce the immune system's activity, reducing the body's ability to fight infection. There are some reports that larger amounts of EPA might increase levels of the "bad"

LDL cholesterol in some people. It may be important to do blood tests periodically to ensure LDL cholesterol is not elevated. One of the biggest concerns is that some fish meats (especially shark, king mackerel, and farm-raised salmon) can be contaminated with mercury and other industrial and environmental chemicals. Usually, fish oil supplements do not contain these contaminants.

CONCLUSION

I would never recommend taking omega-3s as a sole treatment for depression, although it may have a role in improving symptoms. Depression is a serious illness and you should not try to treat it on your own. As I mentioned in the chapter on St. John's wort, I believe that a combination of antidepressant medication and psychotherapy works the best. Be sure to consult with your primary care physician for help.

Although there is evidence for the use of EPA in irregular heartbeats and coronary artery disease, the scientific support is mixed. I would not discourage people from taking it for these problems but I don't routinely add fish oils to the long list of drugs these patients are already taking. Fish oils, omega-3s, and EPA particularly are probably helpful for depression and high triglycerides. I often encourage my patients with these conditions to take them because I believe there is enough scientific evidence to support their use. The good benefit outweighs the cost and risk for side effects. Before adding omega-3s to your treatment plan, it is important to talk it over with your physician. Eating two to four servings of (uncontaminated) fish per week is a good idea.

CHAPTER 33

GLUCOSAMINE FOR OSTEOARTHRITIS

There are a few natural health products that have been associated with a lot of controversy, and glucosamine is one of them. Not surprisingly, most people find it very confusing. I am going to summarize the research, clear up some misunderstandings, and make some recommendations. Patients have been extolling the benefits of glucosamine for years, and I am convinced that it works for a large number of people even though the research is confusing.

Osteoarthritis is a degenerative illness that is generally believed to be a result of the wear and tear of living. It is not as crippling as rheumatoid arthritis, ankylosing spondylitis, or lupus erythematosus, but it causes a great deal of distress and pain. We now believe there is a metabolic process taking place that causes inflammation and subsequent degeneration of the joints. There is increasing loss of cartilage, remodeling of the bone around the joint, and inflammation of the synovial membrane. Osteoarthritis can affect any joint, but the most common are hips, knees, hands, and spine.

There is no known cure for osteoarthritis, and physicians find it difficult to treat. Often nonsteroidal anti-inflammatory drugs like ibuprofen, naproxen, or celecoxib are prescribed. Although relatively safe, these drugs can cause stomach ulcers, kidney damage, and raise blood pressure. Often acetaminophen is prescribed to help relieve pain and enable people to function, but acetaminophen can also cause side effects. In older patients, where osteoarthritis is so prevalent, it is helpful to have other choices to control symptoms. That is where glucosamine comes in. German physicians first reported the use of glucosamine as a therapeutic agent for osteoarthritis in 1969.

HOW GLUCOSAMINE MAY WORK

Glucosamine is an amino monosaccharide, which is a normal constituent of glycosaminoglycans in cartilage matrix and synovial fluid. Since experiments on cultured human chondrocytes have shown that glucosamine increases the production of aggrecans (a major component of cartilage) and reduces the formation of nitric oxide and interleukin in response to interleukin 1ß. It is believed that it may have a protective effect on cartilage and an anti-inflammatory effect. Glucosamine stimulates the synthesis of proteoglycans and the decrease in catabolic activity of chondrocytes by inhibiting the synthesis of proteolytic enzymes and other factors that contribute to cartilage matrix damage and cause the death of these cells. Furthermore, experiments in animals have suggested that circulating glucosamine can localize in cartilage.[1]

STUDIES THAT SHOW GLUCOSAMINE WORKS FOR OSTEOARTHRITIS

McAlindon et al. reviewed fifteen randomly assigned, double-blind, controlled trials of more than four weeks' duration for osteoarthritis of the knee and hip. While the researchers had some concerns about the methodological flaws of many of the studies, they found glucosamine had a positive effect on symptoms.[2]

Richy et al. did a meta-analysis of trials that studied the use of glucosamine and chondroitin for osteoarthritis of the knee and found that glucosamine has a highly significant, beneficial effect on symptoms and joint-space narrowing. Chondroitin was also found to cause a significant improvement in pain and mobility. Safety was excellent for both compounds.[3]

Poolsup et al. did a meta-analysis of double-blind, randomized, placebo-controlled trials that evaluated long-term oral glucosamine treatment in knee osteoarthritis that had been prevalent at least one year. Reported symptom severity and disease progression as assessed by joint-space narrowing were the outcome measures. They concluded that glucosamine sulfate may be effective and safe in delaying the progression and improving the symptoms of knee osteoarthritis.[4]

Another systematic review, which is the basis upon which the Osteoarthritis Research Society International (OARSI) makes recommendations for the management of hip and knee osteoarthritis, gathered results from nineteen randomized, placebo-controlled trials. Sixteen of them used glucosamine sulfate preparations (thirteen oral, two intramuscular, and one intra-articular) and three of them used glucosamine hydrochloride. Based on this review, OARSI recommended the use of glucosamine sulfate but not glucosamine hydrochloride for hip and knee osteoarthritis.[5]

Two methodologically sound, randomized, double-blind, placebo-controlled trials by Reginster et al.[6] and Pavelka et al.[7] followed patients with mild to moderate osteoarthritis of the knee for three years. They both found that the glucosamine-treated group had better functional outcomes and reduced narrowing of the tibio-femoral joint space.

Another meta-analysis reviewed six studies involving 1,502 cases. They assessed the structural efficacies of daily glucosamine sulfate and chondroitin sulfate in patients with knee osteoarthritis on joint space narrowing (JSN). Two studies on glucosamine sulfate and four studies on chondroitin sulfate were included. Although glucosamine sulfate did not show a significant effect versus controls over the first year of treatment, after three years of treatment, glucosamine sulfate revealed a small to moderate protective effect on minimum joint-space narrowing. The same was observed for chondroitin sulfate, which had a small but significant protective effect on minimum joint-space narrowing after two years. Reviewers concluded that glucosamine and chondroitin sulfate may delay radiological progression of osteoarthritis of the knee after daily administration over two or three years.[8]

Two other meta-analyses by Kreder[9] and Denham et al.[10] found that glucosamine had a beneficial effect on osteoarthritis of the knee. Finally, one more study demonstrated that treatment with crystalline glucosamine sulfate is well tolerated and leads to an improvement in complaints related to osteoarthritis accompanied by an increase in quality of life. The use of analgesics could be reduced, and patients reported a progressive improvement of symptoms over the observation period. They concluded that crystalline glucosamine sulfate can be considered an effective and well-tolerated medication.[11]

NEGATIVE STUDIES THAT INDICATE GLUCOSAMINE DOES NOT WORK

There is controversy about the reliability of the meta-analyses. Some say that only mild to moderate osteoarthritis was studied. There was a large dropout rate in the Reginster and Pavelka studies, and a study that included more severe symptoms did not show a difference between placebo and glucosamine.[12]

A study reported in *Arthritis and Rheumatism* in October 2004 found that, in patients who were already on glucosamine, when withdrawn off the substance and followed, there was no difference in the flares of their osteoarthritis of the knee compared to placebo.[13]

Wandel and colleagues analyzed the results of randomized trials with an average of at least one hundred patients with hip or knee osteoarthritis. They found a total of ten trials involving 3,803 patients. They concluded that glucosamine produced no clinically relevant effect on pain or structure.[14]

A meta-analysis of nineteen trials involving 3,159 patients found glucosamine hydrochloride ineffective for pain reduction in patients with knee osteoarthritis. They found that glucosamine sulfate may have function-modifying effects in patients with knee osteoarthritis when administered for more than six months. However, it showed no pain-reduction benefits after six months of therapy.[15]

Perhaps the most important of the negative studies was the one called the GAIT study. This double-blind, placebo-controlled study was conducted at nine sites in the United States. Patients with knee osteoarthritis were divided into five groups over a trial period lasting twenty-four months. Three times daily, Group 1 received glucosamine hydrochloride (500 mg); Group 2 received chondroitin sulfate (400 mg); and Group 3 received a combination of the two (500 and 400 mg respectively). Group 4 received celecoxib 200 mg once daily, and the control group received placebo. Over two years, no treatment (including the nonsteroidal anti-inflammatory drug celecoxib) achieved a clinically important difference in pain or function as compared with placebo. Glucosamine and celecoxib showed beneficial but not significant trends. However, there was a statistically significant benefit in the subgroup of patients with moderate to severe osteoarthritis. Of the 1,583 patients in the trial, 354 (22 percent) fell into this subgroup. Adverse reactions were similar among treatment groups and serious adverse events were rare for all treatments.[16]

Critics also say that because there is no regulation in the production of glucosamine that there may be a wide variation in what is actually present in the products being sold.

SIDE EFFECTS OF GLUCOSAMINE

All studies found that the side effects of glucosamine were no greater than placebo and the benefit of using glucosamine is that it is safer than other choices.

Because altered glucose metabolism can be associated with parenteral administration of large doses of glucosamine in animals, one study looked at the clinical trial data of 3,063 human subjects. Fasting plasma glucose values decreased slightly for subjects after oral glucosamine for sixty-six weeks, but there were no adverse effects of oral glucosamine administration on blood, urine, or fecal parameters and side effects were significantly less common with glucosamine than placebo or nonsteroidal anti-inflammatory drugs. Another study demonstrated that oral glucosamine supplementation does not result in clinically significant alterations in glucose metabolism in patients with Type 2 diabetes mellitus.

Glucosamine recipients had a markedly lower incidence of gastrointestinal disturbances than those receiving ibuprofen. Since glucosamine sulfate is a salt and contains sodium it may increase blood pressure and there have been some case reports of glucosamine causing reversible hypertension. There have also been anecdotal reports of gastrointestinal side effects, aggravation of asthma, kidney problems, palpitations, headaches, and drowsiness. There have been some case reports saying that glucosamine-chondroitin products have been shown to increase the time it takes your blood to clot and potentiate the anticoagulant effects of warfarin, so caution must be used in patients taking blood thinners.

I have one patient, sixty-two-year-old Joan, who suffered from hypothyroidism (an underactive thyroid gland). She developed abnormal thyroid blood levels while taking glucosamine and her dose of thyroid medicine had to be adjusted accordingly.

One study analyzed safety data from two long-term (six-month and three-year, respectively) randomized controlled trials of crystalline glucosamine sulfate. Mean changes in blood pressure, lipids, and glucose were calculated for all patients randomized to crystalline glucosamine sulfate or placebo in either study and for subgroups with abnormally elevated levels of these parameters when the studies were started. They concluded that long-term use of crystalline glucosamine sulfate did not affect blood pressure, lipids, or glucose in patients with osteoarthritis. These findings further support the cardiovascular safety of crystalline glucosamine sulfate.[17]

Glucosamine may be unsafe when used in patients during pregnancy and lactation. Glucosamine is not recommended in children under the age of two years. Patients with shellfish allergies should avoid glucosamine; poor processing during the manufacturing process can lead to traces of intact proteins that can contribute to allergic reactions.

CONCLUSION

In my opinion, there seem to be enough positive clinical studies to warrant the use of glucosamine sulfate for osteoarthritis. Taking pills that contain chondroitin may improve symptom scores. Sometimes it takes four weeks for there to be any clinical improvement. The Cochrane review in 2005 concluded that glucosamine from Rotta Research Laboratorium in Italy was superior to other forms of glucosamine, and that is why studies using Rotta glucosamine generated different results.[18] Also, after reviewing all the literature, I believe that there may be variations in effectiveness between glucosamine sulfate and glucosamine hydrochloride. I recommend using glucosamine sulfate at a dose of 500 mg, three times a day. Most of the positive research has shown its usefulness for osteoarthritis of the knees.

CHAPTER 34

MELATONIN FOR JET LAG

Carol Chan, BScPhm, ACPR, RPh, and Mel Borins, MD

With so many people involved in international business, it is important for traveling professionals to arrive at their destination fully oriented and wide awake. For many years people have been taking melatonin to prevent jet lag, but is there any scientific proof that it works?

WHAT IS MELATONIN?

Deep inside the brain is a pea-sized gland shaped like a pine cone, thus the name *pineal gland*. In some animals, this gland contains a light-responsive structure much like an eye. But humans further evolved to receive light through receptors in the retinal layer of the eyeball. In spite of this, the human's clever pineal gland never forgot its relationship with the rising and setting sun, for amongst its many responsibilities in the biological-functions department, this gland produces (from the amino acid tryptophan) a hormone called melatonin.

Structures inside our brain respond to nerve signals from each retina, producing hormones and neurotransmitters that make us do the things we need to do to support and maintain life. The hormone melatonin regulates our circadian rhythm of sleep and wakefulness. Soon after our brain perceives that darkness is descending, the pineal gland increases its secretion of melatonin, but minutes after we enter the light, particularly very bright light, melatonin secretion is inhibited. Nature has tuned our bodies, therefore, to rise with the sun and go to bed with the sunset. This is all fine and dandy until you hop a jet and fly with the sun for twelve hours, then, exhausted and ready for bed, you emerge to the same dawn that you left behind. No wonder your body gets confused!

DOES MELATONIN WORK?

In 2002, a Cochrane review[1] examined the data from ten studies that met methodological standards of high quality. These are the results they found:

Seventeen participants were flying from San Francisco eastward to London. For three days before their flight, eight participants took a 5 mg daily dose of melatonin, and nine subjects took placebo, at 18:00 local (San Francisco) time, and then at bedtime (London) 22:00–24:00 for the first four days after their return to Britain. Jet lag was significantly less severe among subjects treated with melatonin as rated on day seven after the flight.[2]

Fifty-two participants were flying round-trip from the UK to Australia and New Zealand. Jet lag was self-rated six to seven days after the flight. Mean jet lag ratings for both eastward and westward flights were better after melatonin than placebo.[3]

Twenty participants flew eastward from Auckland to London on a twenty-six-hour flight. They returned on a similar westward flight three weeks later. Participants were randomized to receive either melatonin or placebo on the outward flight and the other substance on the return flight. They took melatonin (5 mg) or placebo between 10:00 and 12:00 (local time) for three days prior to each flight, on the day of flight, and for three days after their arrival, between 22:00 and 24:00 (destination time). Ratings for jet lag and tiredness were significantly less for participants taking melatonin. They took significantly fewer days to establish a normal sleep pattern, to not feel tired during the day, and to reach normal energy levels. The melatonin group also had more vigor activity and less fatigue based on their profile of mood-state (POMS) ratings.[4]

Thirty-six participants were flying westward from Frankfurt to North America, and two weeks later, in the reverse direction. They were divided into three subgroups of twelve people according to the time shift: 6 to 7 hours, 8 to 9 hours, and 10 to 11 hours. After the westbound flight, participants took either melatonin (5 mg) or placebo at bedtime for seven days. After the eastbound flight, they took the same dose for five days. Overall, subjective jet lag ratings were better in all three melatonin subgroups after both west- and eastbound flights, but the differences compared to placebo were not statistically significant.[5]

Thirty participants received melatonin (8 mg) or placebo on the day of flight and at bedtime for the following three days. A significant difference was observed only for evening sleepiness and morning tiredness scores.[6]

Fifty-two airline staff returned to New Zealand from London via Los Angeles. There were three treatment groups. Group 1 (early group) received melatonin 5 mg (at a time corresponding to evening/night at destination) three days before flight until five days after arrival; Group 2 (late group) received placebo for three days before flight and then melatonin 5 mg daily for five days after; Group 3 received placebo. Retrospective ratings on day six showed that participants in the late melatonin group (Group 2) had significantly lower scores of jet lag compared to both the early melatonin and placebo groups. The late melatonin group had significantly less sleep disturbance than the placebo and recovered their energy and alertness faster than the early melatonin group, which reported a worse overall recovery than placebo. Five participants in the early melatonin group reported minor side effects of sleep difficulties, drowsiness, headaches, and feeling depressed. Melatonin taken after arrival resulted in reduced feelings of jet lag and a more rapid recovery of sleep and energy levels.[7]

Two hundred thirty-four subjects flew eastward from America to Europe, and from Europe to Asia. There were four groups: melatonin 0.5 mg fast-release (FR) formulation; melatonin 5 mg FR, melatonin 2 mg controlled-release (CR) formulation; and placebo. All medications were taken once daily at bedtime for four days after the flight. Melatonin 5 mg FR significantly improved self-rated sleep quality, shortened sleep latency, and reduced fatigue and daytime sleepiness. A physiological dose of 0.5 mg was almost as effective as a pharmacological dose of 5 mg; only sleep quality and sleep latency were significantly greater with the 5 mg dose.[8]

One hundred thirty-seven participants flying eastward from America to Switzerland were divided into four groups: melatonin 5 mg, zolpidem 10 mg (a sleeping pill), a combination of melatonin 5 mg and zolpidem 10 mg, and placebo. The medication was taken between 17:00 and 21:00 local time on the day of flight and then for four days post-flight at bedtime. The zolpidem group reported significantly better sleep quality, less jet lag, and rated it as the most effective jet lag medication. Zolpidem and the combination of melatonin + zolpidem were less well tolerated than melatonin alone. Confusion, nausea, and morning sleepiness were reported to be highest in the combination group.[9]

Two hundred fifty-seven Norwegian physicians had visited New York for five days and then traveled back to Oslo, Norway, in an eastward direction. On the returning flight, they were randomized to receive either: melatonin 5 mg at bedtime, 0.5 mg at bedtime, 0.5 mg taken on a shifting schedule, or placebo. Medications were administered on the day of travel and continued daily for five days post-flight. No significant difference in jet lag score was found between the treatment groups. One limitation was that participants had come from Norway to New York and stayed there for only five days before returning to Norway, and the baseline used was not asymptomatic.[10]

Thirty-one sports officials or sports scientists flying from London to Eastern Australia (EA) received melatonin 5 mg or placebo. It was taken on the plane at a time corresponding to 18:00–19:00 in EA, at 22:00–23:00 on evening of arrival in EA, and again for three more evenings. Subjective jet lag and responses to a jet lag questionnaire were measured four times daily for six days post-flight. No significant differences in jet lag ratings, sleep disturbances, and morning alertness over the six days were found between the two groups. The authors concluded that for individuals who followed a busy schedule after arrival (resulting in erratic light exposure) and when alcohol could be drunk in the evening, melatonin had no benefit in alleviating jet lag.[11]

COMPARING CAFFEINE AND MELATONIN

Twenty-seven participants flying from Texas to France were given either 300 mg slow-release caffeine (SRC) taken for five days after the flight at 08:00, 5 mg melatonin, or placebo. These were taken one day before flight at 17:00, on the day of flight at 16:00, and for three days after flight, at 23:00. All participants were prohibited from sleeping during the flight so that they remained awake for thirty-three hours from last awakening in Texas to first sleep in France. SRC participants woke up earlier, slept less, and complained of more awakenings than participants who took melatonin. The melatonin group fell asleep earlier and slept longer than the placebo group. No significant difference was found among the three groups for subjective daytime sleepiness, except on day one where the SRC group was sleepier than the melatonin group, but was less sleepy on subsequent days compared to baseline. The melatonin group felt sleepier than compared to their baseline on day one, but not on days two and three.[12]

SIDE EFFECTS OF MELATONIN

A disorienting "rocking" feeling, increased luteinizing hormone levels, lowered blood pressure, reduced glucose tolerance, and insulin sensitivity have been reported. Other side effects recorded have been allergic reactions/anaphylaxis, autoimmune hepatitis, palpitations, tachycardia, chest pains, mild gastrointestinal upset, increased triglyceride and VLDL levels, neurological effects (including seizures), and depression.

The cytochrome P450 enzyme CYP1A2 plays a major role in the metabolism or breakdown of many commonly used drugs, including clozapine, imipramine, caffeine, fluvoxamine, paracetamol, phenacetin, theophylline, tacrine, and others. Since the metabolism of melatonin is influenced by this enzyme, levels may rise when you take CYP1A2 inhibitors like caffeine, fluvoxamine, and fluoxetine. Melatonin levels may decrease with CYP1A2 inducers like cigarettes and nefedipine. Although melatonin appears to lower blood pressure, it may interact with calcium channel blockers like nefedipine and aggravate blood pressure control. If you are on a calcium channel blocker for hypertension, you should have your blood pressure monitored carefully and dosage adjustment may be necessary. Melatonin may cause increased blood levels of certain sedatives. Caution is advised with driving, operating heavy machinery, pregnancy and lactation, and with warfarin. There is a concern for dependency, which has not yet been borne out in clinical trials.

OTHER USES FOR MELATONIN

There is preliminary research that shows melatonin may be useful in treating Alzheimer's disease,[13] sleep disturbances in Parkinson's disease,[14] high blood pressure,[15, 16] and especially insomnia.[17, 18, 19] Brzezinski et al. did a meta-analyis of seventeen randomized, double-blind, placebo controlled trials involving 284 subjects. Seven trials examined healthy volunteers while seven studied people suffering from insomnia. Melatonin treatment significantly reduced the time to fall asleep, increased sleep efficiency, and increased the total sleep duration compared to placebo.[20]

CONCLUSION

I do recommend melatonin for jet lag. It should be started on the day of travel as close to the target bedtime at the destination as possible and then taken every twenty-four hours at bedtime for several days after arrival. I recommend taking a 1 mg time-release tablet to start and increasing to 6 mg, taking an additional 1 mg each night until restful sleep is obtained. Don't forget melatonin can react with other medication and can have side effects. Always weigh the benefits versus the risk and consult with your physician.

CHAPTER 35
PROBIOTICS FOR YOUR GUT

The gastrointestinal system is a series of tubes, glands, and organs that take food and liquids into the body, break them down, extract useful components, and finally, expel the waste material. When something enters the mouth, a cascade of action begins with saliva release, stomach acid secretion, enzyme activity, and so on. At every stage, food and liquid are moved, filtered, reduced, and distributed to the body. This inner world of transport is full of bacteria—hundreds of different kinds of bacteria that protect the body from disease and help the intestine absorb nutrients. But with the common use of antibiotics and other medications the normal intestinal flora (microorganisms) is disrupted and problems, such as diarrhea, can occur.

To give the body a boost of supportive microorganisms, many people take probiotics, which are naturally found in certain food products. There are different varieties of probiotics such as lactobacillus (found in yogurt), *Bifidobacterium bifidum* (found in non-fermented acidophilus milk), and *Saccharomyces boulardii* (a non-pathogenic yeast found in lychee and mangosteen fruit) that seem to have a beneficial effect on gastrointestinal symptoms.

ANTIBIOTIC-ASSOCIATED DIARRHEA (AAD)

Antibiotics have helped to save millions of lives, and are one of the most important classes of drugs that I prescribe on a daily basis. But like some drugs, there can be side effects. The most common side effect is diarrhea (AAD), and it is reported that 20 percent of people taking antibiotics are affected by AAD. Diarrhea results when the balance between "good" and "bad" bacteria is disrupted. The key word here is balance. Our guts are full of both good and bad bacteria, but when antibiotic medication is sent to fight the inner battle, it cannot discern between good and bad bacteria, so the hero organisms die along with the bandits, and the unhealthy balance inside our bowels leaves us vulnerable to other infections. Infections and drugs can release water into the bowel—water that should not be released. When this happens, a person is experiencing secretory diarrhea. Most people are well familiar with that explosive burst of smelly brown fluid and the feeling of relief when it no longer rumbles around the lower tummy, but gushes out and flushes down into the pot. Diarrhea is uncomfortable, sometimes painful, and it can become a serious problem, leading to dehydration and loss of vitamins and minerals.

PROBIOTICS AS PREVENTIVE TREATMENT FOR AAD

Researchers performed a meta-analysis of nine randomized, double-blind, placebo-controlled trials using *Lactobacillus rhamnosus* and *Saccharmyces boulardii*. Two of the studies investigated the effects of probiotics in children.[1] Four trials used *Saccharomyces boulardii*, four used lactobacilli, and one used a strain of enterococcus that produced lactic acid. Three trials used a combination of probiotic strains of bacteria.[2] Reviewers concluded that compared to placebo, these probiotics were useful in preventing antibiotic-associated diarrhea.

Another meta-analysis of thirty-four studies shows the preventive effect of probiotic supplementation on the incidence of AAD to be relatively consistent across different probiotic species used, with various antibiotic regimens, and infection indications, including *H. pylori* eradication, in both adult and pediatric populations.[3]

I generally recommend that my patients take a high quality probiotic, one tablet twice a day, when they go on an antibiotic, and continue using the probiotic for a few days after finishing the antibiotic.

PROBIOTICS IN THE TREATMENT OF DIARRHEA

Three meta-analyses seem to conclude that probiotics are useful in treating diarrhea once it starts. The first meta-analysis of thirteen trials concluded that lactobacillus was useful in treating infectious diarrhea in infants and children, especially in those infected with rotavirus.[4] The second meta-analysis of eighteen trials in the treatment of acute pediatric diarrhea showed that probiotics reduced the duration of diarrhea by about one day. The researchers concluded that starting treatment early was very important.[5]

Finally, a Cochrane review of twenty-three trials involving 1,917 participants concluded that probiotics reduced the risk of diarrhea at three days and the mean duration of diarrhea by 30.48 hours. They stated that probiotics appear to be a useful adjunct to rehydration therapy in treating acute, infectious diarrhea in both adults and children. They commented that more research is needed to inform the use of particular probiotic regimens in specific patient groups.[6]

There are also some good studies showing probiotics are useful in infantile colic and ulcerative colitis.[7] It would be helpful to work with your family physician to decide which probiotic is best suited for your condition.

PROBIOTICS FOR THE PREVENTION OF DIARRHEA

Although the preventive impact of probiotic therapy against rotavirus is not clear, a mixture of *Bifidobacterium bifidum* and *Streptococcus thermophilus* was used in twenty-nine hospitalized children to prevent rotavirus diarrhea. Only 10 percent of those getting the treatment developed rotaviral diarrhea compared to 38 percent of those getting placebo.[8]

Using probiotics to prevent traveler's diarrhea is not yet proven conclusively. However, one study of 1,016 tourists who were either given *Saccharomyces boulardii* or a placebo showed that 29 percent of those treated with probiotics developed diarrhea. Of those treated with placebo, on the other hand, 39 percent developed diarrhea. No significant side effects were noted.[9]

PROBIOTICS FOR CLOSTRIDIUM DIFFICILE

Clostridium difficile is an anaerobic bacillus (survives only in an oxygen-free environment) that has been colonizing the large intestines of people treated with broad-spectrum antibiotics, especially in hospital populations. It has become a significant public health problem. These pathogenic bacteria may produce toxins that can build up and damage the bowel wall, leading to inflammation. It has been a frequent cause of severe pseudomembranous colitis, which can cause considerable disability and even death. *Clostridium difficile* disease (CDD) can also result in mild diarrhea and nausea.

My mother-in-law was living in a nursing home and had a dental procedure. The dentist put her on the antibiotic clindamycin, and soon afterwards she developed severe bloody diarrhea and nausea, and stopped eating. She had developed *Clostridium difficile*. Because of this illness she remained in hospital for five months and became bedridden. After her long hospital stay she became confined to a wheelchair and was never quite the same again.

There had been controversy about whether taking a probiotic could prevent this very serious infection. A double-blind, placebo-controlled trial looked at 150 consecutive patients who were receiving antibiotic therapy. Upon admission, bowel habit was recorded and fecal samples taken. Within seventy-two hours of having been given a prescription of antibiotics, sixty-nine patients received lactobacillus and bifidobacterium, and sixty-nine patients received placebo. An equal number of patients developed diarrhea, but only 2.9 percent of the probiotic group's samples tested positive for clostridium toxins, versus 7.25 percent of the placebo control group.[10]

A well-performed meta-analysis looked at eleven studies. Most of the studies did not have a large enough number of patients enrolled and so the results were suspect. However, two of the studies showed significantly lower rates of CDD among the probiotic recipients. A meta-analysis of three studies that used a probiotic combination of *Lactobacillus acidophilus* (CL1285) and *Lactobacillus casei* (LBC80R), and a combined analysis of four studies using *Saccharomyces boulardii*, showed lower CDD rates in recipients of probiotics, compared with recipients of placebo.[11] Another meta-analysis of adult hospitalized patients showed that the administration of probiotics along with antibiotics reduced the risk of antibiotic-associated diarrhea by 44 percent and *Clostridium difficile* by 71 percent.[12]

However, another study gave lactobacilli and bifidobacteria to 2,941 inpatients sixty-five years of age and older who were given antibiotics. In this trial, the probiotics did not reduce the incidence of antibiotic associated diarrhea or *C. difficile* rates.[13]

If someone has had a previous *Clostridium difficile* infection, the next time they are prescribed antibiotics, they should have a probiotic given with the antibiotic because this may help to reduce the rate of occurrence. A study that gave *Saccharomyces boulardii* as 500 mg tablet twice a day along with an antibiotic reduced the rate of recurrent CDD by 30 percent.[14]

PROBIOTICS AND IRRITABLE BOWEL SYNDROME

Irritable bowel syndrome (IBS) is a common condition that causes lots of distress. Symptoms of irritable bowel syndrome include constipation, diarrhea, bloating, gas, abdominal pain, and nausea. Although there are many strategies used to help people with this condition, many people continue to suffer. There are a number of research studies that show probiotics can help with symptoms. I will summarize the results of two meta-analyses. Ortiz-Lucas et al. analyzed ten out of twenty-four studies that were deemed suitable for inclusion. They found probiotics had a positive impact on bloating, pain, and gas. However, because there was such a wide variety of probiotics used with varying degrees of success, it was suggested further research should be done to identify which species are good for which symptoms.[15] Another meta-analysis looked at nineteen generally good-quality trials using control groups involving 1,351 patients. Fifteen of the nineteen trials showed that probiotics appear to help improve symptoms in IBS. However the degree of benefit and which species and strains are best is not known.[16]

Brenner et al. looked at sixteen RCTs and found that *Bifidobacterium infantis* showed significant improvement in the composite score for abdominal pain/discomfort, bloating/distention, and/or bowel movement difficulty compared with placebo in two appropriately designed studies. They said that no other probiotic showed significant improvement in IBS symptoms in an appropriately designed study.[17]

PROBIOTICS AND ECZEMA

There is also evidence that probiotics may be useful in the prevention of eczema. When high-risk infants were given *Lactobacillus rhamnosus* during their first six months of age, they had half the development of atopic eczema compared to placebo. The four-year follow-up of this study found that significantly less children developed eczema when taking probiotics.[18]

A meta-analysis looked at six prenatal and four postnatal trials with supplementation of probiotics for the prevention and treatment of pediatric atopic dermatitis. The authors concluded that the current evidence is more convincing for the prevention rather than the treatment of pediatric atopic dermatitis.[19]

Another meta-analysis of fourteen studies found probiotics used during pregnancy and in a child's early life may help avoid atopic dermatitis and immunoglobulin E (IgE) associated atopic dermatitis in infants and young children. The favorable effect was similar regardless of the time of probiotic use (pregnancy or early life) or the subject(s) receiving probiotics (mother, child, or both).[20]

CHALLENGES WITH PROBIOTICS

Perhaps the most difficult decision is which preparation to take. There are significant differences in the active ingredients. Sometimes no active ingredients can be found when analyzed. There are also reports of contamination with extraneous strains not listed on the label. Many experts say that it is important to buy from stores that keep the probiotics in the fridge and to store the containers in the fridge at home because it is only effective as live bacterial cultures. Generally you are advised to consult your pharmacist or health care practitioner to take the best product. Every practitioner must develop expertise in which products are best. The names of the products are continually changing. I recommend probiotics that have had some good-quality research associated with them.

Since there have been reports of complications of infections in immune-compromised patients, there is a suggestion that probiotics should not be used in immune-suppressed patients. This would also apply to patients with HIV disease or those on immunosuppressive drugs. Similarly, patients who have central venous catheters or artificial heart valves should not take probiotics.

CONCLUSION

I recommend that if you are given an antibiotic that you take a probiotic along with it to prevent antibiotic associated diarrhea and potential *C. difficile* infection. If you are traveling to the tropics or countries where diarrhea is commonly acquired, then taking a probiotic preventively may be useful. The diagnosis of irritable bowel syndrome or inflammatory bowel disease usually requires a consultation from a gastrointestinal specialist. Ask the specialist or your primary care physician if a probiotic is advisable. If you are pregnant and there is a history of eczema or allergic dermatitis in you or your children, then, with your doctor's approval, taking probiotics may be a good idea. The most difficult decision is which probiotic to take that has active ingredients and has been proven to be beneficial for the condition you are dealing with.

CHAPTER 36

ZINC FOR THE COMMON COLD

Cheryl Tyler, BScPhm, and Mel Borins, MD

One of the most common reasons for patients to visit their doctor, miss school, and lose valuable days of work is infection with the common cold, usually caused by the rhinovirus. Colds occasionally develop into secondary problems such as middle ear, sinus, and lung infections, and they can exacerbate other reactive conditions of the airways, such as asthma and chronic obstructive lung disease. While no treatment of the common cold has been proven to be an effective therapy, there are some substances that may help to prevent or shorten the duration of the disease when it presents. It has been known for quite some time that zinc inhibits rhinovirus cell reproduction in the laboratory.[1] Many patients take zinc as a treatment for the common cold, in the form of lozenges, nasal spray, syrup, tablet, or in tea preparations with zinc. So what is the evidence?

META-ANALYSIS

A review conducted by Garland and O'Hagmeyer concluded that zinc gluconate lozenges "may be effective in decreasing the duration and severity of cold symptoms." This review included eight trials with a total of 620 participants and found four trials with positive results and four with negative results. Here is a summary of this review:[2]

Studies That Show Zinc Works

Eby et al. conducted a double-blind, placebo-controlled clinical trial for patients with cold symptoms of less than three days. Twenty-eight patients were given placebos and thirty-seven patients were given two zinc gluconate tablets containing 23 mg of elemental zinc to be consecutively dissolved in the mouth as lozenges initially and then one tablet every two wakeful hours until symptoms had disappeared. Eleven percent of patients treated with zinc became asymptomatic within twelve hours. By twenty-four hours, 22 percent of patients were asymptomatic. No patients in the placebo group were asymptomatic during this time frame. By the conclusion of the trial (seven days later), 86 percent of patients in the zinc-treated group were asymptomatic, compared with 46 percent of placebo-treated patients. The trial had poor methodological quality because there was an initial difference in severity between groups at baseline and there was a high dropout rate.[3]

Mossad et al., in a randomized, double-blind, placebo-controlled study, gave fifty patients with cold symptoms for twenty-four hours or less one zinc gluconate lozenge containing 13.3 mg of elemental zinc every two hours while awake for as long as their cold symptoms were present. The median duration of symptoms in the zinc-treated group was found to be 4.4 days compared to 7.6 days in the placebo group. Zinc-treated patients had a lesser duration of coughing, headache, hoarseness, nasal congestion, sore throat, and nasal drainage. The authors concluded that zinc gluconate lozenges decreased the duration of symptoms in patients with the common cold.[4]

A randomized, double-blind, placebo-controlled trial by Prasad et al. assessed the effect of one zinc acetate lozenge containing 12.8 mg elemental zinc given every two to three hours in twenty-five patients who were experiencing signs and symptoms of the common cold for twenty-four hours or less. Patients in the zinc-treated group experienced colds of shorter duration compared to those in the placebo-treated group (4.5 days versus 8.1 days). Half of the patients in the zinc-treated group were asymptomatic within 3.8 days compared to within 7.7 days in the placebo treated group. Patients in the zinc-treated group experienced less severe symptoms by day four of the study compared with patients in the placebo-treated group. The authors concluded that zinc acetate lozenges are effective in decreasing the duration and severity of symptoms of the common cold.[5]

McElroy and Miller conducted a chart review[6] and an open-label single-center phase IV clinical study[7] on the effectiveness of zinc gluconate glycine lozenges in the treatment and prevention of the common cold in children ages twelve to eighteen. Children were given one zinc gluconate glycine lozenge once a day prophylactically during the cold season and were given four lozenges of zinc gluconate glycine daily if they were experiencing at least two signs and symptoms of a common cold on the same day. The authors concluded that the use of zinc gluconate glycine lozenges was effective in decreasing the duration of cold symptoms as well as decreasing the number of colds. This study was neither blinded nor randomized, and so they recommend that further research is needed to support these results.

Hirt et al. examined the effectiveness of zinc gluconate nasal gel in reducing symptoms of the common cold in a randomized, double-blind, placebo-controlled trial. One hundred and eight patients received zinc gluconate nasal gel and 105 received placebo. The gel was to be applied as one spray into each nostril every four hours for as long as symptoms were present. The zinc nasal gel was found to decrease the duration of cold symptoms compared to the placebo-treated group. The average time to resolution of all symptoms was 2.3 days in the zinc-treated group and 9 days in the placebo group. The authors concluded that zinc gluconate nasal gel is effective in reducing the duration of symptoms of the common cold.[8]

META-ANALYSES OF ZINC FOR THE COMMON COLD

A 2013 Cochrane review studied data from sixteen therapeutic trials (1387 participants) and two preventive trials (394 participants). All the trials had been conducted under randomized, double-blind, placebo-controlled conditions. They concluded that zinc administered within twenty-four hours of onset of symptoms reduces the duration of common cold symptoms in healthy people. As the zinc lozenges' formulation has been widely studied and there is a significant reduction in the duration of cold at a dose of ≥ 75 mg/day, for those considering using zinc it would be best to use it at this dose throughout the cold. In 2011 they reported that zinc use was also shown to reduce the number of colds experienced by participants when they took it for five months or more; in 2013 they were unable to make any recommendations regarding prophylactic zinc supplementation because of insufficient data. Researchers reported that people who took the lozenge form of zinc were more likely to experience adverse side effects such as nausea and a bad taste in the mouth. Reviewers cautioned against the use of zinc for people with underlying chronic illness, immunodeficiency, asthma, or other health issues. They believed more research was needed to make qualified recommendations on dose, duration, strength, and formulation of the supplement.[9]

Another meta-analysis looked at seventeen trials involving 2,121 participants. Compared to patients receiving placebo, those receiving zinc had a shorter duration of cold symptoms. They found that studies of adults were successful compared to studies with children. Bad taste and nausea were more common in the zinc group compared to placebo.[10]

STUDIES THAT SHOW ZINC DOES NOT WORK

Smith et al. in a randomized, double-blinded, placebo-controlled study gave eighty-six college-age students with upper respiratory infections an initial dose of four zinc gluconate lozenges containing 11.5 mg of elemental zinc, followed by two lozenges every two hours while awake for seven days or twenty-four hours after the last symptom had subsided. There was no difference in the duration of symptoms of the common cold between groups. There was a decrease in the severity of symptoms on days four to seven of zinc treatment; however, the clinical effect and significance of this decrease was small. The authors concluded that zinc gluconate lozenges were minimally effective in decreasing the severity of symptoms and ineffective in terms of decreasing the duration of symptoms of the common cold.[11]

Farr et al. inoculated two groups of patients with rhinovirus. In the first trial with thirty-two participants, two zinc gluconate lozenges containing 23 mg of elemental zinc were given initially, followed by one lozenge every two hours, to a maximum of eight doses per day. Each lozenge was given thirty-six hours after inoculation with rhinovirus type 39 and continued for five days. In the second trial with forty-one participants, zinc was initiated two hours after inoculation with rhinovirus type 13 and continued for seven days. The authors of this study concluded that zinc gluconate lozenges were not effective at decreasing the rate of viral shedding or in decreasing the severity or duration of symptoms of the common cold.[12]

Macknin et al., in a randomized, double-blind, placebo-controlled trial, gave 249 children in grades one through twelve either zinc gluconate glycine lozenges containing 10 mg of elemental zinc or placebo for the common cold. The authors concluded that zinc gluconate glycine lozenges were ineffective in treating the common cold in this patient population.[13]

Belongia et al. advised patients in a randomized, double-blind, placebo-controlled study to inhale two sprays of zinc sulfate nasal spray containing 0.12 percent zinc sulphate, resulting in 0.011 mg of elemental zinc per dose, four times a day if they had symptoms of the common cold for less than twenty-four hours. Participants were given a viral culture to determine that the symptoms with which they were presenting were actually due to the common cold. No difference was observed in median time to resolution between the zinc and placebo groups. The authors concluded that zinc sulfate nasal spray was ineffective in decreasing the duration or severity of symptoms of the common cold.[14]

In a double-blind, placebo-controlled study, Eby et al. instructed patients to use a 10 mmol zinc gluconate nasal spray two to three times every fifteen to thirty minutes while awake in addition to one zinc orotate lozenge containing 37 mg of elemental zinc every two to three hours while awake. No difference in duration of common cold symptoms was observed between the zinc and placebo groups.[15]

SIDE EFFECTS OF ZINC

Instances of anosmia (loss of smell) have been reported with intranasal use of some products containing zinc gluconate. In September 2003, a maker of intranasal zinc faced lawsuits from users who claimed that the product, a nasal gel containing zinc gluconate and several inactive ingredients, negatively affected their sense of smell and sometimes taste. Some plaintiffs alleged experiencing a strong and very painful burning sensation when they used the product. As already mentioned, bad taste and nausea were the most common side effects reported.

CONCLUSION

I generally recommend patients buy zinc gluconate lozenges (13 mg of elemental zinc) and take them every two to three hours at the first onset of a cold.

CHAPTER 37

L-CARNITINE FOR HEALTH

Carnitine is the generic term for a number of compounds, including L-carnitine, acetyl-L-carnitine, and propionyl-L-carnitine. The Latin *carnus* means flesh, hence the name for this essential compound found mostly in dairy, poultry, and, especially, red meat. Carnitine, a vitamin-like nutrient, is derived from two of the twenty amino acids that are the building blocks of all protein in our body. Protein is needed for skin, muscle, organs, glands, and body fluids.

Two amino acids, lysine and methionine, are precursors of carnitine. Unlike fat, the human body does not store them, so it is important to get a fresh supply every day. Carnitine is needed for almost every cell of the body since a major part of its role is involved with the production of energy. Inside each cell reside oval-shaped energy factories called mitochondria. Something has to carry fuel (long-chain fatty acids) to the factory, and carnitine is the capable transporter that does the job. After it unloads the fatty acid fuel, the industrious carnitine hauls away toxic waste that has built up inside the mitochondrial factory. You can imagine what would happen if a factory ran low on fuel and all its waste material was allowed to fill the hallways.

Some people are born with one of the rare genetic diseases that cause carnitine deficiency. Symptoms usually manifest when the child is about five years of age, with signs of cardiomyopathy (deterioration of heart muscle), skeletal-muscle weakness, and hypoglycemia (low blood sugar). Secondary carnitine deficiencies may occur in chronic renal (kidney) failure, diabetes, and cirrhosis (liver scarring).

L-CARNITINE FOR MENTAL FUNCTION

A meta-analysis of double-blind, placebo-controlled studies focused on trials that used acetyl-L-carnitine for patients with mild cognitive impairment and Alzheimer's disease. In these studies, subjects took 1.5 to 3.0 grams/ day of acetyl-L-carnitine for three to twelve months. After studying all the results, the authors stated that supplements of acetyl-L-carnitine may improve mental function and reduce deterioration in older adults with mild cognitive impairment and Alzheimer's disease.[1]

L-CARNITINE FOR CARDIOVASCULAR DISEASE

A number of early trials showed L-carnitine to have a protective effect on the heart after a heart attack. A randomized placebo-controlled trial found that those patients given L-carnitine after a specific kind of heart attack (acute anterior myocardial infarction) had reduced mortality after five days but no difference in composite death or heart failure at six-month follow-up.[2]

In a randomized, double-blind, placebo-controlled trial, the effects of the administration of oral L-carnitine (2 g/day) for twenty-eight days were compared in the management of fifty-one (carnitine group) and fifty (placebo group) patients with suspected acute myocardial infarction. Infarct size, cardiac enzymes, angina pectoris, heart failure plus left ventricular enlargement, and total arrhythmias were significantly less in the carnitine group compared to placebo. Total cardiac events including cardiac deaths and nonfatal infarction were 15.6 percent in the carnitine group vs. 26.0 percent in the placebo group. The authors said it is possible that L-carnitine supplementation in patients with suspected acute myocardial infarction may be protective against cardiac necrosis and complications during the first twenty-eight days after a heart attack.[3]

A controlled study was carried out on 160 patients of both sexes (age between thirty-nine and eighty-six years) discharged from the Cardiology Department of the Santa Chiara Hospital, Pisa, with a diagnosis of recent myocardial infarction. L-carnitine was randomly administered to eighty-one patients at an oral dose of 4 g/day for twelve months, in addition to the pharmacological treatment generally used. For the whole period of twelve months, these patients showed, in comparison with the controls, an improvement in heart rate and systolic arterial pressure, a decrease of angina attacks, and a clear improvement in the lipid pattern. The above changes were accompanied by a lower mortality in the treated group and in the control group there was a definite prevalence of deaths caused by re-infarction and sudden death. The authors concluded that L-carnitine represents an effective treatment in post-infarction ischemic cardiopathy, since it can improve the clinical evolution of this pathological condition as well as the patient's quality of life and life expectancy.[4]

A double-blind, placebo-controlled, clinical trial in Italy found patients who had suffered a first heart attack and were given supplemental carnitine intravenously for five days, then 6 g/day orally for one year, had reduced heart failure.[5]

Finally, a meta-analysis of thirteen controlled trials involving 1,369 patients looked at the impact of using L-carnitine after an acute heart attack. Compared with placebo or control, L-carnitine was associated with a 27 percent reduction in all-cause mortality, a 65 percent reduction in ventricular arrhythmias, and a 40 percent reduction in angina symptoms in patients experiencing an acute myocardial infarction.[6]

L-CARNITINE FOR CLAUDICATION—LOWER LEG CRAMPS WHEN WALKING

Patients with moderate to severe claudication who were supplemented with 2 g/day of propionyl-L-carnitine for twelve months significantly improved their maximal walking distance and perceived quality of life as compared to subjects receiving the placebo.[7]

A similar trial conducted in the United States and Russia found the same daily dose and form of propionyl-L-carnitine administered for six months in patients with disabling claudication significantly improved walking distance and speed, reduced bodily pain, enhanced physical function, and improved perceived health state as compared to controls.[8]

L-CARNITINE FOR FATIGUE IN CANCER AND MULTIPLE SCLEROSIS

Some cancer patients, who experience fatigue resulting from chemotherapy, radiation treatment, and poor nutritional status, are deficient in carnitine. Those terminal cancer patients supplemented with carnitine 250 mg to 3 g/day experienced less fatigue and improved mood and quality of sleep compared to placebo.[9]

In another study, 4 g/day of carnitine for one week ameliorated fatigue in chemotherapy-treated subjects and restored normal blood levels of carnitine.[10]

In a randomized, double-blind, crossover study thirty-six patients with multiple sclerosis presenting with fatigue were given either 100 mg of amantadine twice daily or 1 gram of acetyl-L-carnitine twice daily for three months. After a three-month washout period, they crossed over to the alternative treatment for three months. Acetyl-L-carnitine was better tolerated and more effective than amantadine for the treatment of MS-related fatigue.[11]

L-CARNITINE FOR DIABETES

A trial involving 333 patients with diabetic neuropathy treated the experimental group with acetyl-L-carnitine 1,000 mg/day intramuscularly for ten days and continued orally at a dosage of 2,000 mg/day for the remaining 355 days of the study. The control group received placebo. Among the 294 patients with impaired electrophysiological parameters at baseline, those treated with acetyl-L-carnitine showed a statistically significant improvement in mean nerve conduction, velocity, and amplitude compared with placebo. After twelve months of treatment, mean scores for pain were significantly reduced from baseline by 39 percent in acetyl-L-carnitine treated patients compared with 8 percent in placebo recipients.[12]

Two randomized, placebo-controlled trials lasting fifty-two weeks tested acetyl-L-carnitine 500 mg and 1,000 mg three times a day on patients with clinical diabetic neuropathy. There were significant improvements in sural (leg calf) nerve fiber numbers and regenerating nerve fiber clusters, vibration perception, and pain in those taking acetyl-L-carnitine.[13]

Twenty-two male and thirteen female Type 2 diabetic patients were randomly assigned to receive 1 g of L-carnitine or placebo orally three times a day for a period of twelve weeks. Fasting plasma glucose decreased significantly in the L-carnitine group. There was a significant increase of triglycerides, Apo A1, and Apo B100. There was no significant change in LDL-C, HDL-C, HbA1C, LP(a), or total cholesterol.[14]

L-CARNITINE FOR CHRONIC RENAL FAILURE AND DIALYSIS

Although there is some evidence that carnitine is beneficial in dialysis patients, the trials that were done were not of sufficient size and quality to reach any firm conclusions about its routine use.

Positive Outcomes with L-Carnitine

In a double-blind, randomized, controlled trial fifty hemodialysis patients were treated intravenously with either 2 g carnitine or placebo for twenty-four weeks. Although there was a large dropout, there was improvement in Medical Outcomes Short Form-36 scores and lower doses of erythropoietin needed in the treatment group compared to controls.[15]

In end-stage renal disease, carnitine insufficiency may contribute to impaired exercise and functional capacities. In one study, patients were administered L-carnitine 20 mg/kg or placebo intravenously at the conclusion of each thrice-weekly dialysis session for twenty-four weeks. In another study, patients were administered intravenous L-carnitine 10 mg/kg, 20 mg/kg, or 40mg/kg, or placebo. Intravenous L-carnitine treatment increased plasma carnitine concentrations, improved patient-assessed fatigue, and seemed to prevent the decline in peak exercise capacity.[16]

Negative Outcomes with L-Carnitine

Sixteen patients were randomized to receive either L-carnitine 20 mg/kg or placebo after each dialysis session for twelve weeks, followed by a

---

CAUTION

A study from the Cleveland Clinic suggests that increased dietary carnitine increases heart disease risk due to its generation of TMAO (timethylamine N-oxide) by gut bacteria. People who regularly eat red meat have an increased colonization of intestinal bacteria that break down the carnitine in red meat into a metabolite that promotes increased cholesterol deposition in the artery wall.[17]

---

six-week washout, then the crossover therapy for twelve weeks. There was no significant effect of L-carnitine on quality of life, irrespective of treatment order. There were also no differences found in any of the secondary outcomes, including incidence of muscle cramping, intradialytic hypotension, erythropoietin requirements, or hemoglobin. Adverse effects consisted of gastrointestinal symptoms, with a similar incidence between L-carnitine and placebo.[18]

CONCLUSION

There is research that suggests L-carnitine may be useful for dementia, heart disease, claudication, fatigue in cancer, multiple sclerosis, diabetes, and chronic renal failure. Because these illnesses are fairly serious, you should consult with your physician before using L-carnitine.

Section VII: Migraines—Alternative Approaches

Scott Forman, MD, and Mel Borins, MD

Although throughout the book I have talked about the different treatments one at a time, because that is the way the research is usually carried out, in reality usually we combine a number of treatments for each condition. To be truly integrative, collaborative, and holistic, multiple approaches are used together to provide successful outcomes. Rarely in clinical practice is just one thing used. For example if you were suffering from depression, your physician might prescribe drugs, do psychotherapy, and maybe add exercise and EPA amino acids and even folic acid. Similarly if you were getting frequent colds you might take American ginseng, Echinacea, and zinc. In this section, preventing migraines is discussed in a more holistic way as a model for the integrative approach.

Some of the therapies discussed in this section have been mentioned elsewhere in the book. Despite risking some repetition, by gathering all the evidence for migraine prevention into this one section, I hope it will prove helpful to those suffering from this type of headache and serve as a model of how multiple strategies are used for one condition. Migraines are a common affliction but modern physicians have yet to find a common cure-all for the condition. Although medical therapy can be successful, not everyone responds to drugs. Most of my patients have found alternative therapies that are useful for the prevention of migraine headaches.

HOW DO I KNOW IT'S A MIGRAINE?

Most common symptoms prior to onset (usually in the twenty-four hours before):

- Aura—prior to onset, the patient may see pulsating lights, spots, or lines in their field of vision. Typically, there is a variation on the theme of an expanding, progressing scintillating series of regular shapes that may remain stationary or move across the visual field leaving a blank area in its wake. This aura lasts for ten to forty minutes and either may be followed by a headache of variable degree or no headache at all ("acephalgic migraine").

- Mood—Sudden change in either direction, to low and depressed or high and even excitable. Mood changes may occur twenty-four hours or more prior to the migraine onset.

- Cravings (i.e., for chocolate)

- Frequent urination

- Excessive yawning

- Migraine may occur in relation to a woman's menses as well ("menstrual migraine")

Most common symptoms after onset:

- Throbbing pain that gets worse upon movement

- Pain can be on only one side of the head

- Pain behind the eye

- Sensitivity to light such as a computer screen or headlights at night or any bright lights

- Sensitivity to noise

- Nausea and/or vomiting

- Generalized dysphoria, or a desire to get away from people and sleep in a dark room

I cannot emphasize enough the importance of lifestyle changes to reduce the incidence of migraines. Sleep hygiene, stress management, regular aerobic exercise, and dietary modification are all key factors that need to be addressed.

DIET AND MIGRAINES

If you have migraines it can be helpful to consider whether there may be any dietary triggers causing the symptoms. The identification of food triggers is an inexpensive way to reduce migraine headaches. I suggest you keep a headache diary and record what foods you ate during the twenty-four-hour period before the onset of symptoms. Although research data surrounding the role of certain foods and substances in triggering headaches has been subject to some controversy, there are subsets of people who may be sensitive to certain substances.[1, 2, 3] It is very important to read labels of prepared foods.

Most Common Food Triggers for Migraines

- Phenylethylamine—present in chocolate and oil of bitter almonds, this amine is also produced naturally in the brain as a neurotransmitter; its action is similar to that of amphetamines.

- Tyramine—an amino acid that stimulates release of the neurotransmitters epinephrine and norepinephrine. It is found in aged cheeses and meats, bananas, nuts, citrus fruits, onions, products containing yeast, and red wine.

- Aspartame—an artificial non-saccharide sweetener used in foods and drinks (also known as NutraSweet, Equal, Spoonful, and Equal-Measure).

- Monosodium glutamate—also known as MSG, this is the sodium salt of glutamate (a naturally occurring amino acid). It is added to foods to balance and enhance flavor. It is commonly added to Chinese food but may be added to prepared foods.

- Nitrates and nitrites—used in food as preservatives, often found in prepared meats like hot dogs, salami, cold cuts, and bacon.

- Alcohol—the darker-colored alcohol is most often cited as a trigger, particularly dark ales, liqueurs, spirits, and red wine.

- Caffeine—found in coffee, black tea, green tea, cola soft drinks, and some over-the-counter headache medications. For some people caffeine can be used to stop headaches, but it has also been found to cause headaches when the caffeine level in the body begins to drop.

- Skipping meals—the importance of eating regularly cannot be overemphasized, as skipping meals can trigger headaches. Skipped meals and fasting were reported as migraine triggers in over 56 percent of cases in a population-based study and 40 to 57 percent in subspecialty clinic-based studies.[4, 5]

- Hypoglycemia (low blood sugar)—could potentially bring on a headache. In healthy people it can be caused by fasting. Diabetics on insulin can get it from an insulin overdose or by not eating enough food after taking insulin. It can also be caused by excessive exercise. Diseases involving the pancreas or liver, and pituitary or adrenal glands, can also cause it. In one study,[6] three quarters of participants with migraine headaches demonstrated five-hour glucose tolerance tests consistent with reactive hypoglycemia.

Other approaches to dealing with migraines may involve taking supplements, herbs, or using other alternative therapies.

COENZYME Q10 FOR MIGRAINES

Coenzyme Q10 is a naturally occurring, fat-soluble, antioxidant enzyme manufactured in the body and is found in fish oils, nuts, meat, and vegetables. It was first identified in heart tissue, where it plays a crucial role in energy production and supporting cardiovascular health. I discussed it in chapter 30 of this book.

In 2005, forty-two migraine patients took part in a trial. The experimental group was given Coenzyme Q10 (3 x 100 mg/day) in a double-blind, randomized, placebo-controlled trial. Results: In the third treatment month CoQ10 was found to be superior to placebo for reducing attack frequency, headache days, and days with nausea, and was well tolerated. The researchers concluded that CoQ10 is efficacious and well tolerated.[7]

FEVERFEW FOR MIGRAINES

Feverfew (*Tanacetum parthenium*) has been used as an antipyretic (fever-reducing), and for the treatment of headaches and arthritis for centuries. Feverfew appears to be a serotonin antagonist and an inhibitor of prostaglandin synthesis. The extract also inhibits platelet aggregation. I mentioned it in chapter 7 but I am summarizing it again.

Two randomly assigned, placebo-controlled trials have shown feverfew to be helpful to reduce migraines. Some patients in the United Kingdom who self-medicate generally eat two to three leaves daily, taken with food or sweetener to relieve the bitter taste. In a BMJ study, patients were given powdered, freeze-dried leaves, about 50 mg/day.[8]

Patients in a study reported in the *Lancet* were given a capsule of dried feverfew leaves (82 mg) per day.[9]

In Canada feverfew is approved by Canada's Health Protection Branch and marketed as Tenacetum at a dosage of 125 mg/day. Four to six weeks of treatment are required to notice a response.

CAUTION

Feverfew should not be used by pregnant or lactating women. It is related to ragweed, and so it has the potential to cause allergy symptoms. Mouth ulcerations are a common side effect; sometimes a more widespread mouth inflammation can occur. Also there can be an increase in headaches (rebound) after feverfew is discontinued.

RIBOFLAVIN THERAPY (VITAMIN B2) FOR MIGRAINES

Vitamin B2 is a precursor for two coenzymes: flavin adenine dinucleotide and flavin mononucleotide. Inside each brain cell are mitochondria, small factories that are fueled by enzymes and produce energy for brain cells to work. These tiny enzymes with giant names are involved in the transfer of electrons in oxidation-reduction reactions, an electron transport chain. There is some evidence that platelet mitochondrial dysfunction may play a role in the cause of migraines. In other words, patients who suffer with migraines may have impaired oxygen metabolism.

In a non-placebo-controlled trial forty-nine patients were given 400 mg/day riboflavin (vitamin B2) in a single oral dose daily for at least three months as a prophylactic (preventive) treatment. Twenty-three patients were also given 75 mg aspirin plus riboflavin. They found riboflavin in both groups to be an effective, low-cost treatment for reducing migraine frequency.[10]

In a randomized, placebo-controlled trial reported in *Neurology*, researchers found that riboflavin was superior to placebo with a 50 percent reduction in number of attacks, and a 59 percent reduction in headache days, compared to only 15 percent reduction in duration for placebo.[11]

An open-label study was conducted with twenty-three migraine patients at a specialized outpatient clinic. Patients received 400 mg riboflavin per day. Headache frequency, duration, and intensity were recorded at baseline, three months, and six months. While intensity and duration showed no significant change, headache frequency was reduced from baseline (of four days per month) to two days per month after the three- and six-month periods. Researchers concluded that riboflavin is a safe and well-tolerated alternative in migraine prevention.[12]

In the studies above, preventive treatments were considered effective if they prevented more than half of migraines in at least 50 percent of patients. Since riboflavin results consistently demonstrated a reduction in migraine frequency, researchers concluded it should be recommended as a first-line preventive treatment option.

MAGNESIUM THERAPY FOR MIGRAINES

Two trials published in *Cephalalgia* in 1996 showed conflicting results. In the first trial, Pfaffenrath et al. found no benefit with magnesium compared to placebo, either in the number of migraine attacks or duration of headache.[13] Ten patients in each randomized group (of thirty-five) responded. Tolerability in the magnesium group was reported as 45.7 percent having mildly adverse events like soft stool and diarrhea, compared to the placebo group who reported only 23.5 percent. This study was discontinued primarily due to a lack of responders.

In the second trial,[14] Peikert et al. found a significant reduction both in attack rate (number of headaches) and duration (days of headache) recorded in weeks nine through twelve of the study, with a 41 percent reduction in attack frequency for the magnesium group (compared to 16 percent reduction for the placebo group). There were a few adverse reactions of gastric irritation (5 percent) and diarrhea (19 percent).

The major difference in these two studies is that the former study utilized 20 mmol daily of magnesium-L-aspartate HCl, whereas the latter study used 24 mmol (600 mg) of magnesium dicitrate. It is postulated there is a difference in bioavailability. I have found consistently good results with my patients using 600 mg of magnesium dicitrate per day in the prevention of migraine.

Several other trials, including one using oral magnesium oxide (MgO) with migraine in children,[15] found benefit in migraine prophylaxis.

Mauskop et al.[16] gave a 1 g intravenous infusion of magnesium sulfate (MgSO4) to forty consecutive patients with acute migraine. Pain reduction of 50 percent or more occurred within fifteen minutes of infusion in thirty-five patients. In twenty-one patients, continued improvement or complete relief persisted for twenty-four hours or more. Of the 44 percent that responded well, 86 percent had low serum-ionized magnesium, whereas only 16 percent of non-responders had low serum-ionized values.

There have been other studies that have shown low magnesium levels in the serum and tissues of patients with migraine. Low levels may predispose patients to vasoconstriction, reduced affinity for serotonin receptors, and lowered threshold for N-CH3-d-aspartate receptors. Researchers concluded that measurement of serum-ionized magnesium levels may be useful in identifying patients who may respond to intravenous infusion of magnesium sulfate. Generally it is suggested to use MgO, Mg diglycinate, and slow-release MgCl, which tend to be well absorbed and tolerated at dosages of between 400 mg and 800 mg daily.

ACUPUNCTURE FOR MIGRAINE PROPHYLAXIS

A recent Cochrane review of twenty-six randomized trials concluded that existing evidence supports using acupuncture for chronic headache, but the quality and amount of evidence were not fully convincing, and that well-planned, large-scale studies were needed.[17]

In 2004, Vickers et al. performed such a trial involving 400 patients, of whom 301 completed the trial, and 31 provided three months' data. At twelve months, scores fell by 34 percent from baseline in the acupuncture group compared to 16 percent of controls. Patients randomized to acupuncture treatment had experienced fewer days with headache, used less medication than controls, made fewer visits to their doctors, and took fewer days away from work. Researchers found that acupuncture, in addition to standard care, resulted in clinically relevant benefits for patients with chronic headache—particularly migraine—compared with controls.[18]

Furthermore, the results of a study published in *Headache* (2002) found acupuncture to be as effective as flunarizine (a calcium-channel blocker) in reducing headache frequency, severity, and analgesic use in migraine without aura. The treatment was given weekly for two months, then monthly for the next four months. Acupuncture was more effective in reducing attack frequency after two and four months of treatment and reducing headache severity after six months of therapy. Fewer side effects were reported with acupuncture.[19]

CHIROPRACTIC TREATMENT FOR MIGRAINES

In two randomized studies chiropractic manipulations reduced migraine frequency and severity.[20, 21]

PSYCHOTHERAPEUTIC TECHNIQUES FOR MIGRAINES

There have been studies of biofeedback where patients exhibited conscious control of physiologic readings such as skin temperature, pulse rate, and EMG.[22]

In a study reported in 2009, biofeedback combined with relaxation instruction was compared with relaxation techniques alone in sixty-four patients. After the first twelve months, 52 percent of the relaxation group reported fewer severe headaches as compared to 57 percent in the biofeedback group.[23]

A meta-analysis of eighteen trials suggested that relaxation training, thermal biofeedback combined with relaxation training, electromyographic (EMG) biofeedback, and cognitive-behavioral therapy are all modestly effective in treating migraine when compared to a wait-list control.[24]

Crystal Hawke and I did a study with high-school students that showed they could improve their migraine headaches using a handheld temperature thermometer, biofeedback, and guided imagery.[25] We taught them how to raise the temperature of a handheld thermometer by biofeedback and guided imagery and then apply this skill when they felt a migraine coming on.

Cognitive-behavioral therapy has also been shown to be useful at improving migraines and has been advocated for migraine prevention based on meta-analysis of the US Headache Consortium and the Canadian Consortium.

INTRAORAL INFLAMMATION ASSOCIATED WITH MIGRAINE

Studies by M. H. Friedman et al.[26] suggest a relationship of migraine and tension-type headache to a local maxillary gingival inflammation. An intraoral zone of tenderness occurs in the maxillary nerve segment accessible inside the mouth. Local tenderness has been palpated consistently in asymptomatic migraine patients and significant migraine relief has been obtained from chilling confined to this area (molar periapical area adjacent to the maxillary second and third molar root apices). This was identified in 93 percent of 1,100 patients—mostly asymptomatic migraineurs and tension-type headaches. Tenderness was present whether or not the patient was experiencing a headache and corresponded to the plexus formed by the posterior superior alveolar branches of the maxillary nerve. In headache-free patients, or those with temporomandibular joint/masticatory muscle pathology (clenched-jaw syndrome), this tenderness is usually absent. When a person has no symptoms, higher recorded temperatures are found in the area of maximal tenderness in unilateral headache in comparison to the contralateral side when a person has no symptoms.

You can palpate with your index finger the maxillary second and third molar periapical areas even if you have no teeth by pressing upward and backward inside the mouth as far as possible along the ridge between the cheek and the alveolar mucosa (mucous membrane that extends below the gingiva) with the mouth partially opened.

A study was done on thirty-five symptomatic patients[27] comparing three randomized conditions of maxillary intraoral chilling (forty minutes), versus 50 mg sumatriptan, versus forty minutes of sham tongue chilling (placebo). Outcome measures were taken post-treatment at two hours, four hours, and twenty-four hours. Significant headache relief was recorded at all four time intervals for both chilling and sumatriptan, while the placebo showed poor relief results. Maxillary chilling was more effective than sumatriptan, and significant relief from nausea was recorded at all four time intervals with the maxillary chilling, whereas some headache and nausea recurrence was noted with the sumatriptan. Researchers concluded that local inflammation was associated with vasodilation and edema, and because chilling resolved the edema, it raised the possibility that intraoral inflammation may be a factor in migraine etiology.

Another study by Friedman, Frishman, and Peterson[28] examined twenty patients with migraine, tension-type, or post-traumatic headache and used a daily application of 20 percent topical ketoprofen gel for the prevention of migraine, tension-type, and post-traumatic headache for sixty days. After thirty days, significant improvement was recorded in headache intensity and duration. Analgesic and headache medication were also significantly reduced from baseline, and side effects were minimal.

CONCLUSION

Dietary approaches, relaxation therapy, the use of magnesium, riboflavin, and Coenzyme Q10 all have some scientific support for their use in preventing migraines. I have found these therapies most useful in my own clinical practice.

Section VIII:
Conclusion—Talk to
Your Doc

Now that we have come to the end of the book, I hope you have gained a better understanding (if you did not already know) of randomly assigned, double-blind, controlled trials and why they are the gold standard in medicine. I am sure the description of each study and meta-analysis was not always fascinating, but I felt it was important to share the details behind some of the recommendations I was making. Perhaps you will gain a better idea of the dilemma facing decisions about treatment for different conditions.

If you read a conservative medical journal you will undoubtedly be left with the idea that what they are reporting is gospel. However, not everything is so black and white. When deciding on a treatment, physicians must weigh the pros and cons, and the benefit versus harm. There is evidence showing that many treatments that the medical profession believed were helpful based on so-called evidence were later found to be of no benefit and sometimes even harmful.[1, 2, 3]

Evidence can change quite rapidly over time both with new treatments and new evidence about how effective existing treatments are.

When you read a health magazine put out by a health-food store or a natural health product manufacturer you may get the idea that all that is natural is good and can do no harm. You may also be told that the natural approaches have been proven to be true through research. I hope now you can judge the difference between reliable research and research that is inadequate. A poorly done clinical trial may not prove very much.

It is important to understand that an open-label trial that is not blinded or placebo-controlled, although interesting, has limited value. Perhaps you will also understand that a small trial is not as powerful as one involving hundreds or thousands of patients. I am sure you appreciate how important it is that the person giving the treatment and the person evaluating the treatment do not know whether placebo or the treatment was given. Often open-label trials and small clinical trials are done before undertaking a large properly done trial both to see if the treatment holds promise and also to deal with all the problems and questions that can emerge before proceeding to a larger costly study.

Some journals are more reliable than others. If results are published in a peer-reviewed journal, then the article and research have been scrutinized, usually by experts in the field. Peer-reviewed journals have their results published in *Pub Med*, which usually means the journal has been accepted by the medical profession as being reliable. So if you hear of research being published in some obscure publication, it might be quite biased and not necessarily reliable.

One of the other challenges facing research in alternative medicine has to do with funding. Pharmaceutical companies develop most drugs, and they expect to market and make money on those drugs that they discover and research. They invest millions of dollars into making sure the drugs work and are safe. The financial benefit of researching natural health products may not be the same. If an herb or natural health product cannot be patented, then it makes sense that no company is willing to foot the bill for research because they may not get anything back on their investment.

I am sure you have heard testimonials and case studies of alternative approaches that sound too good to be true. Often they are. Just because one person has gotten a good result does not mean that there is any proof that it would be helpful for you.

KEEPING AN OPEN MIND

Values are one of the core components of all social constructs such as family, government, religion, or any organization that defines a group of people. Each one of us has individual values that are shown by the choices we make and the way we behave. If we value honesty, for example, we tell the truth and we expect others to do likewise. Basically, whatever we invest our energy, time, and resources in reveals what we value the most.

When we share common values with others, these values become like the glue that bonds us, motivating us to form moral and behavioral parameters that help us to achieve our common goals and protect and nurture what we hold most dear. The walls or building blocks that identify our parameters are called principles. Principles define who we are; they act as guides that inspire, lead, and keep us on track. When a certain choice or behavior does not fulfill our principles, it undermines, and eventually destroys, that which we value.

In the case of medicine, life is what we value, so eliminating disease becomes our common goal, and doing no harm is one of the principles that supports this goal. While the basic tenet sounds simple, very little that involves people and medicine is clear-cut. Cutting off a leg, for example, is normally considered harmful, so we don't do it. But when faced with a severely gangrenous limb, removal saves the life we value. Despite the consequences of losing a leg, in this case, our choice of intervention supports the "do no harm" principle because the patient can heal and live.

A majority of the illnesses I deal with in my medical practice are a result of self-destructive lifestyle practices. Overeating, smoking, excess alcohol, drug addiction, and suicide attempts reflect this self-destructive tendency. We can go a long way to becoming healthy by stopping self-destructive behavior and focusing on health-promoting activities. Exercising regularly, maintaining your ideal body weight, eating a healthy well-balanced diet, taking care of your emotions, and having loving relationships, all contribute to staying healthy. I like the term psychospiritualsomatic medicine to highlight this approach. You are a composite of body, mind, emotions, spirit, and of your place in family and society. When the physical, emotional, spiritual and social aspects of your being are in balance then you are healthy.

We are living in an exciting time. Medicine is racing ahead with DNA mapping, stem cell research, organ transplantation, MRIs, and new diagnostic equipment, as well as newer, more-sophisticated drugs and surgical techniques. While we focus on eliminating symptoms and diseases with all these new tools at our fingertips, sometimes we forget that a person is more than the disease in their body. When we in the medical professions forget that human beings are more than their symptoms or treatment, we undermine our work as healers. We can even risk inadvertently causing harm. To counter this modern tendency, many people in the healing profession have joined the trend back to a more natural, humanistic, and holistic approach. As always, the challenge is to synthesize and integrate the scientific and the humanistic. When that happens, patient and practitioner become a powerful force.

Medicine has always been a conservative profession, which I believe is a positive thing. For the most part, we can be assured today that when some new treatment is accepted by the medical profession, it has been thoroughly researched and tested. Even so, physicians often take years to accept new treatments.

Physicians' cautious mindset can be a defect, as revealed by history. Take, for example, Semmelweis, who, in 1848, introduced the washing of hands and using antiseptic procedures in gynecological wards. His new approach reduced mortality from puerperal fever by a factor of fifteen, yet he was ostracized by his colleagues who were offended at the idea that physicians could be carriers of death! So while we must not drop our scientific ways of dealing with new propositions, at the same time we need to be open to new ideas.

The American Holistic Medical Association developed ten principles to inspire and guide practitioners while reminding them of the core values that motivate true healers. I strongly believe that medical professionals and patients will benefit if they are familiar with and have full understanding of these principles. When you work together as a team, you will feel more empowered and be more likely to achieve a better outcome.

PRINCIPLES OF THE AMERICAN HOLISTIC MEDICAL ASSOCIATION

1. Use a variety of safe, effective options in diagnosis and treatment, including: education for lifestyle changes and self-care, complementary approaches, and conventional drugs and surgery.

2. Searching for underlying causes of disease is preferable to treating symptoms alone.

3. It is important to establish what kind of person has the disease in addition to what kind of disease a person has.

4. Prevention is usually more cost effective.

5. Illness is a manifestation of a dysfunction of the whole person, not an isolated event.

6. A major determinant of healing outcomes is the quality of the relationship established between physician and patient in which patient autonomy is encouraged.

7. The ideal physician-patient relationship considers the needs, desires, awareness, and insight of the patient as well as the physician.

8. Physicians significantly influence patients by their example.

9. Illness, pain, and the dying process can be learning opportunities for patients and physicians.

10. Encourage people to evoke the healing power of love, hope, humor, and enthusiasm and to release the toxic consequences of hostility, shame, greed, depression, prolonged fear, anger, and grief.

11. Unconditional love is life's most powerful medicine. Physicians need to strive to adopt an attitude of unconditional love for patients, themselves, and other practitioners.

12. Optimal health is much more than the absence of sickness. It is the conscious pursuit of the highest qualities of the physical, environmental, mental, emotional, spiritual, and social aspects of the human experience.

TALK TO YOUR DOC

Dr. Heather Boon, a colleague of mine at the University of Toronto, has done research into understanding why patients were taking alternative treatments. She found complementary treatments are used commonly among people diagnosed with chronic or life-threatening conditions.

Patients with AIDS, cancer, and chronic mental-health illness often seek alternative treatments and practitioners because their conditions are not always adequately cured by conventional medicine.

Sometimes people choose alternatives because of their fears of the adverse effects of conventional treatments, lack of efficacy of conventional treatments, and perceived poor doctor-patient interactions. Some people believe that "natural" is better, that Complementary Alternative Medicine (CAM) or Integrative Medicine is safer and its approaches are more congruent with beliefs about the nature of health and illness.

A number of research studies have found that one in three patients routinely use alternative treatments but seven out of ten users of alternative therapies do not tell their physicians. Sometimes patients think that if it is natural then it can do no harm and see no need to tell their doctors. Other patients do not think their physician is interested or knowledgeable about CAM, so there's no point in discussing it. Some physicians may feel defensive or criticized when patients tell them they are seeing a naturopath, acupuncturist, or other health care practitioner. Some patients feel that their physician may feel threatened and refuse to see them or may suggest throwing all that junk in the garbage. Sometimes physicians may have had a bad experience with patients who do not follow their expert advice and may react unfavorably to patients who want to follow their own path in healing. Physicians may get quite frustrated when they offer an approach they know will work but their patient chooses something else.

Some physicians find the doctor-patient relationship difficult when the patient's belief system is different from their own. As a physician it is always helpful to appreciate your patient's ways of thinking about health and treatment and find some common ground where there can be agreement. Rather than attacking a patient's beliefs, it is more helpful to understand where they are coming from and how they developed these misunderstandings and sometimes mistrust of modern medicine. I have learned so much about alternatives just listening to my patients' experiences.

In the real world some physicians are pressed for time and are so busy they are not able to explore all the concerns and questions that patients have. One thing you can do before visiting your doctor is to write your questions down on a piece of paper or in your smartphone so that you will remember to ask the most important things you are interested in exploring. While you are sitting in the waiting room waiting for your physician, use the time to review what you want to get out of the visit. When you are asking about an alternative therapy, it is helpful if you have some scientific studies to back up your questions, so bring this book!

Remember to consult with your physician before undertaking any course of treatment. An herb or natural health product may be interfering with medical drugs or surgery. Sharing what you are doing can only be to your advantage. When patients and doctors work together as a team, health outcomes are better. The future of health care will hopefully be more collaborative. You will be better taken care of when all the health care practitioners who are providing treatments communicate more effectively with each other. When physicians, chiropractors, dieticians, naturopaths, acupuncturists, psychotherapists, physiotherapists, pharmacists, nurses, social workers, dentists, massage therapists, and other allied health professionals talk to each other about what is being done, then the patient will benefit and our care will be truly integrative and collaborative. I hope you have enjoyed reading my book and that you have learned something that is helpful. I am sure you realize by now that there is scientific support for the effectiveness of many alternative approaches. I hope you have gained a new understanding about how to make decisions about complementary treatments from a scientific perspective as opposed to anecdotal information. Perhaps you now have an appreciation of why some physicians are so highly critical of alternatives. My mother Lily used to say that if you have your health then you have everything. Take care and treat yourself lovingly and with compassion.

ENDNOTES

INTRODUCTION

1 Feinberg, Cara, "The placebo phenomenon," *Harvard News*, September-October 2013.
2 Friedman, J.H. and R. Dubinsky, "The placebo effect," *Neurology*, August 26, 2008; 71 (9): e25–e26.

SECTION I: TRADITIONAL HEALING AND HERBAL REMEDIES

1 Akerele, O., "Nature's medicinal bounty: don't throw it away," *World Health Forum*, 1993; 14(4): 390–95.
2 Borins, M., "First world should help third world maintain traditional healing practices," *CMAJ*, 1991; 144(10): 1306–7.
3 Borins, M., "Traditional healing around the world," *Humane Med*, 1990; 6(3): 213–16.
4 Eisenberg, D.M. et al., "Unconventional medicine in the USA," *NEJM*, 1993; 328(4): 246–52.
5 "Self-treatment with herbal and other plant-derived remedies—rural Mississippi, 1993," *MMWR*, 1995; 44(11): 204–7.
6 Kassler, W. et al., "The use of medicinal herbs by AIDS infected patients," *Arch Intern Med*, 1991; 151: 2281–88.

Chapter 1: St. John's Wort for Depression
1 Linde, K. et al., "St. John's Wort for major depression," *Cochrane Database of Systematic Reviews*, 2008, (4): CD000448.
2 Linde, K. et al., "St. John's Wort for depression—an overview and meta-analysis of randomized clinical trials," *BMJ*, 1996; 313: 253–58.
3 Brenner, R. et al., "Comparison of an extract of hypericum (LI 160) and sertraline in the treatment of depression: a double-blind, randomized pilot study," *Clinical Therapeutics*, 2000; 22(4): 411–19.
4 Trautmann-Sponsel, R.D. and A. Dienel, "Safety of hypericum extract in mildly to moderately depressed outpatients: a review based on data from three randomized, placebo-controlled trials," *Journal of Affective Disorders*, 2004; 82(2): 303–7.
5 Gaster B. and J. Holroyd, "St. John's Wort for depression: a systematic review," *Arch Intern Med*, 2000; 160(2): 152–56.

Chapter 2: Echinacea for Upper Respiratory Infections
1 Lindenmuth, G.F. and E.B. Lindenmuth, "The efficacy of echinacea compound herbal tea preparation on the severity and duration of upper respiratory and flu symptoms: a randomized, double-blind placebo-controlled study," *Journal of Alternative & Complementary Medicine*, Aug 2000; 6(4): 327–34.

2 Goel, V. et al., "Efficacy of a standardized echinacea preparation (Echinilin) for the treatment of the common cold: a randomized, double-blind, placebo-controlled trial," *Journal of Clinical Pharmacy and Therapeutics*, 2004; 29(1): 75–83.

3 Cohen, H.A. et al., "Effectiveness of an herbal preparation containing echinacea, propolis, and vitamin C in preventing respiratory tract infections in children: a randomized, double-blind, placebo-controlled, multicenter study," *Arch Pediatr Adolesc Med*, 2004; 158(3): 217–21.

4 Linde, K. et al., "Echinacea for preventing and treating the common cold," *Cochrane Database of Systematic Reviews*, 2006; (1): CD000530.

5 Shah S.A., S. Sander., C.M. White, M. Rinaldi, and C.I. Coleman, "Evaluation of echinacca for the prevention and treatment of the common cold: a meta-analysis," *Lancet Infectious Diseases*, 2007; 7: 473–80.

6 Karsch-Völk, M. et al., "Echinacea for preventing and treating the common cold," *Cochrane Database of Systematic Reviews*, Feb 2014; 20; 2: CD000530.

7 Turner, R.B. et al., "An evaluation of *Echinacea angustifolia* in experimental rhinovirus infections," *NEJM*, 2005; 353(4): 341–48.

8 Yale, S.H. and K. Liu, "Echinacea purpurea therapy for the treatment of the common cold: a randomized, double-blind, placebo-controlled clinical trial," *Arch Intern Med*, 2004; 164(11): 1237–41.

9 Taylor, J.A. et al., "Efficacy and safety of Echinacea in treating upper respiratory tract infections in children: a randomized controlled trial," *JAMA*, 2003; 290(21): 2824–30.

10 Barrett, B.P. et al., "Treatment of the common cold with unrefined Echinacea: a randomized, double-blind, placebo-controlled trial," *Annals of Internal Medicine*, 2002; 137(12): 939–46.

11 Caruso, T.J. and J.M. Gwaltney, Jr. "Treatment of the common cold with Echinacea: a structured review," *Clinical Infectious Diseases*, 2005; 40(6): 807–10.

Chapter 3: Ginger for Nausea and Vomiting and Menstrual Pain

1 Kew Gardens, *Exploring Plant Cultures*. Retrieved November 27, 2012, from: www.kew.org/plant-cultures/plants/ginger_history.html.

2 Ernst, E. and M.H. Pittler, "Efficacy of ginger for nausea and vomiting: a systemic review of randomized clinical trials," *British Journal of Anaesthesia*, 2000; 84/3: 367–71.

3 Borelli, F. et al., "Effectiveness and safety of ginger in the treatment of pregnancy-induced nausea and vomiting," *Obstet Gynecol Surv*, 2005; 105(4): 849–56.

4 http://sogc.org/guidelines/the-management-of-nausea-vomiting-of-pregnancy.

5 Chaiyukunapruk, N. et al., "The efficacy of ginger for the prevention of postoperative nausea and vomiting: a meta-analysis," *Am J Obstet Gynecol*, 2006; 194: 95–99.

6 Nanthakomon, T. and D. Pongrojpaw, "The efficacy of ginger in prevention of postoperative nausea and vomiting after major gynecologic surgery," *J Med Assoc Thai*, Oct 2006; 89; Suppl 4: S130–36.

7 Eberhart, L.H. et al., "Ginger does not prevent postoperative nausea and vomiting after laparoscopic surgery," *Anesth Analg*, 2003; 96(4): 995–98.

8 Hunt, R. et al., "Aromatherapy as treatment for postoperative nausea: a randomized trial," *Anesth Analg*, 2012.

9 Ryan, J. L. et al., "Ginger for chemotherapy-related nausea in cancer patients: A URCC CCOP randomized, double-blind, placebo-controlled clinical trial of 644 cancer patients," *J Clin Oncol*, 2009; 27: 15s (suppl; abstr 9511).

10 Ozgoli, G. et al., "Comparison of effects of ginger, mefenamic acid, and ibuprofen on pain in women with primary dysmenorrhea," *Journal of Alternative & Complementary Medicine*, Feb 2009; 15(2): 129–32.

11 Rahnama, P. et al., "Effect of Zingiber officinale R. rhizomes (ginger) on pain relief in primary dysmenorrhea: a placebo randomized trial," *BMC Complementary and Alternative Medicine*, Jul 10, 2012; 12(1): 92.

Chapter 4: Black Cohosh for Menopausal Symptoms

1 Lloyd, J.U. and C.G. Lloyd, *Drugs and Medicines of North America*, 2 vols. (Cincinnati: J.U. & C.G. Lloyd, 1884–85). Retrieved November 21, 2012, from: www.stevenfoster.com/education/monograph/bkcohosh.html.

2 "Black cohosh: a literature review," *Herbal Gram*, 1999; 45: 35–50. American Botanical Council. Retrieved November 21, 2012, from: http://cms.herbalgram .org/herbalgram/issue45/article2659.html.

3 Borrelli, F. and E. Ernst, "Black cohosh (Cimicifuga racemosa) for menopausal symptoms: a systematic review of its efficacy," *Pharmacological Research*, 2008; 58(1): 8–146.

4 Leach M.J., Moore V., "Black cohosh (Cimicifuga spp.) for menopausal symptoms," *Cochrane Database of Systematic Reviews*, 2012 Sep 12; 9: CD007244.

5 Wuttke, W. et al., "The non-estrogenic alternative for the treatment of climacteric complaints: black cohosh (*Cimicifuga* or *Actaea racemosa*)." *J Steroid Biochem Mol Biol*, Jan 2014: (139) 302–10.

6 Beer, A.M. et al., "Efficacy of black cohosh (*Cimicifuga racemosa*) medicines for treatment of menopausal symptoms—comments on major statements of the Cochrane Collaboration report 2012 black cohosh (*Cimicifuga spp.*) for menopausal symptoms (review)." *Gynecol Endocrinol*, Dec 2013: 29(12): 1022–5.

7 Pockaj, B.A. et al., "Pilot evaluation of black cohosh for the treatment of hot flashes in women," *Cancer Investig*, 2004; 22(4): 515–21.

8 Bodinet, C. "Influence of Cimicifuga racemosa on the proliferation of estrogen receptor-positive human breast cancer cells," *Breast Cancer Res Treat*, 2002; 76(1): 1–10.

9 "Update on black cohosh for hot flashes," *Harvard Women's Health Watch*, 2004; 11: 2–3.

Chapter 5: Red Clover for Menopausal Symptoms

1 Yildiz, F., *Phytoestrogens in Functional Foods* (Boca Raton: CRC Press, 2006): 3–5, 210–11.

2 Johnson, I. and G. Williamson (eds.), *Phytochemical Functional Foods* (Boca Raton: CRC Press, 2003): 66–68.

3 Lethaby, A. et al., "Phytoestrogens for vasomotor menopausal symptoms," *Cochrane Database of Systematic Reviews*, 2007; Issue 4. Art. No: CD001395.

4 Hidalgo, L.A. et al., "The effect of red clover isoflavones on menopausal symptoms, lipids and vaginal cytology in menopausal women: a randomized, double-blind, placebo-controlled study," *Gynecological Endocrinology*, 2005; 21(5): 257–64.

5 Howes, L.G. et al., "Isoflavone therapy for menopausal flashes: a systematic review and meta-analysis," *Maturitas*, 2006; 55: 203–11.

6 Coon, J.T. et al., "Trifolium pratense isoflavones in the treatment of menopausal hot flushes: a systematic review and meta-analysis," *Phytomedicine*, 2007; 14(2–3): 153–59.

7 Van de Weijer, P.H. and R. Barentsen, "Isoflavones from red clover (Promensil) significantly reduce menopausal hot flush symptoms compared with placebo," *Maturitas*, 2002; 42(3): 187–93.

8 Lipovac, M. et al., "The effect of red clover isoflavone supplementation over vasomotor and menopausal symptoms in postmenopausal women," *Gynecological Endocrinology*, 2011; 28(3): 203–7.

9 Lipovac, M. et al., "Improvement of postmenopausal depressive and anxiety symptoms after treatment with isoflavones derived from red clover extracts," *Maturitas*, 2010; 65(3): 258–61.

10 Wu, Q. et al., "Determination of isoflavones in red clover and related species by high-performance liquid chromatography combined with ultraviolet and mass spectrometric detection," *Journal of Chromatography A*, 2003; 1016: 195–209.

11 Shu, X.O. "Soy Food Consumption and Breast Cancer Prognosis: Review of the Epidemiologic Data," presented at the Symposium on Evaluating the Efficacy and Safety of Isoflavones for Postmenopausal Women, Council for Responsible Nutrition; Milan, May 13–14, 2009.

12 Howes, J.B. et al., "Effects of dietary supplementation with isoflavones from red clover on ambulatory blood pressure and endothelial function in postmenopausal type 2 diabetes," *Diabetes Obes Metab*, 2003; 5(5): 325–32.

Chapter 6: Ginseng for Whole Body Health

1 Grafton, E., "The history, the mystery of ginseng," *West Virginia Wildlife Magazine*, South Charleston: West Virginia Division of Natural Resources; (2) Summer 2002. Retrieved December 4, 2012, from: www.wvdnr.gov/wildlife/magazine/archive/02summer/the_history_the_mystery_of_ginseng.shtm.

2 USDA Natural Resources Conservation Service, *Plant Guide: American Ginseng*, 2003.

3 Stuart. M., ed., *Encyclopedia of Herbs and Herbalism* (London: Orbis Publishing, 1979).

4 Grafton, E., 2002.

5 Sumner, J., *Natural History of Medicinal Plants* (Portland: Timber Press, 2000): 191.

6 Grafton, E., 2002.

7 Carrol, C. and D. Apsley, *Growing American Ginseng in Ohio: An Introduction.* (Columbus: The Ohio State University; EFS F-56-04, 2004).

8 Kitts, D. and C. Hu, "Efficacy and safety of Ginseng," *Public Health Nutrition*, 2000; 3(4A): 473–85.

9 Subhasree Ashok Nag et al., "Ginsenosides as anticancer agents: in vitro and in vivo activities, structure–activity relationships, and molecular mechanisms of action," *Front Pharmacol*, 2012; 3: 25.

10 Vuksan, V. et al., "American ginseng reduces postprandial glycemia in non-diabetic and diabetic subjects," *Arch Intern Med*, 2000; 160: 1009–13.

11 Vuksan V. et al., "American ginseng improves glycemia in individuals with normal glucose tolerance: Effect of dose and time escalation," *Journal of the American College of Nutrition*, 2000; 19(6): 738–44.

12 Vuksan V. et al., "Similar postprandial glycemic reductions with escalation of dose and administration time of American ginseng in type 2 diabetes," *Diabetes Care*, 2000; 23(9):1221–26.

13 "Mayo Clinic-led study finds Ginseng fights fatigue in cancer patients," Retrieved December 6, 2012, from: www.mayoclinic.org/news2012-rst/6907.html.

14 Predy, G.N. et al., "Efficacy of an extract of North American ginseng containing poly-furanosyl-pyranosyl-saccharides for preventing upper respiratory tract infections: a randomized controlled trial," *CMAJ*, 2005; 173(9): 1051–2.

15 McElhaney, J.E., A. E. Simor, S. McNeil et al., "Efficacy and safety of CVT-E002, a proprietary extract of Panax quinquefolius in the prevention of respiratory infections in influenza-vaccinated community-dwelling adults: a multicenter, randomized, double-blind, and placebo-controlled trial," *Influenza Res Treat*, 2011; article ID 759051.

16 McElhaney, J.E. et al., "A placebo-controlled trial of a proprietary extract of North American ginseng (CVT-E002) to prevent acute respiratory illness in institutionalized older adults," *J Am Geriatr Soc.* Jan 2004; 52(1): 13–19.

17 Choi, J., T.H. Kim, T.Y. Choi, and M.S. Lee, "Ginseng for health care: a systematic review of randomized controlled trials in Korean literature," *PLoS One.* 2013; 8(4): e59978. doi: 10.1371/journal.pone.0059978. Epub Apr 1, 2013.

18 Kolber, M.R., and J. McCormack, "COLD FX[R] evidence: consistently reported inconsistently," in: *Tools for Practice* [newsletter]. Edmonton (AB): Alberta College of Family Physicians; 2011.

19 Seida, J.K., T. Durec, and S. Kuhle, "North American (Panax quinquefolius) and Asian Ginseng (Panax ginseng) preparations for prevention of the common cold in healthy adults: a systematic review," *Evid Based Complement Alternat Med* 2011: 282151.

20 Allan, M.G. and B. Arroll, "Prevention and treatment of the common cold: making sense of the evidence," *CMAJ*, 186.3 (Feb 18, 2014): 190.

21 Nguyen, A. and V. Slavik, "Cold FX," *Can Fam Phys*, 2007; 53(3): 481–82.

Chapter 7: Feverfew for Migraine

1 Murphy, J.J. et al., "Randomized double-blind placebo controlled trial of feverfew in migraine prevention," *Lancet*, 1988; i: 189–92.

2 Johnson, E.S. et al., "Efficacy of feverfew as prophylactic treatment of migraine," *BMJ*, 1985; 291: 569–73.

3 Cady, R.K. et al., "A double-blind placebo-controlled pilot study of sublingual feverfew and ginger (LipiGesic) in the treatment of migraine," *Headache*, 2011; 51(7): 1078–86.

4 Pittler, M.H. and E. Ernst, "Feverfew for preventing migraine," *Cochrane Database of Systematic Reviews*, 2004; (1): CD002286.

5 Pfaffentreath, V. et al., "The efficacy and safety of *Tanacetum parthenium* (feverfew) in migraine prophylaxis—a double-blind, multicentre, randomized placebo-controlled dose-response study," *Cephalalgia*, 2002; 22: 523–32.

6 Diener, H.C. et al., "Efficacy and safety of 6.25 mg tid feverfew CO2 extract (MIG-99) in migraine prevention—a randomized, double-blind, multicenter, placebo-controlled study," *Cephalalgia*, 2005; 25: 1031–41.

7 Heptinstall, S. et al., "Parthenolide content and bioactivity of feverfew (*Tanacetum parthenium* L.) (Schultz-Bip.). Estimation of commercial and authenticated feverfew products," *J Pharm Pharmacol*, 1992; 44(5): 391–95.

Chapter 8: Ginkgo Biloba for Dementia, Vascular Disorders, and Stroke

1 "Introduction to the gingkoales," Berkeley, University of California Museum of Palentology; Retrieved November 17, 2012, from www.ucmp.berkeley.edu/seedplants/ginkgoales/gonkgo.html.

2 "Ginkgoes," Berkeley, University of California Museum of Palentology; Retrieved November 16, 2012, from www.ucmp.berkeley.edu/IB181/VPL/CorCon/CorCon2.html.

3 Le Bars, P.L. et al., "Placebo-controlled, double-blind, randomized trial of extract of Gingko Biloba for dementia," *JAMA*, 1997; 278: 1327–32.

4 Le Bars, P.L. et al., "A 26-week analysis of a double-blind, placebo-controlled trial of the ginkgo biloba extract EGb 761 in dementia," *Dementia & Geriatric Cognitive Disorders*, 2000; 11(4): 230–37.

5 Gavrilova, S.I., U.W. Preuss, J.W. Wong, R. Hoerr, R. Kaschel, and N. Bachinskaya, "The GIMCIPlus Study Group. Efficacy and safety of Ginkgo biloba extract EGb 761® in mild cognitive impairment with neuropsychiatric symptoms: a randomized, placebo-controlled, double-blind, multi-center trial," *Int J Geriatr Psychiatry*, Mar 16, 2014.

6 Ihl, R, "Effects of Ginkgo biloba extract EGb 761® in dementia with neuropsychiatric features: review of recently completed randomised, controlled trials," *Int J Psychiatry Clin Pract.* Nov 2013; 17 Suppl 1:8–14.

7 "Peripheral Artery Occlusive Disease," Brigham and Women's Hospital, Harvard Medical School, Boston. Retrieved November 19, 2012, from: http://brighamandwomens.org/Departments_and_Services/surgery/services/vascularsurgery/Services/PeripheralVascular.aspx.

8 Pittler, M.H. and E. Ernst, "Ginkgo biloba extract for the treatment of intermittent claudication: a meta-analysis of randomized trials," *American Journal of Medicine*, 2000; 108(4): 341–42.

9 Schweizer, J. and C. Hautmann, "Comparison of two dosages of ginkgo biloba extract EGb 761 in patients with peripheral arterial occlusive disease Fontaine's stage IIb: a randomised, double-blind, multicentric clinical trial," *Arzneimittel-Forschung*, 1999; 49(11): 900–904.

10 Zeng, X. et al., "*Ginkgo biloba* for acute ischaemic stroke," *Cochrane Database of Systematic Reviews*, 2005; (4): CD003691.

11 Kleijnen, J. et al., "Gingko Biloba," *Lancet*, 1992; 340: 1136–39.

Chapter 9: Horse Chestnut Seed Extract for Veins

1 Fleming, V., "America's historic horse chestnut tree," *D.A.R. Magazine*, 1926; Retrieved December 12, 2012, from: http://historicalwoods.com/storage/HorseChestnutTree%20pdf.pdf.

2 "Anne Frank's beautiful tree felled by Amsterdam storm," *The Scotsman,* Aug 2010; Retrieved December 12, 2012, from: http://news.scotsman.com/news/Anne-Frank39s-39beautiful39-tree-felled.6490345.jp.

3 Pittler, M.H. and E. Ernst, "Horse chestnut seed extract for chronic venous insufficiency," *Cochrane Database of Systematic Reviews,* 2006; (1): CD003230.

4 Tiffany, N. et al., "Horse chestnut: a multidisciplinary clinical review," *J Herb Pharmacother,* 2002; 2(1): 71–85.

5 Siebert, U. et al., "Efficacy, routine effectiveness, and safety of horse chestnut seed extract in the treatment of chronic venous insufficiency: a meta-analysis of randomized controlled trials and large observational studies," *Int Angiol,* 2002; 21(4): 305–15.

6 "Horse Chestnut," U.S. National Library of Medicine, National Institutes of Health. *Medline Plus.* Retrieved December 12, 2012, from: www.nlm.nih.gov/medlineplus/druginfo/natural/1055.html.

Chapter 10: Tea Tree Oil for Infections

1 Kamenev, M., "Top 10 Aboriginal bush medicines," *Australian Geographic,* 2011; Retrieved November 29, 2012, from: www.australiangeographic.com.au/journal/view-image.htm?gid=8346.

2 "Australian Tea Tree Oil," *ATTIA,* 2010; Retrieved November 28, 2012, from: www.attia.org.au/teatree_about.php.

3 "Oil from tea-tree," *Central Queensland Herald,* May 31, 1934; Rockhampton, Qld.: 54.

4 Syed, T.A. et al., "Treatment of toenail onychomycosis with 2% butenafine and 5% *Melaleuca alternifolia* (tea tree) oil in cream," *Trop Med Int Health,* 1999; 4(4): 284–87.

5 Buck, D.S. et al., "Comparison of two topical preparations for the treatment of oncychomycosis: *Melaleuca alternifolia* and clotrimazole," *J Fam Prac,* 1994; 38: 601–5.

6 Groppo, F.C. et al., "Antimicrobial activity of garlic, tea tree oil, and chlorhexidine against oral microorganisms," *Int Dent J,* 2002; 52(6): 433–37.

7 Jandourek, A. et al., "Efficacy of melaleuca oral solution for the treatment of fluconazole refractory oral candidiasis in AIDS patients," *AIDS,* 1998; 12(9): 1033–37.

8 Vazquez, J.A. and A.A. Zawawi, "Efficacy of alcohol-based and alcohol-free melaleuca oral solution for the treatment of fluconazole-refractory oropharyngeal candidiasis in patients with AIDS," *HIV Clinical Trials,* 2002; 3(5): 379–85.

9 Satchell, A.C. et al., "Treatment of interdigital tinea pedis with 25% and 50% tea tree oil solution: a randomized, placebo-controlled, blinded study," *Australasian Journal of Dermatology,* 2002; 43: 175–78.

10 "Tea Tree Oil," *U.S. National Library of Medicine,* 2012; Retrieved December 2, 2012, from: www.nlm.nih.gov/medlineplus/druginfo/natural/113.html.

11 "Tea Tree Oil Treatments and Side Effects," *American Cancer Society,* 2008; Retrieved November 28, 2012, from: www.cancer.org/treatment/treatmentsandsideeffects/complementaryandalternativemedicine/herbsvitaminsandminerals/tea-tree-oil.

12 "Anticancer activity of tea tree oil," *Rural Industries Research and Development Corporation*, Kingston, ACT, Australia, 2010; RIRDC Publication No.: 10/060.

Chapter 11: Herbal Treatment for Back Pain

1 "*Harpagophytum procumbens* (Devil's claw)," *Alternative Medicine Review*, 2008; 13(3): 248–52. Retrieved December 28, 2012, from: www.altmedrev.com/publications/13/3/248.pdf.

2 "Plants & Fungi, *Harpagophytum procumbens* (devil's claw)," *Kew Royal Botanic Gardens*. Retrieved December 16, 2012, from: www.kew.org/plants-fungi/Harpagophytum-procumbens.htm.

3 Ibid.

4 Gagnier, J.J. et al., "Herbal medicine for low back pain: a Cochrane review," *Spine*, 2007; 32(1): 82–92.

5 Chrubasik, S. et al., "Effectiveness of Harpagophytum extract WS1531 in the treatment of exacerbation of low back pain: a randomized, placebo-controlled, double blind study," *Eur J Anaesthesiol*, 1999; 16: 118–29.

6 Chrubasik, S. et al., "Effectiveness of Harpagophytum procumbens in the treatment of acute low back pain," *Phytomedicine*, 1996; 3: 1–10.

7 WebMD Network, "Devil's Claw Side Effects," emedicine health, Retrieved December 18, 2012, from: www.emedicinehealth.com/drug-devils_claw/article_em.htm.

8 Stuart, M., (ed.) *Encyclopedia of Herbs and Herbalism* (London: Orbis Publishing, 1979).

9 Mahdi, J.G. et al., "The historical analysis of aspirin discovery, its relation to the willow tree and antiproliferative and anticancer potential," *Cell Proliferation*, 2006; 39: 147–55.

10 Chrubasik, S. et al., "Treatment of low back pain exacerbations with willow bark extract: a randomized double-blind study," *American Journal of Medicine*, 2000; 109: 9–14.

11 Chrubasik, S. et al., "A randomized double-blind pilot study comparing Dolotefin and Vioxx in the treatment of low back pain," *Rheumatology*, 2003; 42: 141–48.

12 AISLE7, "Cayenne," *Tallahassee Memorial Hospital*, 2012; Retrieved December 18, 2012, from: www.tmh.org/body.cfm?xyzpdqabc=0&id=223&action=detail&AEProductID=HW_CAM&AEArticleID=hn-2065009.

13 Keitel, W. et al., "Capsicum pain plaster in chronic non-specific low back pain," *Arzneimittel-forschung*, 2001; 51: 896–903.

14 Frerick, H. et al., "Topical treatment of chronic low back pain with a Capsicum plaster," *Pain*, 2003; 106: 59–64.

Chapter 12: Problems with Herbs

1 Farnsworth, N. et al., "Medicinal plants in therapy," *Bulletin of WHO*, 1985; 63(6): 965–81.

2 Saxe, T., "Toxicity of medicinal herbal preparations," *Am Fam Phys*, 1987; 35: 135–42.

3 Ng, T.H.K. et al., "Encephalopathy and neuropathy following ingestion of a Chinese herbal broth containing podophyllin," *J Neurol Sci*, 1991; 101: 107–13.

4 Lindberg, J., "Kola, ginseng and mislabeled herbs," *JAMA*, 1977; 237: 24.

5 Fox, D.W. et al., "Pyrrolizidine intoxication mimicking Reye syndrome," *J Pediatr*, 1978; 93: 980–82.

6 Tyler, V., "Herbal Medicine in America," *Planta Medica*, 1987; 1–3.

7 Chan, T.Y. et al., "Chinese herbal medicines revisited: a Hong Kong perspective," *Lancet*, 1993; 342. 1532–34.

8 Dupont, R.L. and S. Bogema, "Benzodiazepines in a health-catalog product," *JAMA*, 1990; 264: 695.

9 Tay, C.H. et al., "Arsenic poisoning from anti-asthmatic herbal preparations," *Med J Aust*, 1975; 2: 424–28.

10 Baker, D. et al., "Cadmium and lead exposure associates with pharmaceuticals imported from Asia-Texas," *MMWR*, 1989; 38: 612–14.

11 Goldman, J., "Chinese herbal medicine: camouflaged prescription antiinflammatory drugs, corticosteroids, and lead," *Arthritis and Rheumatism*, 1991; 34(9): 1207.

12 Ries, C. and M. Sahud, "Agranulocytosis caused by Chinese herbal medicines," *JAMA*, 1975; 231: 352–55.

13 Canadian Adverse Drug Reaction Monitoring Program, "Herbal preparations: potential toxicity," *CMAJ*, 1994; 151(1): 65.

14 Centers for Disease Control, "Folk remedy-associated lead poisoning in Hmong children—Minnesota," *MMWR*, 1983; 32: 555–56.

15 D'Alauro, F. et al., "Toxic metal contamination of folk remedy," *JAMA*, 1984; 252: 3127.

16 Centers for Disease Control, "Use of lead tetroxide as a folk remedy for gastrointestinal illness," *MMWR*, 1981; 30: 546–47.

17 Baer, R.D. and A. Ackerman, "Toxic Mexican folk remedies for the treatment of empacho," *J Ethnopharmacology*, 1988; 24: 31–39.

18 Levitt, C. et al., "Sources of lead poisoning," *JAMA*, 1984; 252: 3127–28.

19 Bose, A. et al., "Azarcon por empacho—another case of lead toxicity," *Pediatrics*, 1983; 72: 106–8.

20 Borins, M., "Traditional medicine of India," *Can Fam Phys*, 1987; 33: 1061–65.

21 CDC, "Lead poisoning associated death from Asian Indian folk remedies—Florida," *MMWR*, 1984; 33: 638–45.

22 Zayas, L.H. and P.O. Ozuah, "Mercury use in Espiritismo: a survey of botanicals," *Am J Pub Health*, 1996; 86: 111–12.

23 Pontifex, A. and A. Garg, "Lead poisoning from an Asian Indian folk remedy," *CMAJ*, 1985; 133: 1227–28.

24 Dunbabin, D. et al., "Lead poisoning from Indian herbal medicine (Ayurvedic)," *Med J Aust*, 1992; 157: 835–36.

25 Markowitz, S.B. et al., "Lead poisoning due to hai ge fen," *JAMA*, 1994; 271(12): 932–34.

26 Rosti, L. et al., "Toxic effects of a herbal tea mixture in two newborns," *Acta Paediatr*, 1994; 83: 683.

27 Sayre, J.W. and S. Kaymakcalan, "Cyanide poisoning from apricot seeds among children in central Turkey," *NEJM*, 1964; 270: 1113–15.

28 Bannister, B. et al., "Cardiac arrest due to licorice-induced hypokalemia," *BMJ*, 1977; 2: 738–39.

29 Segelman, A.B. et al., "Sassafras and herb tea: potential health hazards," *JAMA*, 1976; 236: 477.

30 Chan, T.K. et al., "Aconite poisoning following the ingestion of Chinese herbal medicines: a report of eight cases," *Aust NZ J Med*, 1993; 23: 268–71.

31 Vanherwehhem, J. et al., "Rapidly progressive interstitial renal fibrosis in young women: association with slimming regimen including Chinese herbs," *Lancet*, 1993; 341: 387–91.

32 Siegel, R., "Ginseng abuse syndrome," *JAMA*, 1979, 241: 1614.

33 Dubick, M., "Historical perspectives on the use of herbal preparations to promote health," *J Nutr*, 1986; 116: 1348–54.

34 Siegel, R.K., "Herbal intoxication," *JAMA*, 1976; 236: 473–76.

35 Michaels, E., "Canada lags in acceptance, regulation of herbal remedies," *CMAJ*, 1986; 135: 547–48.

36 Benner, M. and H.J. Lee, "Anaphylactic reaction to chamomile tea," *Allergy Clin Immunol*, 1973; 52: 307–8.

37 Casterline, C.L., "Allergy to chamomile tea," *JAMA*, 1980; 244: 330.

38 Mills, S., "Are herbs safe?," *Br J Phyto*, 1991; 2: 76–83.

39 Roitman, J., "Comfrey and liver damage," *Lancet*, 1981: 944.

40 Anderson, R., "Comfrey in the Chinese Materia Medica," *Asian Med Newsletter*, 1992; 2: 7–11.

41 Bach, N. et al., "Comfrey herb tea-induced hepatic veno-occlusive disease," *American Journal of Medicine*, 1989; 87: 97–98.

42 Larrey, D. et al., "Hepatitis after germander administration: another instance of herbal hepatotoxicity," *Annals of Internal Medicine*, 1992; 117: 129–32.

43 Harvey, J. and D.G. Colin-Jones, "Mistletoe hepatitis," *BMJ*, 1981; 282: 186–87.

44 Katz, M. and F. Saibil, "Herbal hepatitis: subacute hepatic necrosis secondary to chaparral leaf," *J Clin Gastro*, 1990; 12(2): 203–6.

45 Macgregor, F. et al., "Hepatotoxicity of herbal remedies," *BMJ*, 1989; 299: 1156–57.

46 Yeung, C.Y. et al., "Effect of a popular Chinese herb on neonatal bilirubin protein binding," *Biol Neonate*, 1990; 58: 98–103.

SECTION II: ACUPUNCTURE

1 Hyvarinen, J. and M. Karisson, "Low resistance skin points that may coincide with acupuncture loci," *Medical Biolog*, 1977; 55(2): 88–94.

2 Gunn, C.C. et al., "Acupuncture loci: a proposal for their classification according to their relationship to known neural structures," *Am J Chin Med*, 1976; 4(2): 183–95.

3 Melzack, R. et al., "Trigger points and acupuncture points for pain: correlations and implications," *Pain*, 1977; 3: 3–23.

4 Cheng, R.S.S. and B. Pomeranz, "Electroacupuncture analgesia is mediated by at least two pain-relieving mechanisms: endorphin and non-endorphin systems," *Life Sci*, 1979; 25(23): 1957–62.

5 Cheng, R. et al., "Electroacupuncture elevates blood cortisol levels in naive horses," *Int J Neurosci*, 1980; 10: 95–97.

6 Yi, C.C. et al., "A study of the release of H3-5-hydroxytryptamine from brain during acupuncture and morphine analgesia," *Sci.Sin*, 1977; 20: 113–24.

7 Langevin, H.M. "Connective Tissue: A body-wide signaling network?" *Medical Hypotheses* (2006) 66, 1074.

8 Zhang, Z-J. et al., "Neural Acupuncture Unit: A New Concept for Interpreting Effects and Mechanisms of Acupuncture," *Evid Based Complement Alternat Med* Volume 2012, Article ID 429412, 23 pages.

9 Zhi-Qi Zhao, "Neural mechanism underlying acupuncture analgesia," *Progress in Neurobiology* 85 (2008) 355–75.

10 Goldman, N., M. Chen, T. Fujita et al., "Adenosine A1 receptors mediate local anti-nociceptive effects of acupuncture," *Nature Neuroscience*, 2010; 13 (7): 883–88.

11 Cho, Z. H., S. C. Hwang, E. K. Wong, et al., "Neural substrates, experimental evidences and functional hypothesis of acupuncture mechanisms," *Acta Neurologica Scandinavica*, 2006; 113 (6): 370–77.

12 Kagitani, F., S. Uchida, and H. Hotta, "Afferent nerve fibers and acupuncture," *Autonomic Neuroscience*, 2010; 157 (1-2): 2–8.

13 Noguchi, E., "Acupuncture regulates gut motility and secretion via nerve reflexes," *Autonomic Neuroscience*, 2010; 156 (1-2): 15–18.

14 Lewith, G.T. and D. Machin, "On the evaluation of the clinical effects of acupuncture," *Pain*, 1983; 16: 111–27.

15 Richardson, P.H. and C. A. Vincent, "Acupuncture for the treatment of pain: a review of evaluative research," *Pain*, 1986; 24: 15–40.

16 Gunn, C.C. et al., "Dry needling of muscle motor points for chronic low back pain," *Pain*, 1986; 26: 277–90.

17 Christensen, P. et al., "Acupuncture and bronchial asthma," *Allergy*, 1984; 39(5): 379–85.

18 Dundee, J. et al., "Non-invasive stimulation of the P6 antiemetic acupuncture point in cancer chemotherapy," *J Royal Soc Med*, 1991; 84: 210–12.

19 Vickers, A.J. et al., "Acupuncture for chronic pain: individual patient data meta-analysis," *Arch Intern Med.* 2012; 172(19): 1444–53.

20 Xiao, L., B. Li, Y.H. Du, J. Xiong, and X. Gao, "Systematic evaluation of the randomized controlled trials about acupuncture and moxibustion treatment of allergic rhinitis," *Zhongguo Zhen Jiu*, 2009; 29 (6): 512–16.

21 Lee, S., M.H. Pittler, B.C. Shin, J.I. Kim, and E. Ernst, "Acupuncture for allergic rhinitis: a systematic review," *Annals of Allergy, Asthma and Immunology*, 2009; 102 (4): 269–79.

22 Brinkhaus, C., M. Witt, S. Jena, B. Liecker, K. Wegscheider, and S. N. Willich, "Acupuncture in patients with allergic rhinitis: a pragmatic randomized trial," *Annals of Allergy, Asthma and Immunology*, 2008; 101 (5): 535–43.

23 Zhang, Z. J., H.Y. Chen, K.C. Yip, R. Ng, and V.T. Wong, "The effectiveness and safety of acupuncture therapy in depressive disorders: systematic review and meta-analysis," *Journal of Affective Disorders*, 2010; 124 (1-2): 9–21.

24 Wu, J., A.S. Yeung, R. Schnyer, Y. Wang, and D. Mischoulon, "Acupuncture for depression: a review of clinical applications," *Can J Psychiatry*, July 2012; 57(7): 397–405.

25 Du, W.F., L. Yu, X.K.Yan, and F.C. Wang, "Meta-analysis on randomized controlled clinical trials of acupuncture and moxibustion on constipation," *Zhongguo Zhen Jiu*, January 2012; 32(1): 92–96.

26 Mu, J.P., H.G. Wu, Z.Q. Zhang, H.R. Liu, Y. Zhu, Z. Shi, and X.M. Wang, "Meta-analysis on acupuncture and moxibustion for treatment of ulcerative colitis," *Zhongguo Zhen Jiu*, September 2007; 27(9): 687–90.

Chapter 13: Acupuncture for Osteoarthritis of the Knee

1 Medical Advisory Secretariat, "Arthroscopic lavage and debridement for osteoarthritis of the knee: an evidence-based analysis," *Ontario Health Technology Assessment Series*, 2005; 5(12).
2 Gaw, A.C. et al., "Efficacy of acupuncture on osteoarthritic pain. A controlled, double-blind study," *NEJM*, 1975; 293: 375-78.
3 Takeda, W. and J. Wessel, "Acupuncture for the treatment of pain of osteoarthritic knees," *Arthritis Care Res*, 1994; 7: 118–22.
4 Berman, B.M. et al., "Effectiveness of acupuncture as adjunctive therapy in osteoarthritis of the knee: a randomized, controlled trial," *Annals of Internal Medicine*, 2004; 141(12): 901–10.
5 White, A. et al., "Acupuncture treatment for chronic knee pain: a systematic review," *Rheumatology* (Oxford), 2007; 46(3): 384–90.

Chapter 14: Acupuncture for Nausea and Vomiting

1 Lee, A. and L.T.Y. Fan, "Stimulation of the wrist acupuncture point P6 for preventing postoperative nausea and vomiting," *Cochrane Database of Systematic Reviews*, 2009; (2): CD003281.
2 Suh, E.E., "The effects of P6 acupressure and nurse-provided counseling on chemotherapy-induced nausea and vomiting in patients with breast cancer," *Oncol Nurs Forum*, 2012; 39(1): E1–9.
3 Roscoe, J.A. et al., "Acupressure bands are effective in reducing radiation therapy-related nausea," *Journal of Pain and Symptom Management*, 38(3): 381–89.
4 Yoo, S.S. et al., "Modulation of cerebellar activities by acupuncture stimulation: evidence from fMRI study," *Neuroimage*, 2004; 22(2): 932–40.
5 Lee, A. and M. Done, "Stimulation of the wrist acupuncture point P6 for preventing postoperative nausea and vomiting," *Cochrane Database of Systematic Reviews*, 2004; (3): CD003281.
6 Alkaissi, A. et al., "P6 acupressure may relieve nausea and vomiting after gynecological surgery: an effectiveness study in 410 women," *Can J Anaesth*, 2002; 49(10): 1034–39.
7 Wang, Shu-Ming and N.K. Zeev, "P6 acupoint injections are as effective as droperidol in controlling early postoperative nausea and vomiting in children," *Anesthesiology*, 2002; 97: 359–66.
8 Rosen, T. et al., "A randomized controlled trial of nerve stimulation for relief of nausea and vomiting in pregnancy," *Obstet Gynecol*, 2003; 102(1): 129–35.
9 Miller, K.E. and E.R. Muth, "Efficacy of acupressure and acustimulation bands for the prevention of motion sickness," *Aviat Space Environ Med*, 2004; 75: 227–34.
10 Josefson, A. and M. Kreuter, "Acupuncture to reduce nausea during chemotherapy treatment of rheumatic diseases," *Rheumatology* (Oxford), 2003; 42(10): 1149–54.
11 Lu, D.P. et al., "Acupuncture/acupressure to treat gagging dental patients: a clinical study of anti-gagging effects," *Gen Dent*, 2000; 48(4): 446–52.

Chapter 15: Acupuncture for Tennis Elbow

1 Fink, M. et al., "Acupuncture in chronic epicondylitis: a randomized controlled trial," *Rheumatology* (Oxford), 2002; 41(2): 205–9.
2 Fink, M. et al., "Chronic epicondylitis: effects of real and sham acupuncture treatment: a randomised controlled patient- and examiner-blinded long-term trial," *Forsch Komplementarmed Klass Naturheilkd*, 2002; 9(4): 210–15.
3 Green, S. et al., "Acupuncture for lateral elbow pain," *Cochrane Database of Systematic Reviews*, 2002; (1): CD003527.
4 Trinh, K.V. et al., "Acupuncture for the alleviation of lateral epicondyle pain: a systematic review," *Rheumatology*, 2004; 43(9): 1085–90.

Chapter 16: Acupuncture for Neck Pain

1 White, A.R. and E. Ernst, "A systematic review of randomized controlled trials of acupuncture for neck pain," *Rheumatology* (Oxford), 1999; 38(2): 143–47.
2 Trinh, K. et al., Cervical Overview Group, "Acupuncture for neck disorders," *Cochrane Database of Systematic Reviews*, 2006; (3): CD004870.
3 Vas, J. et al., "Efficacy and safety of acupuncture for chronic uncomplicated neck pain: a randomized controlled study," *Pain*, 2006; 126(1-3): 245–55.
4 Witt, C.M. et al., "Acupuncture for patients with chronic neck pain," *Pain*, 2006; 125(1-2): 98–106.
5 Willich, S.N. et al., "Cost-effectiveness of acupuncture treatment in patients with chronic neck pain," *Pain*, 2006; 125(1-2): 107–13.

Chapter 17: Acupuncture for Headache

1 Melchart, D. et al., "Acupuncture for idiopathic headache," *Cochrane Database of Systematic Reviews*, 2001; (1): CD001218.
2 Manias, P. et al., "Acupuncture in headache: a critical review," *Clin J Pain*, 2000; 16(4): 334–39.
3 Griggs, C. and J. Jensen, "Effectiveness of acupuncture for migraine: critical literature review," *Journal of Advanced Nursing*, 2006; 54(4): 491–501.
4 Streng, A. et al., "Effectiveness and tolerability of acupuncture compared with metoprolol in migraine prophylaxis," *Headache*, 2006; 46(10): 1492–1502.
5 Coeytaux, R.R. et al., "A randomized, controlled trial of acupuncture for chronic daily headache," *Headache*, 2005; 45: 1113–23.
6 Vickers, A. et al., "Acupuncture for chronic headache in primary care: large, pragmatic, randomised trial," *BMJ*, 2004; 328: 744.
7 Allais, G., "Acupuncture in the prophylactic treatment of migraine without aura: a comparison with flunarizine," *Headache*, 2002; 42: 855–61.
8 Ebneshahidi, N.S. et al., "The effects of laser acupuncture on chronic tension headache—a randomised controlled trial," *Acupunct Med*, 2005; 23(1): 13–18.
9 Linde, K. et al., "Acupuncture for patients with migraine: a randomized controlled trial," *JAMA*, 2005; 293(17): 2118–25.

SECTION III: PHYSICAL THERAPIES

Chapter 18: Yoga for Back Pain

1 Saper, R. et al., "Prevalence and patterns of adult yoga use in the United States: results of a national survey," *Altern Ther Health Med*, 2004; 10(2): 44–49.

2 Chaya, M. et al., "The effect of long term combined yoga practice on the basal metabolic rate of healthy adults," *BMC Complementary and Alternative Medicine*, 2006; 6: 28.

3 Williams, K. et al., "Effect of Iyengar yoga therapy for chronic low back pain," *Pain*, 2005; 115(1–2): 107–17.

4 Sherman, K. et al., "Comparing yoga, exercise, and a self-care book for chronic low back pain: A randomized, controlled trial," *Annals of Internal Medicine*, 2005; 143(12): 849–56.

5 Sherman, K. et al., "A randomized trial comparing yoga, stretching, and a self-care book for chronic low back pain," *Arch Intern Med*, 2011; 171(22): 2019–26.

Chapter 19: Manipulation for Back Pain

1 Cyriax, J., *Textbook of Orthopaedic Medicine: Treatment by Manipulation, Massage and Injection* (London: Balliere Tindall, 1978).

2 Meade, T.W. et al., "Low back pain of mechanical origin: randomized comparison of chiropractic and hospital outpatient treatment," *BMJ*, 1990; 300: 1431–37.

3 Hass, M., "A practice-based study of patients with acute and chronic low back pain attending primary care and chiropractic physicians: two week to 48-month follow-up," *J Manip Physiol Ther*, 2004; 27(3): 160–69.

4 Hertzman-Miller et al., "Comparing the satisfaction of low back pain patients randomized to receive medical or chiropractic care: results from the UCLA low-back pain study," *Am J Pub Health*, 2002; 92(10): 1628–33.

5 Hoiriis, K.T. et al., "A randomized clinical trial comparing chiropractic adjustments to muscle relaxants for subacute low back pain," *J Manip Physiol Ther*, 2004; 27(6): 388–98.

6 Giles, L.G. and R. Muller, "Chronic spinal pain: a randomized clinical trial comparing medication, acupuncture, and spinal manipulation," *Spine*, 2003; 28(14): 1490–1503.

7 Koes, B.W. et al., "Spinal manipulation and mobilization for back and neck pain: an indexed review," *BMJ*, 1991; 303: 1298–1303.

8 Ernst, E., "Manual therapies for pain control: chiropractic and massage," *Clin J Pain*, 2004; 20(1): 8–12.

9 Rubinstein, S.M., C.B. Terwee, W.J. Assendelft, M.R. de Boer, and M.W. van Tulder, "Spinal manipulative therapy for acute low-back pain," *Cochrane Database of Systematic Reviews*, September 12, 2012; 9: CD008880.

10 Koes, B.W. et al., "Clinical guidelines for the management of low back pain in primary care: an international comparison," *Spine*, 2002; 27(14): 1590.

11 Koes, B.W. et al., "An updated overview of clinical guidelines for the management of non-specific back pain in primary care," *Eur Spine J*, 2010; 19(12): 2075–94.

12 S. Dagenais, A.C. Tricco, and S. Haldeman, "Synthesis of recommendations for the assessment and management of low back pain from recent clinical practice guidelines," *Spine*, J 2010; 10:514–29.

13 Williams, L.S., and J. Biller, "Vertebrobasilar dissection and cervical spine manipulation: a complex pain in the neck," *Neurology*, 2003; 60: 1408–9, and Smith, W.S. et al., "Spinal manipulative therapy is an independent risk factor for vertebral artery dissection," *Neurology*, 2003; 60: 1424–28.

14 Rothwell, D.M. et al., "Chiropractic manipulation and stroke: a population-based case-control study," *Stroke*, 2001; 32: 1054–60.

15 Cassidy J.D., E. Boyle, P. Côté, Y. He, S. Hogg-Johnson, F.L. Silver, and S.J. Bondy," *J Manip Physiol Ther*, 2009; 32(2 Suppl): S201–8.

16 Oliphant, D., "Safety of spinal manipulation in the treatment of lumbar disk herniations: a systematic review and risk assessment," *J Manip Physiol Ther*, 2004; 27(3): 197–210.

17 Coyer, A.B. and I.H. Curwen, "Low back pain treated by manipulation—a controlled series," *BMJ*, 1955; 1(4915): 705–7.

Chapter 20: Manipulation for Asthma

1 Fowler, C.T., "Human health impacts of forest fires in the southern United States: a literature review," *JEA*, 2003; 7: 39–63.

2 Mayo Clinic, "Secondhand smoke: Avoid dangers in the air," retrieved February 27, 2013 from: www.mayoclinic.com/health/second-handsmoke/CC00023.

3 Sibbald, B. et al., "A family study of the genetic basis of asthma and wheezy bronchitis," *Archive of Diseases in Childhood*, 1980; 55: 254–57.

4 Balon, J. et al., "A randomized controlled trial of chiropractic manipulation as an adjunctive treatment for childhood asthma," *NEJM*, 1998; 339: 1013–20.

5 Nielsen, N.H. et al., "Chronic asthma and chiropractic spinal manipulation: a randomized clinical trial," *Clin Exp Allergy*, 1995; 25: 80–88.

6 Bronfort, G. et al., "Chronic pediatric asthma and chiropractic spinal manipulation: A prospective clinical series and randomized clinical pilot study," *J Manip Physiol Ther*, 2001; 24: 369–77.

7 Gibbs, A., "Chiropractic co-management of medically treated asthma," *Clinical Chiropractic*, 2005; 8: 140–44.

8 Hviid, C., "A comparison of the effect of chiropractic treatment on respiratory function in patients with respiratory distress symptoms and patients without," *Bull Eur Chiropractors Union*, 1978; 26: 14–34.

9 Jamison, J.R. et al., "Asthma in a chiropractic clinic: a pilot study," *J Aust Chiropractors Assoc*, 1986; 16: 137–43.

10 Ernst, E., "Spinal manipulation for asthma: a systematic review of randomised clinical trials," *Respiratory Medicine*, 2009; 103(12): 1791–95.

Chapter 21: Massage Therapy

1 Jäkel A, and P. von Hauenschild, "A systematic review to evaluate the clinical benefits of craniosacral therapy," *Complement Ther Med*, Dec 2012; 20 (6): 456–65.

2 Wolsko, P. et al., "Patterns and perceptions of care of back and neck pain," *Spine*, 2003; 28(3): 293–98.

3 Field T., "Massage Therapy Effects," *American Psychologist*, 1998; 53(12): 1270–81.

4 Moyer, C. et al., "A meta-analysis of massage therapy research," *Psychological Bulletin*, 2004; 130(1): 3–18.

5 Dunn, C. et al., "Sensing an improvement: an experimental study to evaluate the use of aromatherapy, massage, and periods of rest in an intensive care unit," *Journal of Advanced Nursing*, 1995; 21: 34–40.

6 Field, T. et al., "Massage reduces anxiety in child and adolescent psychiatric patients," *J Am Acad Child Adolesc Psychiatry*, 1992; 31: 125–31.

7 Preyde, M., "Effectiveness of massage therapy for subacute low-back pain: a randomized controlled trial," *CMAJ*, 2000; 162(13): 1815–20.

8 Netchanok S., M. Wendy, C. Marie, and O. Siobhan, "The effectiveness of Swedish massage and traditional Thai massage in treating chronic low back pain: a review of the literature," *Complement Ther Clin Pract,* Nov 2012; 18(4): 227–34.

9 Furlan, A.D. et al., "Massage for low-back pain: A updated systematic review within the framework of the Cochrane Collaboration Back Review Group," *Spine,* July 15, 2009; 34(16): 1669–84.

10 Kumar S., K. Beaton, and T. Hughes, "The effectiveness of massage therapy for the treatment of nonspecific low back pain: a systematic review of systematic reviews," *Int J Gen Med,* Sept 4, 2013; 6: 733–41.

11 Brosseau L., et al., "Ottawa Panel evidence-based clinical practice guidelines on therapeutic massage for low back pain," *J Bodyw Mov Ther,* Oct 2012; 16 (4): 424–55.

12 Hernandez-Reif, M. et al., "Migraine headaches are reduced by massage therapy," *Int J Neurosci,* 1998; 96: 1–11.

13 Cheng, Y.H., and G.C. Huang, "Efficacy of massage therapy on pain and dysfunction in patients with neck pain: a systematic review and meta-analysis," *Evid Based Complement Alternat Med,* 2014; 2014: 204360. Epub Feb 20, 2014.

14 Patel, K.C., et al., "Massage for mechanical neck disorders," *Cochrane Database of Systematic Reviews,* Sept 12, 2012; 9: CD004871.

15 Lee, M.S., et al., "Massage therapy for children with autism spectrum disorders: a systematic review," *J Clin Psychiatry,* March 2011; 72(3): 406–11.

16 Hou, W.H., P.T. Chiang, T.Y. Hsu, S.Y. Chiu, and Y.C.Yen, "Treatment effects of massage therapy in depressed people: a meta-analysis," *J Clin Psychiatry.* Jul 2010; 71(7): 894–901.

17 Wilkinson S., K. Barnes, and L. Storey, "Massage for symptom relief in patients with cancer: systematic review," *Journal of Advanced Nursing,* Sept 2008; 63 (5): 430–39.

18 Li, Y.H., F.Y. Wang, C.Q. Feng, X.F. Yang, and Y.H. Sun, "Massage therapy for fibromyalgia: a systematic review and meta-analysis of randomized controlled trials," *PLoS One.* Feb 20, 2014; 9(2): e89304.

Chapter 22: Exercise for Depression

1 WHO, "Depression," October 2012, fact sheet No. 369, retrieved March 1, 2013 from: www.who.int/mediacentre/factsheets/fs369/en/index.html.

2 North, T.C. et al., "Effect of exercise on depression," *Exerc Sport Sci Rev,* 1990; 18: 379–415.

3 Cooney G.M. et al., "Exercise for depression," *Cochrane Database of Systematic Reviews* Sept 12, 2013; 9: CD004366.

4 Lawlor, D.A. and S.W. Hopker, "The effectiveness of exercise as an intervention in the management of depression: systematic review and meta-regression analysis of randomised controlled trials," *BMJ,* 2001; 322(7289): 763–67.

5 Martinsen, E.W. and T. Stephens, "Exercise and mental health in clinical and free-living populations," *Human Kinetics,* 1994: 55–72.

6 Babyak, M. et al., "Exercise treatment for major depression: maintenance of therapeutic benefit at 10 months," *Psychosomatic Medicine,* 2000; 62(5): 633–38.

7 McNeil, J.K. et al., "The effect of exercise on depressive symptoms in the moderately depressed elderly," *Psychol Aging,* 1991; 6: 487–88.

8 Singh, N.A. et al., "The efficacy of exercise as a long-term antidepressant in elderly subjects: a randomized, controlled trial," *Journals of Gerontology Series A— Biological Sciences & Medical Sciences*, 2001; 56(8): M497–504.

9 Partonen, T. et al., "Randomized trial of physical exercise alone or combined with bright light on mood and health-related quality of life," *Psychological Medicine*, 1998; 28(6):1359–64.

10 Ratey, John J., *Spark: The Revolutionary New Science of Exercise and the Brain* (New York: Little Brown, 2008).

SECTION IV: PSYCHOLOGICAL THERAPIES

Chapter 23: Eye Movement Desensitizing & Reprocessing (EMDR) for PTSD

1 Shepherd, J. et al., "Eye movement desensitization and reprocessing in the treatment of post-traumatic stress disorder: a review of an emerging therapy," *Psychological Medicine*, 2000; 30(4): 863–71.

2 Shapiro, F., "Eye Movement Desensitization and Reprocessing (EMDR) and the anxiety disorders: clinical and research implications of an integrated psychotherapy treatment," *Journal of Anxiety Disorders*, 1999; 13(1–2): 35–67.

3 Devilly, G.J. and S.H. Spence, "The relative efficacy and treatment distress of EMDR and a cognitive-behavior trauma treatment protocol in the amelioration of posttraumatic stress disorder," *Journal of Anxiety Disorders*, 1999; 13(1–2): 131–57.

4 Davidson, P.R. and K.C. Parker, "Eye movement desensitization and reprocessing (EMDR): a meta-analysis," *Journal of Consulting & Clinical Psychology*, 2001; 69(2): 305–16.

5 Schubert, S. et al., "The efficacy and psychophysiological correlates of dual-attention tasks in eye movement desensitization and reprocessing (EMDR)," *Journal of Anxiety Disorders*, 2011; 25(1): 1–11.

6 Bisson, J. and M. Andrew, "Psychological treatment of post-traumatic stress disorder (PTSD)," *Cochrane Database of Systematic Reviews*, 2007; (3): CD003388.

Chapter 24: Mindfulness-Based Stress Reduction (MBSR)

1 Kabat-Zinn, J., *Full Catastrophe Living: Using the Wisdom of Your Body and Mind to Face Stress, Pain, and Illness.* (New York: Delacorte, 1990).

2 Kabat-Zinn, J., "An outpatient program in behavioral medicine for chronic pain patients based on the practice of mindfulness meditation," *Gen Hosp Psych*, 1982; 4: 33–47.

3 Kabat-Zinn, J. et al., "The clinical use of mindfulness meditation for the self-regulation of chronic pain," *J Behave Med*, 1985; 8(2): 163–90.

4 Astin, J.A., "Stress reduction through mindfulness meditation: effects on psychological symptomatology, sense of control, and spiritual experiences," *Psychother Psychosom*, 1997; 66(2): 97–106.

5 Shapiro, S.L. et al., "Effects of mindfulness-based stress reduction on medical and premedical students," *J Behav Med*, 1998; 21(6): 581–99.

6 Williams, K.A. et al., "Evaluation of a wellness-based mindfulness stress-reduction intervention: a controlled trial," *Am J Health Promot*, 2001; 15(6): 422–32.

7 Carlson, L.E. et al., "The effects of a mindfulness meditation-based stress reduction program on mood and symptoms of stress in cancer outpatients: six-month follow-up," *Support Care Cancer*, 2001; 9(2): 112–23.

8 Carlson, L. E. et al., "MSBR in relation to quality of life, mood, symptoms of stress and immune parameters in breast and prostate cancer outpatients," *Psychosomatic Medicine*, 2003; 65: 571–81.

9 Goyal, M. et al., "Meditation programs for psychological stress and well-being—a systemic review and meta-analysis," *JAMA Intern Med*, 2014; 174(3): 357–68.

10 Kabat-Zinn, J. et al., "Influence of a mindfulness meditation-based stress reduction intervention on rates of skin clearing in patients with moderate to severe psoriasis undergoing phototherapy (UVB) and photochemotherapy (PUVA)," *Psychosomatic Medicine*, 1998; 60(5): 625–32.

11 Davidson, R.J. et al., "Alterations in brain and immune function produced by mindfulness meditation," *Psychosomatic Medicine*, 2003; 65(4): 564–70.

12 Bedard, M. et al., "Pilot evaluation of a mindfulness-based intervention to improve quality of life among individuals who sustained traumatic brain injuries," *Disabil Rehabil*, 2003; 25(13): 722–31.

13 Jain, S. et al., "A randomized controlled trial of mindfulness meditation versus relaxation training: effects on distress, positive states of mind, rumination, and distraction," *Ann Behave Med*, 2007; 33(1): 11–21.

14 Hofmann, S.G. et al., "The effect of mindfulness-based therapy on anxiety and depression: a meta-analytic review," *Journal of Consulting & Clinical Psychology*, 2010; 78(2): 169–83.

15 Chiesa, A., and A. Seretti, "Mindfulness-based stress reduction for stress management in healthy people: a review and meta-analysis," *Journal of Alternative & Complementary Medicine*, 2009; 15(5): 593–600.

Chapter 25: Laughter Is the Jest Medicine

1 Hankins, G.D., and C. Hankins, *Prescription for Anger: Coping with Angry Feelings and Angry People* (Newberg, OR: Barclay Press, 2000), 185.

2 Averill, J., "Autonomic response patterns during sadness and mirth," *Pathophysiology*, 1969; 5(4): 399–414.

3 Cogan, R. et al., "Effects of laughter and relaxation in discomfort thresholds," *J Behave Med*, 1987; 10: 139–44.

4 Cousins, N., "Anatomy of an illness (as perceived by the patient)," *NEJM*, 1976; 295: 1458–63.

5 Dillon, K.M. et al., "Positive emotional states and enhancement of the immune system," *Int J Psychiatr Med*, 1985–86; 15(1): 13–18.

6 Berk, L. et al., "Immune system changes during humour associated laughter," *Clinical Research*, 1991; 39: (124a).

7 George, M. et al., "Brain activity during transient sadness and happiness in healthy women," *Am J Psychiatry*, 1995; 152 (3): 341–51.

8 Said at a workshop he gave in Toronto Sept 22, 1988, Power of Laughter and Play Convention.

9 Grau. M., "Berlin Laughter Project," (YouTube 07/12/2011) retrieved March 13, 2013 from www.youtube.com/watch?v=EeauvE1M7qc.

10 The Miller Early Childhood Initiative of a World of Difference Institute, "How do children learn prejudice?" Anti-Defamation League, retrieved March 12, 2012 from http://archive.adl.org/education/miller/q_a/answer1.asp?sectionvar=1.

11 Sluder, A., "Children and laughter: the elementary school counselor's role," *Elementary School Guidance and Counseling*, 1986; 21(2): 120–27.

12 Shaw, G.B., *The Doctor's Dilemma: A Tragedy*, published June 30, 1950, Penguin Books.

13 Walker. G., "Laugh, teacher, laugh," *Education Digest*, 1990; 55(9): 43–44.

14 Otto, B.K., *Fools Are Everywhere: The Court Jester around the World* (Chicago: University of Chicago Press, 2001), 113.

15 Bryant, J., and D. Zillman, "Using humour to promote learning in the classroom," *Journal of Children in Contemporary Society*, 1988; 20(1): 49–78.

16 Crane, Alison, "Why sickness can be a laughing matter," *RN*, Feb 1987: 41–42.

17 Simonton, O. et al., *Getting Well Again*, (Los Angeles: J. P. Tarcher, 1978).

18 *Tales of the Ramayana*, as told by Aubrey Menon (New York: Scribner's, 1954) 276.

19 LeBlanc, Miriam, "Friedrich Froebel: His life and influence on education," Community Playthings, http://www.communityplaythings.co.uk/resources/articles/friedrich-froebel.html.

SECTION V: HOMEOPATHIC MEDICINE

1 Morrell, P., "Tobacco: two royal anecdotes," *BMJ*, 2001; 322: 203.

2 Ullman, D., *The Homeopathic Revolution: Why Famous People and Cultural Heroes Choose Homeopathy* (Berkeley: North Atlantic, 2007).

3 Ernst, E., "Homeopathic prophylaxis for headache and migraine? A systematic review," *Journal of Pain and Symptom Management*, 1999; 18: 353–57.

4 Linde, K., and K.A. Jobst, "Homeopathy for chronic asthma," *Cochrane Database of Systematic Reviews*, 2000; (2): CD000353.

5 Ernst E., "Efficacy of homeopathic arnica," *Arch Surg*, 1998; 133: 1187–90.

6 Ernst E., "A systematic review of systematic reviews of homeopathy," *Br J Clin Pharmacol*, 2002; 54(6): 577–82.

7 Barnes, J. B. et al., "Homeopathy for postoperative ileus?: a meta-analysis," *J Clin Gastro*, 1997; 25(4): 628–33.

8 Vickers, A.J. and C. Smith, "Homeopathic oscillococcinum for preventing and treating influenza and influenza-like syndromes," *Cochrane Database of Systematic Reviews*, 2000; (2): CD001957.

9 Weiser, M. et al., "Homeopathic vs conventional treatment of vertigo: a randomized double-blind controlled clinical study," *Arch Otolaryngol Head Neck Surg*, 1998; 124(8): 879–85.

10 Jacobs, J. et al., "Homeopathic treatment of acute otitis media in children: a preliminary randomized placebo controlled trial," *Pediatr Infect Dis J*, 2001; 20: 177–83.

11 Wiesenauer, M. and R. Ludtke, "A meta-analysis of homeopathic treatment of pollinosis with *Galphimia glauca*," *Forsch Komplementarmed Klass Naturheilkd*, 1996; 3: 230–36.

12 Jacobs, J. et al., "Treatment of acute childhood diarrhea with homeopathic medicine: a randomized clinical trial in Nicaragua," *Pediatrics*, 1994; 93(5): 719–25.

13 Taylor, M.A. et al., "Randomized controlled trial of homeopathy versus placebo in perennial allergic rhinitis with overview of four trial series," *BMJ,* 2000; 321: 471–75.

14 Riley, D.T. et al., "Is homeopathy a placebo response? Controlled trial of homeopathic potency, with pollen in hay fever as model," *Lancet,* 1986; 18: 881–86.

15 Chapman, E.H. et al., "Homeopathic treatment of mild traumatic brain injury: a randomized double-blind placebo-controlled trial," *J Head Trauma Rehabil,* 1991; 14: 521–42.

16 Bracho, G., et al., "Large-scale application of highly-diluted bacteria for Leptospirosis epidemic control," *Homeopathy,* July 2010; 99(3):156–66.

17 Frass M. et al., "Influence of potassium dichromate on tracheal secretions in critically ill patients," *Chest,* Mar 2005; 127(3): 936–41.

18 Kleijnen, J. et al., "Clinical trials of homeopathy," *BMJ,* 1991; 302: 316–23.

19 Linde, K. et al., "Are the clinical effects of homeopathy placebo effects? A meta-analysis of placebo-controlled trials," *Lancet,* 1997; 350: 834–43.

20 Linde, K. and D. Melchart, "Randomized controlled trials of individualized homeopathy: a state of the art review," *Journal of Alternative & Complementary Medicine,* 1998; 4(4): 371–88.

21 Cucherat, M. et al., "Evidence of clinical homeopathy," *Eur J Clin Pharmacol,* 2000; 56: 27–33.

22 Belon, P. et al., "Histamine dilutions modulate basophil activation," *Inflamm Res,* 2004; 53: 181–88.

23 Bornhöft G., and P. Matthiessen, "Homeopathy in Healthcare: Effectiveness, Appropriateness, Safety, Costs," 2012, Springer; http://www.homeovet. cl/BRIONES/Homeopathy%20in%20Healthcare%20Effectiveness,%20 Appropriateness,%20Safety,%20Costs.pdf.

24 Smith, H.M., "What's this? The rebirth of homeopathy?," *M.D.,* 1985; (5): 15–16.

Chapter 26: Homeopathic Oscillococcinum for Treatment of Flu

1 Ferley, J.P. et al., "A controlled evaluation of a homoeopathic preparation in the treatment of influenza-like syndromes," *Br J Clin Pharmacol,* 1989; 27: 329–35.

2 Mathie, R.T. et al., "Homoeopathic oscillococcinum for preventing and treating influenza and influenza-like illness," *Cochrane Database of Systematic Reviews,* 2012; (12): CD001957.

3 Jonas, W. et al., "A critical overview of homeopathy," *Annals of Internal Medicine,* 2003; 138: 393–99.

SECTION VI: NATURAL HEALTH PRODUCTS

Chapter 27: Vitamin D—The Sunshine Supplement

1 Holick, M.F., "Environmental factors that influence the cutaneous production of vitamin D," *Am J Clin Nutr,* 1995; 61(3S): 638S–45S.

2 Ginde A.A. et al., "Prospective study of serum 25-hydroxyvitamin D level, cardiovascular disease mortality, and all-cause mortality in older U.S. adults," *J Am Geriatr Soc,* Sep 2009; 57(9): 1595–1603.

3 Schöttker B. et al., "Strong associations of 25-hydroxyvitamin D concentrations with all-cause, cardiovascular, cancer, and respiratory disease mortality in a large cohort study," *Am J Clin Nutr,* Apr 2013; 97(4): 782–93.

4 Zittermann A. et al., "Vitamin D deficiency and mortality risk in the general population: a meta-analysis of prospective cohort studies," *Am J Clin Nutr,* Jan 2012; 95(1): 91–100.

5 Bjelakovic G., et al., "Vitamin D supplementation for prevention of mortality in adults," *Cochrane Database of Systematic Reviews,* Jan 10, 2014; 1: CD007470.

6 Combs, G.F., "Vitamins," In: Mahan, L.K. and Escott-Stump, S. (eds.) *Krause's Food, Nutrition and Diet Therapy* (Philadelphia: W.B. Saunders Company, 2000), 67–109.

7 Calvo, M.S. et al., "Vitamin D fortification in the United States and Canada: current status and data needs," *Am J Clin Nutr,* 2004; 80: 1710S–16S.

8 Calvo, M.S. and S.J. Whiting, "Prevalence of vitamin D insufficiency in Canada and the United States: importance to health status and efficacy of current food fortification and dietary supplement use," *Nutr Rev,* 2003; 61: 107–13.

9 Vieth, R. et al., "Wintertime vitamin D insufficiency is common in young Canadian women, and their vitamin D intake does not prevent it," *Eur J Clin Nutr,* 2001; 55: 1091–97.

10 Rucker, D. et al., "Vitamin D insufficiency in a population of healthy western Canadians," *CMAJ,* 2002; 166: 1517–24.

11 Looker, A.C. et al., "Serum 25-hydroxyvitamin D status of adolescents and adults in two seasonal subpopulations from NHANES III," *Bone,* 2002; 30: 771–77.

12 Gordon, C.M. et al., "Prevalence of vitamin D deficiency among healthy adolescents," *Arch Pediatr Adolesc Med,* 2004; 158: 531–37.

13 Jones, G. et al., "Vitamin D insufficiency in adolescent males in Southern Tasmania: prevalence, determinants, and relationship to bone turnover markers," *Osteoporos Int,* 2005; 16: 636–41.

14 Nesby-O'Dell, S. et al., "Hypovitaminosis D prevalence and determinants among African American and white women of reproductive age: third National Health and Nutrition Examination Survey, 1988–1994," *Am J Clin Nutr,* 2002; 76: 187–92.

15 Roth, D.E. et al., "Risk of vitamin D deficiency in Canadian children and adolescents is weight-dependent: Canadian guidelines provide insufficient vitamin D to maintain adequate blood levels," Unpublished.

16 Holick, M.F., "Sunlight and vitamin D for bone health and prevention of autoimmune diseases, cancers, and cardiovascular disease," *Am J Clin Nutr,* 2004; 80 (Suppl): 1678S–88S.

17 Ziegler, E.E. et al., "Vitamin D deficiency in breastfed infants in Iowa," *Pediatrics,* 2006; 118(2): 603–10.

18 Hypponen, E. et al., "Intake of vitamin D and risk of type 1 diabetes: a birth-cohort study," *Lancet,* 2001; 358(9292): 1500–503.

19 "Vitamin D supplement in early childhood and risk for Type I (insulin-dependent) diabetes mellitus. The EURODIAB Substudy 2 Study Group," *Diabetelogia,* 1999; 42(1): 51–54.

20 Stene, L.C. and G. Joner, Norwegian Childhood Diabetes Study Group, "Use of cod liver oil during the first year of life is associated with lower risk of childhood-onset type 1 diabetes: a large, population-based, case-control study," *Am J Clin Nutr,* 2003; 78(6): 1128–34.

21 Stene, L.C. et al., "Use of cod liver oil during pregnancy associated with lower risk of type I diabetes in the offspring," *Diabetelogia*, 2000; 43(9): 1093–98.

22 Bischoff-Ferrari, H.A. et al., "Effect of vitamin D on falls: a meta-analysis," *JAMA*, 2004; 291(16): 1999–2006.

23 Sato, Y. et al., "Low-dose vitamin D prevents muscular atrophy and reduces falls and hip fractures in women after stroke: a randomized controlled trial," *Cerebro Vasc Dis*, 2005; 20(3): 187–92.

24 Bischoff-Ferrari, H.A. et al., "Effect of cholecalciferol plus calcium on falling in ambulatory older men and women: a 3-year randomized controlled trial," *Arch Intern Med*, 2006; 166(4): 424–30.

25 Flicker, L. et al., "Serum vitamin D and falls in older women in residential care in Australia," *J Am Geriatr Soc*, 2003; 51(11): 1533–38.

26 Dhesi, J.K, et al., "A rationale for vitamin D prescribing in a falls clinic population," *Age Aging*, 2002; 31(4): 267–71.

27 Kalyani, R.R., et al., "Vitamin D treatment for the prevention of falls in older adults: systematic review and meta-analysis," *J Am Geriatr Soc* 2010; 58(7): 1299–310.

28 Cameron I.D., et al., "Interventions for preventing falls in older people in nursing care facilities and hospitals," *Cochrane Database of Systematic Reviews* 2010; (1): CD005465.

29 Bischoff-Ferrari, H.A. et al., "Fracture prevention with vitamin D supplementation: a meta-analysis of randomized controlled trials," *JAMA*, 2005; 293(18): 2257–64.

30 De Torrente de la Jara, G. et al., "Musculoskeletal pain in female asylum seekers and hypovitaminosis D3," *BMJ*, 2004; 329(7458): 156–57.

31 Plotnikoff, G.A. and J.M. Quigley, "Prevalence of severe hypovitaminosis D in patients with persistent, nonspecific musculoskeletal pain," *Mayo Clin Proc*, 2003; 78(12): 1463–70.

Chapter 28: Vitamins & Lutein for Age-Related Macular Degeneration

1 Richer, S. et al., "Double-masked, placebo-controlled, randomized trial of lutein and antioxidant supplementation in the intervention of atrophic age-related macular degeneration: the Veterans LAST study (Lutein Antioxidant Supplementation Trial)," *Optometry*, 2004; 75(4): 216–30.

2 Cho, E. et al., "Prospective study of intake of fruits, vegetables, vitamins, and carotenoids and risk of age-related maculopathy," *Arch Ophthalmol*, 2004; 122(6): 883–92.

3 Evans, J.R. and J. G. Lawrenson, "Antioxidant vitamin and mineral supplements for slowing the progression of age-related macular degeneration," *Cochrane Database of Systematic Reviews*, Nov 14, 2012; 11: CD000254.

4 "The Age-Related Eye Disease Study (AREDS): A randomized, placebo-controlled clinical trial of high-dose supplementation with vitamins C and E, beta carotene and zinc for age-related macular degeneration and vision loss," *Arch Ophthalmol*, 2001; 119: 1417–36.

5 Chang, C.W. et al., "Current use of dietary supplementation in patients with age-related macular degeneration," *Can J Ophthalmol*, 2003; 38(1): 27–32.

6 Bjelakovic G. et al., "Antioxidant supplements for prevention of mortality in healthy participants and patients with various diseases," *Cochrane Database of Systematic Reviews*, Mar 14, 2012; 3: CD007176.

Chapter 29: Vitamin E for Non-Alcoholic Fatty Liver Disease

1 "Nonalcoholic Steatohepatitis," *National Digestive Diseases Information Clearing House (NDDIC)*, US Department of Health and Human Services, 2006; NIH Publication: No. 07–4921.

2 von Herbay, A., W. Stahl, C. Niederau, and H. Sies, "Vitamin E improves the aminotransferase status of patients suffering from viral hepatitis C: a randomized, double-blind, placebo-controlled study," *Free Radic Res*, December 1997; 27(6): 599–605.

3 Dufour, J.F. et al., "A randomized placebo-controlled study testing UDCA in combination with vitamin E to treat NASH," *Journal of Hepatology*, 2005; 42: 4–5.

4 Sanyal, A.J. et al., "A pilot study of vitamin E versus vitamin E and pioglitazone for the treatment of nonalcoholic steatohepatitis," *Clin Gastroenterol Hepatol*, 2004; 2(12): 1107–15.

5 Harrison, S.A. et al., "TI: Vitamin E and vitamin C treatment improves fibrosis in patients with nonalcoholic steatohepatitis," *American Journal of Gastroenterology*, 2003; 98(11): 2485–90.

6 Harrison, S.A. et al., "The role of vitamin E and C therapy in NASH," *American Journal of Gastroenterology*, 2004; 99(9): 1862.

7 Kugelmas, M. et al., "CJTI: Cytokines and NASH: a pilot study of the effects of lifestyle modification and vitamin E," *Hepatology*, 2003; 38(2): 413–19.

8 Bugianesi, E. et al., "A randomized controlled trial of metformin versus vitamin E or prescriptive diet in nonalcoholic fatty liver disease," *American Journal of Gastroenterology*, 2005; 100(5): 1082–90.

Chapter 30: Coenzyme Q10 for Health

1 Rosenfeldt, F. et al., "Systematic review of effect of coenzyme Q10 in physical exercise, hypertension, and heart failure," *Biofactors*, 2003; 18(1-4): 91–100.

2 Keogh, A. et al., "Randomised double-blind, placebo-controlled trial of coenzyme Q, therapy in class II and III systolic heart failure," *Heart Lung Circ.* 2003; 12(3): 135–41.

3 Kocharian, A. et al., "Coenzyme Q10 improves diastolic function in children with idiopathic dilated cardiomyopathy," *Cardiol Young*, September 2009; 19(5): 501–6. doi: 10.1017/S1047951109990795. Epub August 29, 2009.

4 Burke, B.E. et al., "Randomized, double-blind, placebo-controlled trial of coenzyme Q10 in isolated systolic hypertension," *South Med J*, 2001; 94(11): 1112–17.

5 Rosenfeldt, F.L., et al., "Coenzyme Q10 in the treatment of hypertension: a meta-analysis of the clinical trials," *J Hum Hypertens*, April 2007; 21(4): 297–306. Epub February 8, 2007.

6 Rosenfeldt, F. et al., "Coenzyme Q10 therapy before cardiac surgery improves mitochondrial function and in vitro contractility of myocardial tissue," *J Thorac Cardiovasc Surg*, January 2005; 129(1): 25–32.

7 Berman, M. et al., "Coenzyme Q10 in patients with end-stage heart failure awaiting cardiac transplantation: A randomized, placebo-controlled study," *Clin Cardiol*, 2004; 27:295–98.

8 Singh, R.B. et al., "Effect of coenzyme Q10 on risk of atherosclerosis in patients with recent myocardial infarction," *Mol Cell Biochem*, 2003; 246(1-2): 75–82.

9 Hodgson, J.M. et al., "Coenzyme Q10 improves blood pressure and glycaemic control: a controlled trial in subjects with type 2 diabetes," *Eur J Clin Nutr*, 2002; 56(11): 1137–42.

10 Sandor, P.S. et al., "Efficacy of coenzyme Q10 in migraine prophylaxis: a randomized controlled trial," *Neurology*, 2005; 64(4): 713–15.

11 Liu, J., L. Wang, S.Y. Zhan, Y. Xia, "Coenzyme Q10 for Parkinson's disease," *Cochrane Database of Systematic Reviews*, December 7, 2011; (12): CD008150.

Chapter 31: Folic Acid for Depression

1 Reynolds, E.H., "Folic acid, ageing, depression, and dementia," *BMJ*, 2002; 324(7352): 1512–15.

2 Taylor, M.J. et al., "Folate for depressive disorders: Systematic review and meta-analysis of randomized controlled trials," *J Psychopharmacol*, 2004; 18(2): 251–56.

3 Bottiglieri, T. et al., "Homocysteine, folate, methylation and monoamine metabolism in depression," *J Neurol Neurosurg Psychiatry*, 2000; 69: 228–32.

4 Reynolds, E.H., 2002.

5 Ibid.

6 Coppen, A. et al., "Folic acid enhances lithium prophylaxis," *Journal of Affective Disorders*, 1986; 10: 9–13.

7 Coppen, A. and J. Bailey, "Enhancement of the antidepressant action of fluoxitine by folic acid: a randomised, placebo controlled trial," *Journal of Affective Disorders*, 2000; 60: 121–30.

8 Godfrey, P.S.A. et al., "Enhancement of recovery from psychiatric illness by methyl folate," *Lancet*, 1990; 336: 392–95.

9 Alpert, J. E. et al., "Folinic acid (Leucovorin) as an adjunctive treatment for SSRI-refractory depression," *Ann Clin Psychiatr*, 2002; 14: 33–38.

10 Coppen, A. and C. Bolander-Gouaille, "Treatment of depression: Time to consider folic acid and vitamin B12," *J Psychopharmacol*, 2005; 19(1): 59–65.

Chapter 32: Omega-3 Fatty Acids

1 Matthan, N.R. et al., "A systematic review and meta-analysis of the impact of omega-3 fatty acids on selected arrhythmia outcomes in animal models," *Metabolism*, 2005; 54(12):1557–65.

2 Rodrigo, R., P. Korantzopoulos, M. Cereceda, R. Asenjo, J. Zamorano, E. Villalabeitia, C. Baeza, R. Aguayo, R. Castillo, R. Carrasco, J.G. Gormaz, "A randomized controlled trial to prevent post-operative atrial fibrillation by antioxidant reinforcement," *J Am Coll Cardiol*, Oct 15, 2013; 62(16): 1457–65.

3 Costanzo, S., V. di Niro, A. Di Castelnuovo, F. Gianfagna, M.B. Donati, G. de Gaetano, L. Iacoviello, "Prevention of postoperative atrial fibrillation in open heart surgery patients by preoperative supplementation of n-3 polyunsaturated fatty acids: an updated meta-analysis," *J Thorac Cardiovasc Surg*, Oct 2013; 146(4): 906–11.

4 Mariani, J., H.C. Doval, D. Nul, S. Varini, H. Grancelli, D. Ferrante, G. Tognoni, A. Macchia, "N-3 polyunsaturated acids to prevent atrial fibrillation: updated systematic review and meta-analysis of randomized controlled trials," *J Am Heart Assoc*, February 19, 2013; 2(1): e005033.

5 Khoueiry, G., N. Abi Rafeh, E. Sullivan, F. Saiful, Z. Jaffery, D.N. Kenigsberg, S.C. Krishnan, S. Khanal, S. Bekheit, M. Kowalski, "Do omega-3 polyunsaturated fatty acids reduce risk of sudden cardiac death and ventricular arrhythmias? A meta-analysis of randomized trials," *Heart Lung*, July–Aug 2013; 42(4): 251–56.

6 Raitt, M.H. et al., "Fish oil supplementation and risk of ventricular tachycardia and ventricular fibrillation in patients with implantable defibrillators: a randomized controlled trial," *JAMA*, 2005; 293(23): 2884–91.

7 Brouwer, I.A. et al., "Effect of fish oil on ventricular tachyarrythmia and death in patients with implantable cardio defibrillators: the study on omega-3 fatty acids and ventricular arrhythmia (SOFA) randomized trial," *JAMA*, 2006; 295(22): 2613–19.

8 Yzebe, D. and M. Lievre, "Fish oils in the care of coronary heart disease patients: a meta-analysis of randomized controlled trials," *Fundam Clin Pharmacol*, 2004; 18(5): 581–92.

9 Harper, C.R. and T.A. Jacobson, "Usefulness of omega-3 fatty acids and the prevention of coronary heart disease," *Am J Cardiol*, 2005; 96(11): 1521–29.

10 GISSI-Prevenzione, "Dietary supplementation with n–3 polyunsaturated fatty acids and vitamin E after myocardial infarction: results of the GISSI-Prevenzione trial," Gruppo Italiano per lo Studio della Sopravvivenza nell'Infarto miocardico [see comments], *Lancet*, 1999; 354: 447–55.

11 Breslow, Jan, "n–3 Fatty acids and cardiovascular disease," *Am J Clin Nutr*, June 2006; 83 (6): S1477–82S.

12 Saito Y. et al., "Effects of EPA on coronary artery disease in hypercholesterolemic patients with multiple risk factors: sub-analysis of primary prevention cases from the Japan EPA Lipid Intervention Study (JELIS)," *Atherosclerosis*, Sep 2008; 200(1): 135–40. doi: 10.1016/j.atherosclerosis.2008.06.003.

13 Risk and Prevention Study Collaborative Group, Roncaglioni, M.C. et al, "n-3 fatty acids in patients with multiple cardiovascular risk factors," *NEJM*, May 9, 2013; 368(19): 1800–808. doi: 10.1056/NEJMoa1205409.

14 Balk, E.M. et al., "Effects of omega-3 fatty acids on coronary restenosis, intima-media thickness, and exercise tolerance: a systematic review," *Atherosclerosis*, 2006; 184(2): 237–46.

15 Holub, B., "EPA/DHA omega-3 fatty acids in the primary and secondary prevention of cardiovascular disease and the modification of risk factors," University of Guelph, 2009; Retrieved March 27, 2013 from www.uoguelph.ca/~bholub/2010omega-3cardioreview2009-1.pdf.

16 Hooper, L. et al., "Omega 3 fatty acids for prevention and treatment of cardiovascular disease," *Cochrane Database of Systematic Reviews*, 2005; (4): CD003177.

17 Casula, M., D. Soranna, A.L. Catapano, G. Corrao. "Long-term effect of high dose omega-3 fatty acid supplementation for secondary prevention of cardiovascular outcomes: A meta-analysis of randomized, double blind, placebo controlled trials." *Atheroscler Suppl*, Aug 2013; 14(2): 243–51.

18 McKelvie, R.S. et al.,"The 2012 Canadian Cardiovascular Society heart failure management guidelines update: focus on acute and chronic heart failure," *Can J Cardiol*, Feb 2013; 29(2): 168–81.

19 Lewis, A. et al., "Treatment of hypertriglyceridemia with omega-3 fatty acids: a systematic review," *J Am Acad Nurse Pract*, 2004; 16(9): 384–95.

20 Skerrett, P.J. and C.H. Hennekens, "Consumption of fish and fish oils and decreased risk of stroke," *Prev Cardiol*, 2003; 6(1): 38–41.

21 Issa, A.M. et al., "The efficacy of omega-3 fatty acids on cognitive function in aging and dementia: A systematic review," *Dementia and Geriatric Cognitive Disorders*, 2005; 21(2): 88 96.

22 Udell, T. et al., "The effect of alpha-linolenic acid and lenoleic acid on the growth and development of formula-fed infants: a systematic review and meta-analysis of randomized controlled trials," *Lipids*, 2005; 40(1): 1–11.

23 Parker, G., N.A. Gibson, H. Brotchie, G. Heruc, A.M. Rees, D. Hadzi-Pavlovic, "Omega-3 fatty acids and mood disorders," *Am J Psychiatry*, June 2006; 163(6): 969–78.

24 Sublette, M.E. et al., "Meta-analysis: Effects of cicosapentaenoic acid in clinical trials in depression." *J Clin Psychiatry*, 2011; 72(12): 1577–84.

25 Sarris, J., D. Mischoulon, I. Schweitzer, "Omega-3 for bipolar disorder: meta-analyses of use in mania and bipolar depression," *J Clin Psychiatry*, Jan 2012; 73(1): 81–86.

26 Sarris, J., N. Schoendorfer, D.J. Kavanagh. "Major depressive disorder and nutritional medicine: a review of monotherapies and adjuvant treatments," *Nutr Rev*, March 2009; 67(3): 125–31.

27 "Comparison of therapeutic effects of omega-3 fatty acid eicosapentaenoic acid and fluoxetine, separately and in combination, in major depressive disorder," *Aust NZ J Psychiatry*, March 2008; 42(3): 192–98.

Chapter 33: Glucosamine for Osteoarthritis

1 Manson, J. and A. Rahman, "This house believes that we should advise our patients with osteoarthritis of the knee to take glucosamine," *Rheumatology*, 2004; 43: 100–101.

2 McAlindon, T.E. et al., "Glucosamine and chondroitin for treatment of osteoarthritis: a systematic quality assessment and meta-analysis," *JAMA*, 2000; 283(11): 1469–75.

3 Richy, F. et al., "Structural and symptomatic efficacy of glucosamine and chondroitin in knee osteoarthritis: a comprehensive meta-analysis," *Arch Intern Med*, 2003; 163(13): 1514–22.

4 Poolsup, N. et al., "Glucosamine long-term treatment and the progression of knee osteoarthritis: systematic review of randomized controlled trials," *Ann Pharmacother*, 2005; 39(6): 1080–87.

5 Zhang, W. et al., "OARSI recommendations for the management of hip and knee osteoarthritis: part III: Changes in evidence following systematic cumulative update of research published through January 2009," *Osteoarthritis Cartilage*, 2010; 18(4): 476–99.

6 Reginster, J.Y. et al., "Long term effects of glucosamine sulfate on osteoarthritis progression: a randomised, placebo-controlled clinical trial," *Lancet*, 2001; 357(9252): 251–56.

7 Pavelka, K. et al., "Glucosamine sulfate use and delay of progression of knee osteoarthritis: a 3-year, randomized, placebo-controlled, double-blind study," *Arch Intern Med*, 2002; 162(18): 2113–23.

8 Lee, Y.H. et al., "Effect of glucosamine or chondroitin sulfate on the osteoarthritis progression. a meta-analysis," *Rheumatol Int*, 2010; 30(3): 357–63.

9 Kreder, H. J., "Glucosamine and chondroitin were found to improve outcomes in patients with osteoarthritis," *J Bone Joint Surg Am*, 2000; 82(9): 1323.

10 Denham, A. C. and W.P. Newton, "Are glucosamine and chondroitin effective in treating osteoarthritis?" *J Fam Prac*, 2000; 49(6): 571–72.

11 Heisel, J. and C. Kipshoven, "Treatment of osteoarthritis with cristalline glucosamine sulfate. Results of the IDEAL-study," *MMW Fortschr Med*, 2011; 153 Suppl 3: 95–100.

12 Hughes, R. and A. Carr, "A randomized, double-blind, placebo-controlled trial of glucosamine sulfate as an analgesic in osteoarthritis of the knee," *Rheumatology*, 2002; 41(3): 279–84.

13 Cibere, J. et al., "Randomized, double-blind, placebo-controlled glucosamine discontinuation trial in knee osteoarthritis," *Arthritis and Rheumatism*, 2004; 51(5): 738–45.

14 Wandel, S. et al., "Effects of glucosamine, chondroitin, or placebo in patients with osteoarthritis of hip or knee: network meta-analysis," *BMJ*, 2010; 341: c4675.

15 Wu, D. Huang, Y. Gu, W. Y. Fan, "Efficacies of different preparations of glucosamine for the treatment of osteoarthritis: a meta-analysis of randomised, double-blind, placebo-controlled trials," *International Journal of Clinical Practice*, June 2013; 67(6): 585–94.

16 Sawitzke, A.D. et al., "Clinical efficacy and safety of glucosamine, chondroitin sulphate, their combination, celecoxib or placebo taken to treat osteoarthritis of the knee: 2-year results from GAIT," *Ann Rheum Dis*, 2010; 69(8): 1459–64.

17 dos Reis, R.P. et al., "Crystalline glucosamine sulfate in the treatment of osteoarthritis: Evidence of long-term cardiovascular safety from clinical trials," *Open Rheumatology Journal*, 2011; 5 (1): 69–77.

18 Towheed, T. et al., "Glucosamine therapy for treating osteoarthritis," *Cochrane Database of Systematic Reviews*, 2005; (2): CD002946.

Chapter 34: Melatonin for Jet Lag

1 Herxheimer, A. and K.J. Petrie, "Melatonin for the prevention and treatment of jet lag," *Cochrane Database of Systematic Reviews*, 2002; (2): CD001520.

2 Arendt, J. et al., "Alleviation of jet lag by melatonin: preliminary results of controlled double blind trial," *BMJ*, 1986; 292: 1170.

3 Arendt, J. and M. Aldhous, "Further evaluation of the treatment of jet lag by melatonin: a double blind crossover study," *Annual Review of Chronopharmacology*, 1988; 5: 53–55.

4 Petrie, K. et al., "Effect of melatonin on jet lag after long haul flights," *BMJ*, 1989; 298: 705–7.

5 Nickelsen, T. et al., "The effect of 6-, 9-, and 11-hour time shifts on circadian rhythms: adaptation of sleep parameters and hormonal patterns following the intake of melatonin or placebo," *Advances in Pineal Research*, Vol. 5, Arendt, J. (ed.) (London: John Libbey & Co., 1991); 303–6.

6 Claustrat, B. et al., "Melatonin and jet lag: Confirmatory result using a simplified protocol," *Biological Psychiatry*, 1992; 32: 705–11.

7 Petrie, K. et al., "A double-blind trial of melatonin as a treatment for jet lag in international cabin crew," *Biological Psychiatry*, 1993; 33: 526–30.

8 Suhner, A. et al., "Comparative study to determine the optimal melatonin dosage form for the alleviation of jet lag," *Chronobiology International*, 1998; 15(6): 655–66.

9 Suhner, A. et al., "Effectiveness and tolerability of melatonin and zolpidem for the alleviation of jet-lag," *Aviat Space Environ Med*, 2001; 72(7): 638–46.

10 Spitzer, R.L. et al., "Jet lag: clinical features, validation of a new syndrome-specific scale, and lack of response to melatonin in a randomized double-blind trial," *Am J Psychiatry*, 1999; 156: 1392–96.

11 Edwards, B.J. et al., "Use of melatonin in recovery from jet-lag following an eastward flight across 10 time-zones," *Ergonomics*, 2000; 43: 1501–13.

12 Beaumont, M. et al., "Caffeine or melatonin effects on sleep and sleepiness after rapid eastward transmeridian travel," *J Appl Physiol*, 2004; 96: 50–58.

13 Asayama, K. et al., "Double blind study of melatonin effects on the sleep-wake rhythm, cognitive and non-cognitive functions in Alzheimer type dementia," *J Nippon Med Sch*, 2003; 70(4): 334–41.

14 Medeiros, C.A. et al., "Effect of exogenous melatonin on sleep and motor dysfunction in Parkinson's disease. A randomized, double blind, placebo-controlled study," *J Neurol*, 2007; 254: 459–64.

15 Simko, F. and L. Paulis, "Melatonin as a potential antihypertensive treatment," *J Pineal Res*, 2007; 42(4): 319–22.

16 Grossman, E. et al., "Effect of melatonin on nocturnal blood pressure: meta-analysis of randomized controlled trials," *Vasc Health Risk Manag*, 2011; 7: 577–84.

17 Lemoine, P. et al., "Prolonged-release melatonin improves sleep quality and morning alertness in insomnia patients aged 55 years and older and has no withdrawal effects," *J Sleep Res*, 2007; 16(4): 372–80.

18 Suresh Kumar, P.N. et al., "Melatonin in schizophrenic outpatients with insomnia: a double-blind, placebo-controlled study," *J Clin Psychiatry*, 2007; 68(2): 237–41.

19 Bendz, L.M. and A.C. Scates, "Melatonin treatment for insomnia in pediatric patients with attention-deficit/hyperactivity disorder," *Ann Pharmacother*, 2010; 44(1): 185–91.

20 Brzezinski A., M.G. Vangel, R.J. Wurtman, G. Norrie, I. Zhdanova, A. Ben-Shushan, and I. Ford, "Effects of exogenous melatonin on sleep: a meta-analysis," *Sleep Med Rev*, Feb 2005; 9(1): 41–50.

Chapter 35: Probiotics for Your Gut

1 Reimer, R.A., "Pro- and prebiotics: Significance and impact in clinical practice," *Clinical Nutrition Rounds*, 2004; 4(3): 2.

2 D'Souza, A. L. et al., "Probiotics in prevention of antibiotic associated diarrhoea: meta-analysis," *BMJ*, 2002; 324: 1361.

3 Videlock, E.J. and F. Creminini, "Meta-analysis: probiotics in antibiotic-associated diarrhoea," *Aliment Pharmacol Ther*, 2012; 35(12): 1355–69.

4 Szajewska, H. and J.Z. Mrukowicz, "Probiotics in the treatment and prevention of acute infectious diarrhea in infants and children: a systematic review of published randomized, double-blind, placebo-controlled trials," *J Pediatr Gastroenterol Nutr*, 2001; 33 Suppl 2: S17–25.

5 Huang, J. S. et al., "Efficacy of probiotic use in acute diarrhea in children: a meta-analysis," *Dig Dis Sci*, 2002; 47(11): 2625–34.

6 Allen, S.J. et al., "Probiotics for treating infectious diarrhea (Review)," *Cochrane Database of Systematic Reviews*, 2003; (4): CD003048.

7 Fedorak, R.N., "Probiotics in the management of ulcerative colitis," *Gastroenterol Hepatol (NY)*, November 2010; 6(11): 688–90.

8 Saavedra, J. M., "Feeding of *Bifidobacterium bifidum* and *Streptococcus thermophilus* to infants in hospital for prevention of diarrhoea and shedding of rotavirus," *Lancet*, 1994; 344(8929): 1046–49.

9 Kollaritsch, H. et al., "Prevention of traveler's diarrhea with the *Saccarimyces boulardii*: results of a placebo controlled double-blind study," *Fortschr Med*, 1993; 111: 152–56.

10 Plummer, S. et al., "*Clostridium difficile* pilot study: effects of probiotic supplementation on the incidence of *C. difficile* diarrhoea," *Int Micro*, 2004; 7: 59–62.

11 Johnson, S. et al., "Is primary prevention of *Clostridium difficile* infection possible with specific probiotics?," *Int J Infect Dis*, 2012; 16(11): e786–92.

12 Avadhani, A. and H. Miley, "Probiotics for prevention of antibiotic-associated diarrhea and *Clostridium difficile*-associated disease in hospitalized adults—a meta-analysis," *J Am Acad Nurse Pract*, 2011; 23(6): 269–74.

13 Allen, S.J., et al., "Lactobacilli and bifidobacteria in the prevention of antibiotic-associated diarrhoea and Clostridium difficile diarrhoea in older inpatients (PLACIDE): a randomised, double-blind, placebo-controlled, multicentre trial," *Lancet*, Oct 12, 2013; 382(9900): 1249–57.

14 McFarland, L. V. et al., "A randomized placebo-controlled trial of *Saccharomyces boulardii* in combination with standard antibiotics for *Clostridium difficile* disease," *JAMA*, 1994; 271(24): 1913–18.

15 Ortiz-Lucas, M. et al., "Effect of probiotic species on irritable bowel syndrome symptoms: A bring up to date meta-analysis," *Rev Esp Enferm Dig*, January 2013; 105(1): 19–36.

16 Moavvedi, P. et al., "The efficacy of probiotics in the therapy of irritable bowel syndrome: a systematic review," *Gut*, March 2010; 59(3): 325–32.

17 Brenner, D.M., M.J. Moeller, W.D. Chey, and P.S. Schoenfeld, "The utility of probiotics in the treatment of irritable bowel syndrome: a systematic review," *American Journal of Gastroenterology*, Apr 2009; 104(4): 1033–49.

18 Kalliomaki, M. et al., "Probiotics in the prevention of atopic eczema: 4-year follow-up of a randomised placebo-controlled trial," *Lancet*, 2003; 361(9372): 1869–71.

19 Lee, J. et al., "Meta-analysis of clinical trials of probiotics for prevention and treatment of pediatric atopic dermatitis," *J Allergy Clin Immunol*, 2008; 121: 116–21.

20 Pelucchi, C. et al., "Probiotics supplementation during pregnancy or infancy for the prevention of atopic dermatitis: a meta-analysis," *Epidemiology*, May 2012; 23(3): 402–14.

Chapter 36: Zinc for the Common Cold

1 Korant, B.D. and B.E. Butterworth, "Inhibition by zinc of rhinovirus protein cleavage: interaction of zinc with capsid polypeptides," *J Virol*, 1976; 18(1): 298–306.

2 Garland, M.L. and K. O'Hagmeyer, "The role of zinc lozenges in treatment of the common cold," *Ann Pharmacother*, 1998; 32: 63–69.

3 Eby, G.A. et al., "Reduction in duration of common colds by zinc gluconate lozenges in a double-blind study," *Antimicrob Agents Chemother*, 1984; (1): 20–24.

4 Mossad, S.B. et al., "Zinc gluconate lozenges for treating the common cold," *Annals of Internal Medicine*, 1996; 125(2): 81–88.

5 Prasad, A.S. et al., "Duration of symptoms and plasma cytokine levels in patients with the common cold treated with zinc acetate," *Annals of Internal Medicine*, 2000; 133(4): 245–52.

6 Howell-McElroy B. and S. Porter Miller, "Effectiveness of zinc gluconate glycine lozenges (Cold-Eeze) against the common cold in school-aged subjects: a retrospective chart review." *Am J Ther*, 2002; 9(6): 472–75.

7 Howell-McElroy, B. and S. Porter Miller, "An open-label, single-centre, phase IV clinical study of the effectiveness of zinc gluconate glycine lozenges (Cold-Eeze) in reducing the duration and symptoms of the common cold in school-aged subjects," *Am J Ther*, 2003; 10: 324–29.

8 Hirt, M. et al., "Zinc nasal gel for the treatment of common cold symptoms: a double-blind, placebo-controlled trial," *Ear Nose Throat J*, 2000; 79(10): 778–82.

9 Singh, M. and R.R. Das, "Zinc for the common cold," *Cochrane Database of Systematic Reviews*, Jun 18, 2013; 6: CD001364.

10 Science, M., J. Johnstone, D.E. Roth, G. Guyatt, and M. Loeb, "Zinc for the treatment of the common cold: a systematic review and meta-analysis of randomized controlled trials," *CMAJ*, Jul 10, 2012; 184(10): E551-61. doi: 10.1503/cmaj.111990. Epub May 7, 2012.

11 Smith, D.S. et al., "Failure of zinc gluconate in treatment of acute upper respiratory tract infections," *Antimicrob Agents Chemother*, 1989; 33(5): 646–48.

12 Farr, B.M. et al., "Two randomized controlled trials of zinc gluconate lozenge therapy of experimentally induced rhinovirus colds," *Antimicrob Agents Chemother*, 1987; (8): 1183–87.

13 Macknin, M.L. et al., "Zinc gluconate lozenges for treating the common cold in children," *JAMA*, 1998; 279(24): 1962–67.

14 Belongia, E.A. et al., "A randomized trial of zinc nasal spray for the treatment of upper respiratory illness in adults," *American Journal of Medicine*, 2001; 111(2): 103–8.

15 Eby, G.A. and W.W. Halcomb, "Ineffectiveness of zinc gluconate nasal spray and zinc orotate lozenges in common-cold treatment," *Altern Ther Health Med*, 2006; 12(1): 34–38.

Chapter 37: L-Carnitine for Health

1 Montgomery, S.A. et al., "Meta-analysis of double blind randomized controlled clinical trials of acetyl-L-carnitine versus placebo in the treatment of mild cognitive impairment and mild Alzheimer's disease," *Int Clin Psychopharmacol*, 2003; 18(2): 61–71.

2 Tarantini, G. et al., "Metabolic treatment with L-carnitine in acute anterior ST segment elevation myocardial infarction. A randomized controlled trial," *Cardiology*, 2006; 106(4): 215–23.

3 Singh, R.B. et al., "A randomised, double-blind, placebo-controlled trial of L-carnitine in suspected acute myocardial infarction," *Postgrad Med J*, January 1996; 72(843): 45–50.

4 Davini, P., "Controlled study on L-carnitine therapeutic efficacy in post-infarction," *Drugs Exp Clin Res*, 1992; 18(8): 355–65.

5 Iliceto, S. et al., "Effects of L-carnitine administration on left ventricular remodeling after acute anterior myocardial infarction: the L-carnitine ecocardiografia Digitalizzata Infarto Miocardico (CEDIM) Trial," *J Am Coll Cardiol*, 1995; 26(2): 380–87.

6 Dinicolantonio, J.J. et al., "L-Carnitine in the Secondary Prevention of Cardiovascular Disease: Systematic Review and Meta-analysis," *Mayo Clin Proc*, June 2013; 88(6): 544–51. doi: 10.1016/j.mayocp.2013.02.007. Epub April 15, 2013.

7 Brevetti, G., et al., "European multicenter study on propionyl-L-carnitine in intermittent claudication," *J Am Coll Cardiol*, 1999; 34(5): 1618–24.

8 Hiatt, W.R. et al., "Propionyl-L-carnitine improves exercise performance and functional status in patients with claudication," *American Journal of Medicine*, 2001; 110(8): 616–22.

9 Cruciani, R.A. et al., "L-carnitine supplementation for the treatment of fatigue and depressed mood in cancer patients with carnitine deficiency: a preliminary analysis," *Ann NY Acad Sci*, 2004; 1033: 168–76.

10 Graziano, F. et al., "Potential role of levocarnitine supplementation for the treatment of chemotherapy-induced fatigue in non-anaemic cancer patients," *Br J Cancer*, 2002; 86: 1854–57.

11 Tomassini, V. et al., "Comparison of the effects of acetyl L-carnitine and amantadine for the treatment of fatigue in multiple sclerosis: results of a pilot, randomised, double-blind, crossover trial," *J Neurol Sci*, 2004; 218(1-2): 103–8.

12 DeGrandis, D. and C. Minardi, "Acetyl-L-carnitine (levacecarnine) in the treatment of diabetic neuropathy. A long-term, randomised, double-blind, placebo-controlled study," *Drugs R D*, 2002; 3(4): 223–31.

13 Sima, A.A.F. et al., "Acetyl-L-carnitine improves pain, nerve regeneration, and vibratory perception in patients with chronic diabetic neuropathy: an analysis of two randomized placebo-controlled trials," *Diabetes Care*, 2005; 28: 89–94.

14 Rahbar, A. R. et al., "Effect of L-carnitine on plasma glycemic and lipidemic profile in patients with type II diabetes mellitus," *Eur J Clin Nutr*, 2005; 59(4): 592–96.

15 Steiber, A.L. et al., "Carnitine treatment improved quality-of-life measure in a sample of Midwestern hemodialysis patients," *J Parenter Enteral Nutr*, 2006; 30(1): 10–15.

16 Brass, E.P. et al., "Intravenous L-carnitine increases plasma carnitine, reduces fatigue, and may preserve exercise capacity in hemodialysis patients," *Am J Kidney Dis*, 2001; 37(5): 1018–28.

17 Koeth, R.A. et al., "Intestinal microbiota metabolism of L-carnitine, a nutrient in red meat, promotes atherosclerosis," *Nat Med*, May 2013; 19(5): 576–85. doi: 10.1038/nm.3145. Epub April 7, 2013.

18 Semeniuk, J. et al., "Evaluation of the effect of intravenous l-carnitine on quality of life in chronic hemodialysis patients," *Clin Nephrol*, 2000; 54(6): 470–77.

SECTION VII: MIGRAINES—ALTERNATIVE APPROACHES

1 Camboim, Rockett F. et al., "Perceived migraine triggers: do dietary factors play a role?" *Nutr Hosp*, Mar-Apr 2012; 27(2): 483–89.

2 Sun-Edelstein, C., and A. Mauskop, "Foods and supplements in the management of migraine headaches," *Clin J Pain*, Jun 2009; 25(5): 446–52.

3 Finocchi, C., and G. Sivori, "Food as trigger and aggravating factor of migraine," *Neurol Sci*, May 2012; 33 Suppl 1: S77–80.

4 Turner, L.C. et al., "Migraine trigger factors in non-clinical Mexican-American population in San Diego county: implications for etiology," *Cephalalgia*, 1995; 15: 523–30.

5 Kelman, L., "The triggers or precipitants of the acute migraine attack," *Cephalalgia*, 2007; 27: 394–402.

6 Dexter, J.D. et al., "The five-hour glucose tolerance test and effect of low sucrose diet in migraine," *Headache*, 1978; 18: 91–94.

7 Sandor, P.S. et al., "Efficacy of coenzyme Q10 in migraine prophylaxis: a randomized controlled trial," *Neurology*, 2005; 64(4): 713–15.

8 Johnson, E.S. et al., "Efficacy of feverfew as prophylactic treatment of migraine," *BMJ*, 1985; 291: 569–73.

9 Murphy, J.J. et al., "Randomized double-blind placebo-controlled trial of feverfew in migraine prevention," *Lancet*, 1988; ii: 189–92.

10 Schoenen, J. et al., "High dose riboflavin as a prophylactic treatment of migraine: results of an open pilot study," *Cephalalgia*, 1994; 14: 328–29.

11 Schoenen, J. et al., "Effectiveness of high-dose riboflavin in migraine prophylaxis: a randomized control trial," *Neurology*, 1998; 50(2): 466–70.

12 Boehnke, C. et al., "High-dose riboflavin treatment is efficacious in migraine prophylaxis: an open study in a tertiary care centre," *Eur J Neurol*, 2004; 11(7): 475–77.

13 Pfaffenrath, V. et al., "Magnesium in the prophylaxis of migraine—a double-blind placebo-controlled study," *Cephalalgia*, 1996; 16(6): 436–40.

14 Peikert, A. et al., "Prophylaxis of migraine with oral magnesium: results from a prospective, multi-center, placebo-controlled and double-blind randomized study," *Cephalalgia*, 1996; 16(4): 257–63.

15 Wang, F. et al., "Oral magnesium oxide prophylaxis of frequent migrainous headache in children: a randomized, double-blind, placebo-controlled trial," *Headache*, 2003; 43(6): 601–10.

16 Mauskop, A. et al., "Intravenous magnesium sulphate relieves migraine attacks in patients with low serum ionized magnesium levels: a pilot study," *Clin Sci (Lond)*, 1995; 89(6): 633–36.

17 Melchart, D. et al., "Acupuncture for idiopathic headache," *Cochrane Database of Systematic Reviews*, 2001; (1): CD001218.

18 Vickers, A.J. et al., "Acupuncture for chronic headache in primary care: large, pragmatic, randomised trial," *BMJ*, 2004; 328: 744.

19 Allias, G. et al., "Acupuncture in the prophylactic treatment of migraine without aura: a comparison with flunarizine," *Headache*, 2002; 42(9): 855–61.

20 Parker, G.B. et al., "A controlled trial of cervical manipulation of migraine," *Aust NZ J Med*, 1978; 8: 589–93.

21 Parker, G.B. et al., "Why does migraine improve after a clinical trial? Further results from a trial of cervical manipulation of migraine," *Aust NZ J Med*, 1980; 10: 193–94.

22 Mullinix, J. et al., "Skin temperature biofeedback and migraine," *Headache*, 1978; 17: 242–44.

23 Mullaly, W.J. et al., "Efficacy of biofeedback in the treatment of migraine and tension type headaches," *Pain Physician*, 2009; 12(6): 1005–11.

24 Goslin, R.E. et al., "Behavioral and physical treatments for migraine headache," Rockville (MD): Agency for Health Care Policy and Research (US); *Technical Reviews*, 1999; No. 2.2. Available from: www.ncbi.nlm.nih.gov/books/NBK45267.

25 Borins, M. and C. Croll-Young, "Biofeedback, relaxation techniques and attitudinal changes in adolescents with migraines," *Can Fam Phys*, 1987; 33: 417–21.

26 Friedman, M.H., "Local inflammation as a mediator of migraine and tension-type headache," *Headache*, 2004; 44(8): 767–71.

27 Friedman, M.H. et al., "Intraoral chilling versus oral sumatriptan for acute migraine," *Heart Disease*, 2001; 3(6): 357–61.

28 Friedman, M. H. et al., "Intraoral topical nonsteroidal antiinflammatory drug application for headache prevention," *Heart Disease*, 2002; 4(4): 212–15.

SECTION VIII: CONCLUSION—TALK TO YOUR DOC

1 Prasad, V. et al., "A decade of reversal: an analysis of 146 contradicted medical practices," *Mayo Clin Proc*, Aug 2013; 88(8): 790–98.

2 Smith, R., "Where is the wisdom...?" *BMJ*, Oct 5, 1991; 303(6806): 798–99.

3 Ladouceur, R., "Ups and downs of evidence and practice guidelines," *Can Fam Phys*, Nov 2013; 59(11): 1143.

INDEX

ABOUT THE AUTHOR

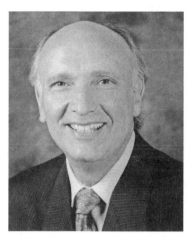

Mel Borins, MD, is a family physician in private practice and has been active for more than two decades in training physicians in complementary and alternative medicine, counseling and psychotherapy, stress management, and communication. He is an associate professor in the Faculty of Medicine at the University of Toronto and on staff at St. Joseph's Health Center. He is a fellow of the College of Family Physicians of Canada and author of the books *An Apple A Day—A Holistic Health Primer* and *Go Away Just for the Health of It*. He has lectured in the United States, Canada, India, Indonesia, China, Taiwan, Korea, New Zealand, and Hong Kong on health and healing. In addition to his private practice, Dr. Borins is a sought-after speaker who has appeared on television and radio across North America. He lives in Toronto, Canada. Visit him at www.melborins.com.